Care on the

Every boater matters

Sister Mary Ward. BEM.

Consultant Sister to long-distance boatmen and families,
British Canals, Stoke Bruerne on the Grand Union / Grand Junction Canal

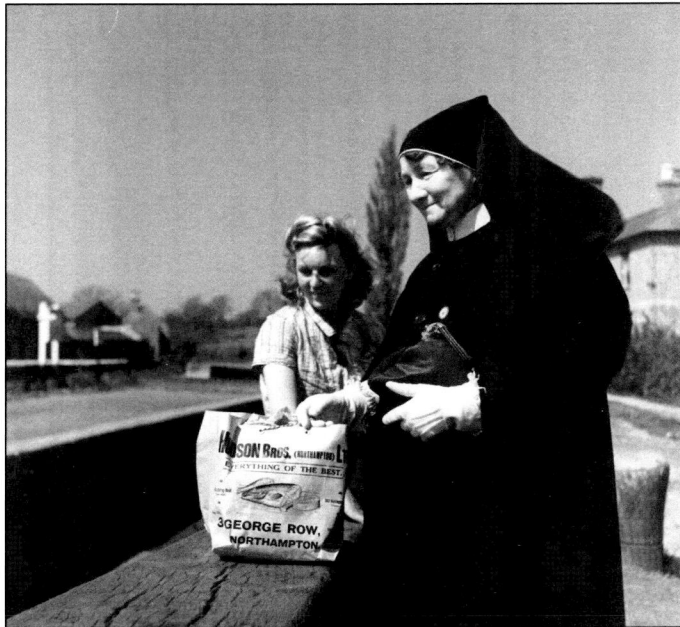

by

Della Sadler-Moore, Lorna York and Christopher M Jones

with 137 Illustrations and 40 Tables

Published by: Del-Lor-Chris Publishing Co

This book is dedicated to:

The hundreds of *boat families* who travelled back and forth,
along the Grand Junction / Grand Union Canal carrying goods.

Front and Back Cover: Christopher M Jones

Title Page: Sister Mary with Evelyn Hunt at top-lock Stoke Bruerne

(Source: Waterways' Archive. Monnington collection)

First published 2015 by: Del-Lor-Chris Publishing Company

©2015

ISBN 978-0-9933780-0-3

Design and layout by Mark Smith - mark@marksart.graphics

Printed in England

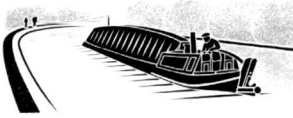

Acknowledgments

This book has been made possible through the award of a post-doctoral Early Researcher Award Scheme (ERAS) fellowship from the University of Wolverhampton titled *Care on the CUT*. Initial thanks therefore go to the University for supporting the research and for extending the funding to enable the publishing of this first edition. The funding awarded to the *Care on the Cut* project enabled the authors to pay for archival services (scanning, copyright and photocopying), a permanent and portable display in Stoke Bruerne Canal Museum as well as other costs (purchase of the ISBN) incurred during preparation of the manuscript.

David Blagrove, M.B.E, local resident, canal historian and Chairman of the *Friends of Stoke Bruerne Museum,* where do we begin to thank you?. A casual email inquiring about Sister Mary led to you agreeing to allow me access to a number of her original case books / ledgers, primary research data which is rare and a privilege to be entrusted with. We hope the book meets with your approval and thank you.

We would also like to thank staff from a number of archives visited in the course of undertaking the research. As the book is essentially about one village in Northamptonshire, Northampton Record Office (NRO) has been a tremendous source of information. Archivist Scott Pettit initially pointed us in the right direction, subsequently Daniel Williams, Archive Development Manager and his front and back-stage team. Over the last two years Daniel and your team patiently enabled us to view a large amount of archival material, special thanks go to Daniel for advice on additional holdings which proved invaluable, also for your help with interpreting many of these.

The Waterway's Archive at Ellesmere Port has been a most useful source of material. Thanks go to Archivist Linda Barley and the team of volunteers who found nothing too much trouble to locate. Jon-Paul Carr, Northamptonshire Studies Manager at Northampton Central Library you were particularly helpful and prompt in managing the digitization of images dispersed across this book, as well as advising on local newspaper holdings. I'm sure we will call upon your services again.

Other individuals who have been most generous in our search for information include Brian Collings. Thank you Brian for allowing us to include images of two paintings of Blisworth Hill Road and for kindly creating an impression of Mr Amos's rope walk, as well as allowing Lorna access to Robert Pettifer's original blacksmith records. We also thank Brian's wife, Janet Collings and her mom for providing a first hand account of Sister Mary.

Jenny Glynn (nee Littlemore) you have been so kind to us since we mentioned we were researching Sister Mary. Thank you for initially sharing your memories of Sister Mary on the towing path at Braunston Canal festival (2014), you kind words convinced us a book would be a valuable addition to canal heritage resources. We also thank you for the photographic images included in the concluding chapter.

Christopher R Jones and ex boatman Philip Garrett, thank you for allowing us to reproduce photographic images from your private collections, and for spending time searching the family archives in pursuit of answers to some difficult questions. Richard Thomas (the steamer man) your web site has been an extremely useful source of research data thank you for allowing us to reproduce some material from this.

Louise Stockwin, Manager Stoke Bruerne Canal Museum, your back-stage role chasing up sources and acting as go-between enabled us to access additional resources which have contributed significantly to the book, best wishes for all your hard work. Thanks specifically go to the couple who anonymous loaned us an additional Nurse Ward *Surgery Dressing Book*, containing entries which provided insight into her role whilst in Earls Barton, as well as the early period when Sister Mary set up her canal-side surgery in Stoke Bruerne. Access to this primary data provided more *pieces in the jigsaw puzzle* leading the authors to new lines of inquiry which enabled us to fill gaps in our research and to extend the period of verifiable evidence about Sister Mary's life and nursing work. On several visits to Earls Barton Hilary Bailey and Glenys Ingram were helpful in the early stages of the research, thank you both.

Roy Hallam for allowing me to stay on *Gerald* in Little Venice, enabling daily visits to the Public Record Office at Kew, without which the time and cost would have precluded such in-depth research. I also thank you for traveling to Stoke Bruerne for a week and, again *putting me up* which allowed a somewhat circuitous tour of venues in Northamptonshire.

Thanks go to Professor Laura Serrant, Director of the Centre for Health and Social Care Improvement (CHSCI) for your mentorship during the initial research with itinerant boaters and for travelling to Stoke Bruerne to meet with David Blagrove to discuss the issues surrounding this aspect of the fellowship. Colleagues in the office we share at Wolverhampton University (Sue Talbot, Chris Lyle, Denise Bellingham-Young and Deborah Richardson) I thank you for keeping me motivated with regards to completing the book and not to forget Emma Hall, Assistant Accountant in the University for all your diligent help and support in managing the ERAS budget.

List of Figures
(Including illustrations, photographs and maps)

The watershed continues for the Amos family

The inter war years - father calls

List of Tables

List of Appendices

Declaration of Anonymity and Confidentiality

Five Sister Mary case books / ledgers became available during the research, a description of each, and how the data was managed is provided in Appendix 1. All data from the case books has been anonymised when re-presented throughout this book, to preserve the confidentiality of Sister Mary's work and in respect of the requirements of the Data Protection Act, where medical records are required to remain confidential for 100 years following the date of the last entry. No boat, boater or boat family is named in associated with a particular medical condition treated by Sister Mary, with one exception. This is where a document is already in the public domain, for example some letters written by Sister Mary have been published before or are available from archives. The *Care on the Cut* research was approved by the ethics committee of the Institute of Health Professionals at the University of Wolverhampton.

Stern of Horse Drawn Narrow Boat with Living Cabin

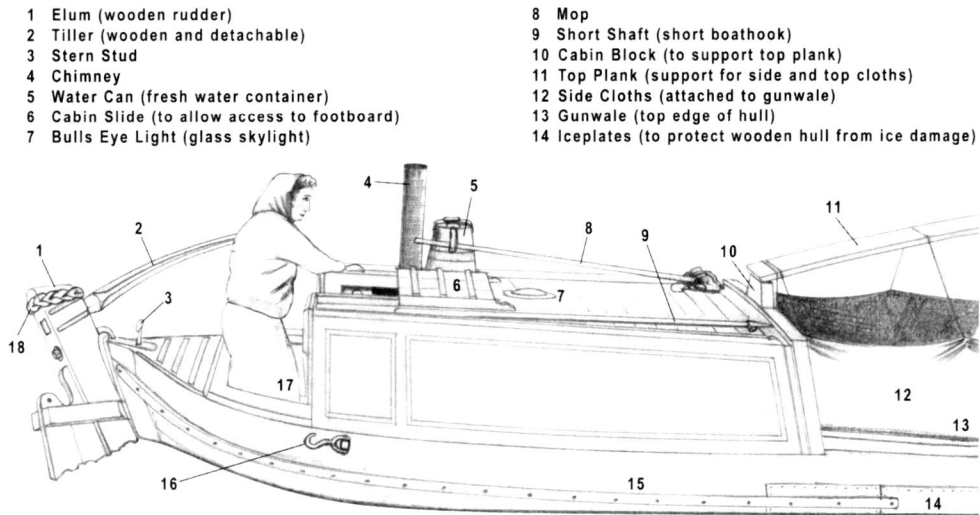

1 Elum (wooden rudder)
2 Tiller (wooden and detachable)
3 Stern Stud
4 Chimney
5 Water Can (fresh water container)
6 Cabin Slide (to allow access to footboard)
7 Bulls Eye Light (glass skylight)

8 Mop
9 Short Shaft (short boathook)
10 Cabin Block (to support top plank)
11 Top Plank (support for side and top cloths)
12 Side Cloths (attached to gunwale)
13 Gunwale (top edge of hull)
14 Iceplates (to protect wooden hull from ice damage)

15 Rubbing Guard (iron strip to protect hull from wear)
16 Hook and Anser Pin (pin is bolted to hull for attaching iron towing hook or shackle)
17 Hatches (well deck and entrance to cabin or door hole, and steering position or footboard)
18 Turks Head (decorative woven rope band)

Figure   1   Stern of Horse Drawn Narrow Boat with Living Cabin (Christopher M Jones)

Stern of Motor Boat with Living Cabin

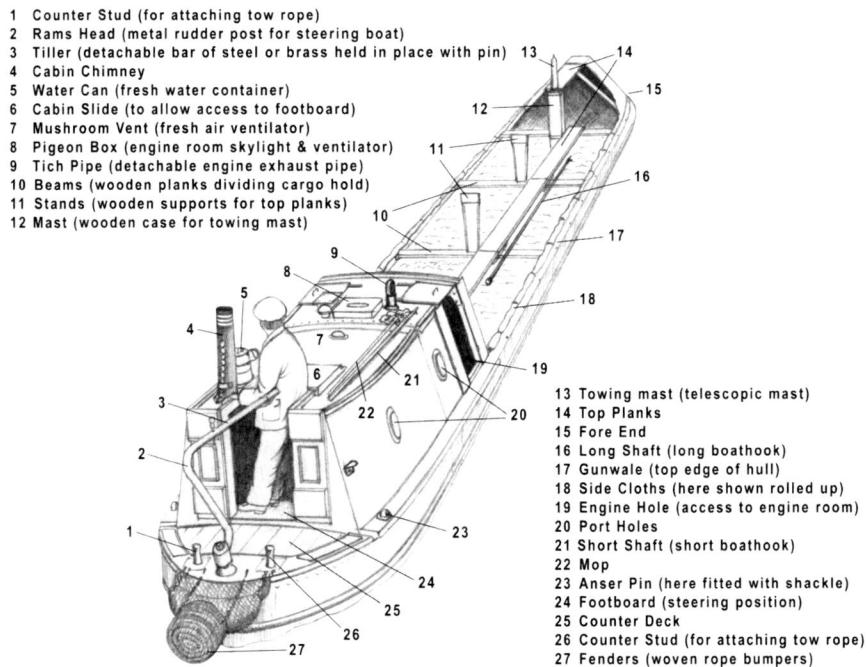

1 Counter Stud (for attaching tow rope)
2 Rams Head (metal rudder post for steering boat)
3 Tiller (detachable bar of steel or brass held in place with pin)
4 Cabin Chimney
5 Water Can (fresh water container)
6 Cabin Slide (to allow access to footboard)
7 Mushroom Vent (fresh air ventilator)
8 Pigeon Box (engine room skylight & ventilator)
9 Tich Pipe (detachable engine exhaust pipe)
10 Beams (wooden planks dividing cargo hold)
11 Stands (wooden supports for top planks)
12 Mast (wooden case for towing mast)

13 Towing mast (telescopic mast)
14 Top Planks
15 Fore End
16 Long Shaft (long boathook)
17 Gunwale (top edge of hull)
18 Side Cloths (here shown rolled up)
19 Engine Hole (access to engine room)
20 Port Holes
21 Short Shaft (short boathook)
22 Mop
23 Anser Pin (here fitted with shackle)
24 Footboard (steering position)
25 Counter Deck
26 Counter Stud (for attaching tow rope)
27 Fenders (woven rope bumpers)

Figure   2   Stern of Motor Boat with Living Cabin (Christopher M Jones)

13

Fore End of Motor Boat with Living Cabin

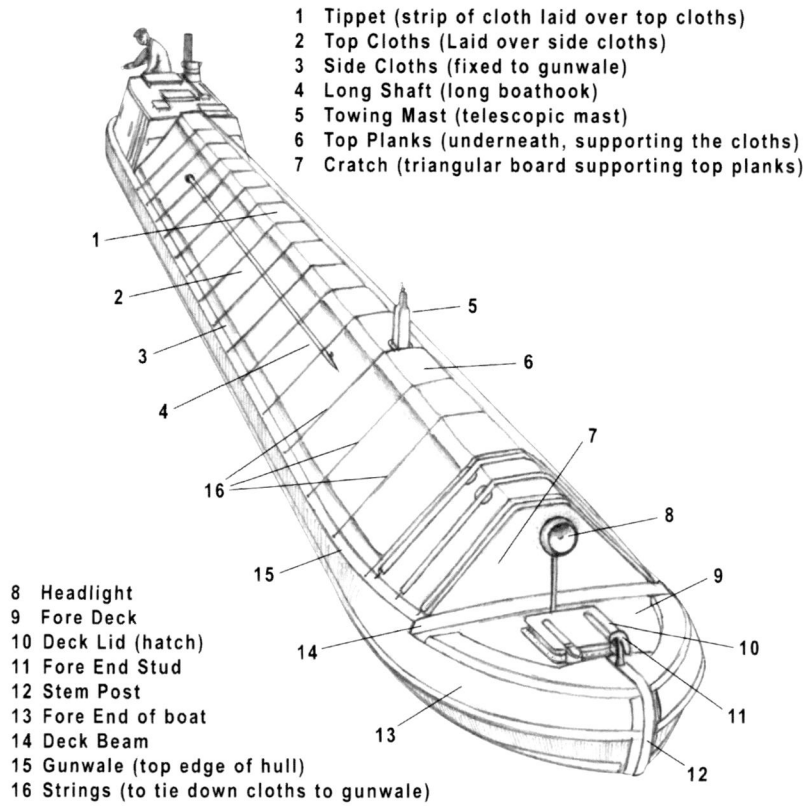

1 Tippet (strip of cloth laid over top cloths)
2 Top Cloths (Laid over side cloths)
3 Side Cloths (fixed to gunwale)
4 Long Shaft (long boathook)
5 Towing Mast (telescopic mast)
6 Top Planks (underneath, supporting the cloths)
7 Cratch (triangular board supporting top planks)

8 Headlight
9 Fore Deck
10 Deck Lid (hatch)
11 Fore End Stud
12 Stem Post
13 Fore End of boat
14 Deck Beam
15 Gunwale (top edge of hull)
16 Strings (to tie down cloths to gunwale)

Figure   3   Fore End of Motor Boat with Living Cabin (Christopher M Jones)

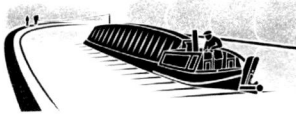

Introduction

From the mid 1750's a new form of transport began in England to serve the growing industrial revolution, the canals. These man-made, still-water inland highway's, were *cut* through the landscape and put in water for the sole purpose of carrying goods commercially by boat. From the beginning of commercial carrying on England's inland waterway's there evolved live-aboard, *family* [narrow] *boaters*. This book focuses on the boat families who earned their living by going back and forth along the Grand Junction Canal, which later became known as the Grand Union Canal.

For most of the history of the English canals, narrow boats were towed on a rope line either by animals, and to a much lesser extent by humans. Initially these craft were used singly then as larger quantities of cargo were required due to the growing economy, narrow boats started working in pairs with the trailing boat called a butty. The Grand Junction Canal was ideal for this method of working as the locks could easily accommodate two boats side-by-side. From the middle of the 19th century steam power was gradually introduced, but only for a relatively small number of vessels mainly express cargo carrying craft working night and day. Independently powered craft like this were powerful enough to tow an unpowered former horse drawn boat behind as its butty. In the first decade of the 20th century internal combustion engined boats appeared, which only started to become commonplace during the 1920's. Even so horse power was used along the Grand Union Canal well into the mid-1930's, then motor and butty pairs reigned until the end of long distance carrying in 1970. *Figure 1* shows the stern of a horse drawn narrow boat indicating its noticeable features, whilst *Figure 2* and *Figure 3* identify the significant parts of a motor powered narrow boat.

The *Care on the Cut* project came about when one author was awarded a fellowship to study *contemporary live-aboard itinerant boaters experiences of accessing health care and welfare services*. Having located itinerant live-aboard boaters and gained their trust to interview them, the time came to write up and publish the research findings. After reviewing published literature to see where and how boaters' health and welfare needs were met, Sister Mary was regularly referred to, but, on deeper analysis of the literature little was revealed about her life and nursing work, although it was evident she was iconic in the canal community for her ministering to the boat people as they passed through the Northamptonshire village of Stoke Bruerne. Tom Rolt referring to Sister Mary as *having an understanding of human nature*[1] ...

> As a general rule the boaters are somewhat mistrustful of the medical profession who, through failure to understand their mentality, seem seldom to be able to win their confidence. An exception is the district nurse at a certain canal-side village in Northamptonshire. Not

only do the boatmen come to her with all their ills, but she has become their unfailing guide, philosopher and friend. Though there should be more like her, to find her equal would not be easy because her success is due, not so much to medical training as to an understanding of human nature which is rare to-day because it cannot be taught out of a first-aid textbook.

Curiosity about Sister Mary led to an enquiry to David Blagrove asking if he knew the whereabouts of additional material which would shed light on her role within the boating community. David replied he was *custodian of a number of (as yet unanalysed) Sister Mary Case Books*, given to him by her grandson on the sale of the family's canal-side cottage in Stoke Bruerne. After meeting with David he kindly allowed me to analyse the case books, this is where the book began.

A wealth of publications exist on diverse aspects of English canals. Dispersed across this specialist literature are accounts of live-aboard *family boaters*, but there is no single source which focuses on the floating populations health, well-being and welfare during the lengthy period of commercial carrying. This book is therefore about *one* canal; the Grand Junction Canal (subsequently the Grand Union Canal), which cut through the south of *one* county, Northamptonshire. The canal was cut through the centre of *one* South Northamptonshire village, Stoke Bruerne, after which the village evolved into a canal community. In Stoke Bruerne five generations of Sister Mary's family had a presence with *family boaters* throughout commercial carrying, commencing in 1850 when John and Elizabeth Amos (Sister Mary's Grandparents), with their first son William, moved from Long Buckby Wharf to Stoke Bruerne. The family's presence in the village came to a close when Sister Mary's grandson sold the family canal-side cottage c1984. An overview of the five generations of Sister Mary's family is shown in *Figure 4*.

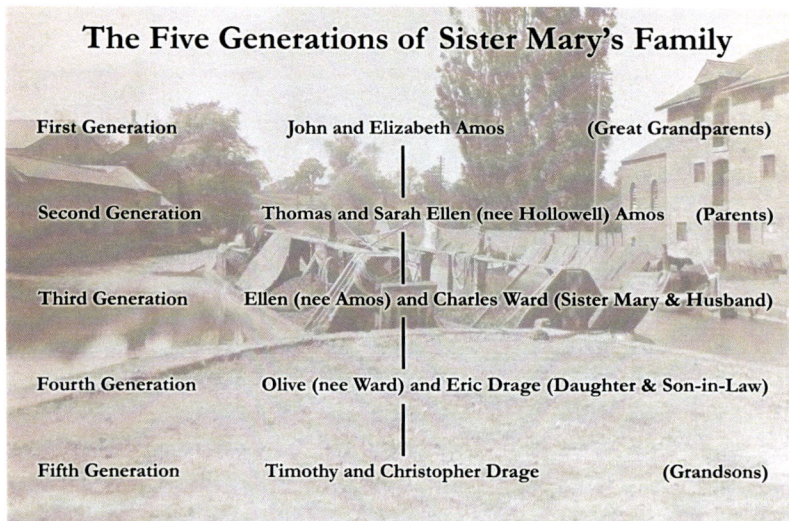

The Five Generations of Sister Mary's Family

First Generation	John and Elizabeth Amos	(Great Grandparents)
Second Generation	Thomas and Sarah Ellen (nee Hollowell) Amos	(Parents)
Third Generation	Ellen (nee Amos) and Charles Ward (Sister Mary & Husband)
Fourth Generation	Olive (nee Ward) and Eric Drage (Daughter & Son-in-Law)
Fifth Generation	Timothy and Christopher Drage	(Grandsons)

Figure 4   The *Five Generations of Sister Mary's Family* on a backdrop of canal boats outside Stoke Bruerne mill building c1920's (Christopher M Jones and Waterway's Archive)

Three authors (DSM, LY & CMJ) have brought together their expertise on Sister Mary, Stoke Bruerne, family boater's, the canal and commercial carrying. Thanks to David Blagrove's support the data now reported is from verifiable sources gathered from archives across England, and from *the connections* two authors have (LY & CMJ) within the canal community.

The kinship / family history research on boaters, boat families, and the individuals and families from Stoke Bruerne and beyond are re-presented by Lorna York, Canal Boat Families Historian. As we go to print Lorna has researched over 9,000 boatmen using an *Evidence Based Family History* approach[2]. The illustrations and detailed accounts of commercial carrying are re-presented thanks to Canal Historian, Artist and Illustrator Christopher M Jones, whose talents and expertise are published in the quarterly specialist journal *NarrowBoat*. Chris's contribution to the book is extensive; illustrations, accounts of canal carrying and verification of facts from archival materials accrued over the last 30 years. As this book is aimed at a wider audience than canal enthusiasts Chris's publications we hope will be increasingly recognised for their excellence by the next generation who enjoy England's inland waterway's www.chrismjones1artist.com My contribution is that of a Registered Nurse and Nursing Academic who specialises in ethnographic research. My interest in Sister Mary's role and *caring virtues* originates from being raised in a household with my aunt Nurse Elsie May Moore, a Triple Nurse[3], who shared many similarities with Sister Mary. All three authors have a boat family heritage. Lorna York is related to the *Yarnall and Wenlock* families originating from Worcestershire. Christopher M Jones the *Firkins* family from Birmingham, and Della Sadler-Moore the *Stokes, Hollis and Webb* families from Brierley Hill.

It is easy to *romanticise* boating life and commercial carrying, this book provides a down to earth, accessible account of the realities of life for family boaters and those working in canal related occupations. The chapters logically take the reader on a journey from the late eighteenth century to 1972. As the writer is an ethnographic researcher, the voices of those at the time when events took place, are where possible, re-presented as quotations to engender a sense of *being there*. The re-presented voices are from a number of different people; reporters, travel writers, clergymen, campaigners, scribes, witnesses, boaters, the Amos family and Sister Mary. The book is a timely edition to canal resources and is an essential read as today's new custodians of our canals (the Canal and River Trust) move towards greater charitable and leisure agendas. As Professor's Willis and Trondman in their manifesto for ethnography remind us …

> … it is an increasing imperative for all social groups to find and make their roots, routes and 'lived' meanings in societies undergoing profound processes of re-structuration and de-traditionalization, processes which are eroding the certainties of previous transitions and inherited cultures, as well as inciting them to re-establish themselves in new forms[4]

The first edition is published in 2015 which would be Sister Mary's 120th year. All profits from the sale of the book go to the *Friends of the Museum* at Stoke Bruerne, an arrangement I am sure Sister Mary would approve of. When the book went to print we acknowledge more data could come to light regarding Sister Mary's life and nursing work, therefore we invite all who wish to contribute additional information to contact us so we can include it in the second edition.

Dr Della Sadler-Moore.
August 2015.

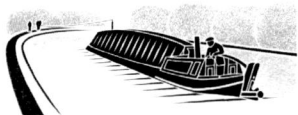

The First Sixty Years

The pack-horse was the mainstay for transporting goods across England before the introduction of artificial canals. Horse's carried goods along *bad roads … being at once loose, rough, and perishable, expensive, tedious and dangerous to travel on, and very costly to repair,* from these conditions *canals saved the country*[5]. To transport raw materials used in production processes and finished goods for the export market, and to distribute imported goods the earliest Inland Waterway route between the major economic centres of trade in England (London and the Midlands) opened in 1789. The journey took a boater along the Staffordshire and Worcestershire Canal, the River Severn and the Stroudwater Canal, which joined the River Thames at Lechlade. In total the journey was 280 miles with 130 locks and numerous navigable weirs. In 1790 the Oxford Canal created a further route, and although a slightly shorter journey (248 miles with 109 locks) it was more circuitous.

Both inland waterway's routes shown in Figure 5, proved unsatisfactory to meet the ever increasing demands for *commercially viable* goods transportation, therefore a more direct route was sought. The new route materialised when parliament authorized a Royal Assent in April 1793 to create the wide gauge Grand Junction Canal, beginning at the Braunston Junction with the Oxford Canal and ending at Brentford, the gateway to the River Thames[6], the route would pass through the counties of Middlesex, Hertfordshire, Buckinghamshire and Northamptonshire. Construction of the Grand Junction Canal was an ambitious project due to the substantial engineering works required to negotiate summits at Tring, Blisworth and Braunston as well as a valley between Wolverton and Cosgrove.

The Third Duke of Grafton, Augustus Henry FitzRoy supported the new canal route by selling his land in South Northamptonshire to the Company of Proprietors of the Grand Junction Canal, which enabled the company to *cut the line of the canal and its' associated structures*[7]. The Duke received staged payments for the land totalling £2,722 18s 7d[8], in exchange for 29 plots shown in Figure 6, plots 17-28 being in the Parish of Stoke Bruerne. Details of each of the Stoke Bruerne plots sold by the Duke are given in Table 1[9]. Construction of the canal commenced the same year as Royal Assent was awarded, with the Grand Junction Canal opening in parts as each section was completed. Before the canal arrived in the rural village of Stoke Bruerne it had at it's centre Saint Mary the Blessed Virgin, with it's rectory and a number of fish ponds, presided over by Rev. Stalman. The Parish comprised a number of farms with their associated buildings, and on the hill looking towards Blisworth was a Mill[10], when the Grand Junction Canal Act was passed Stoke Bruerne was a one street settlement.

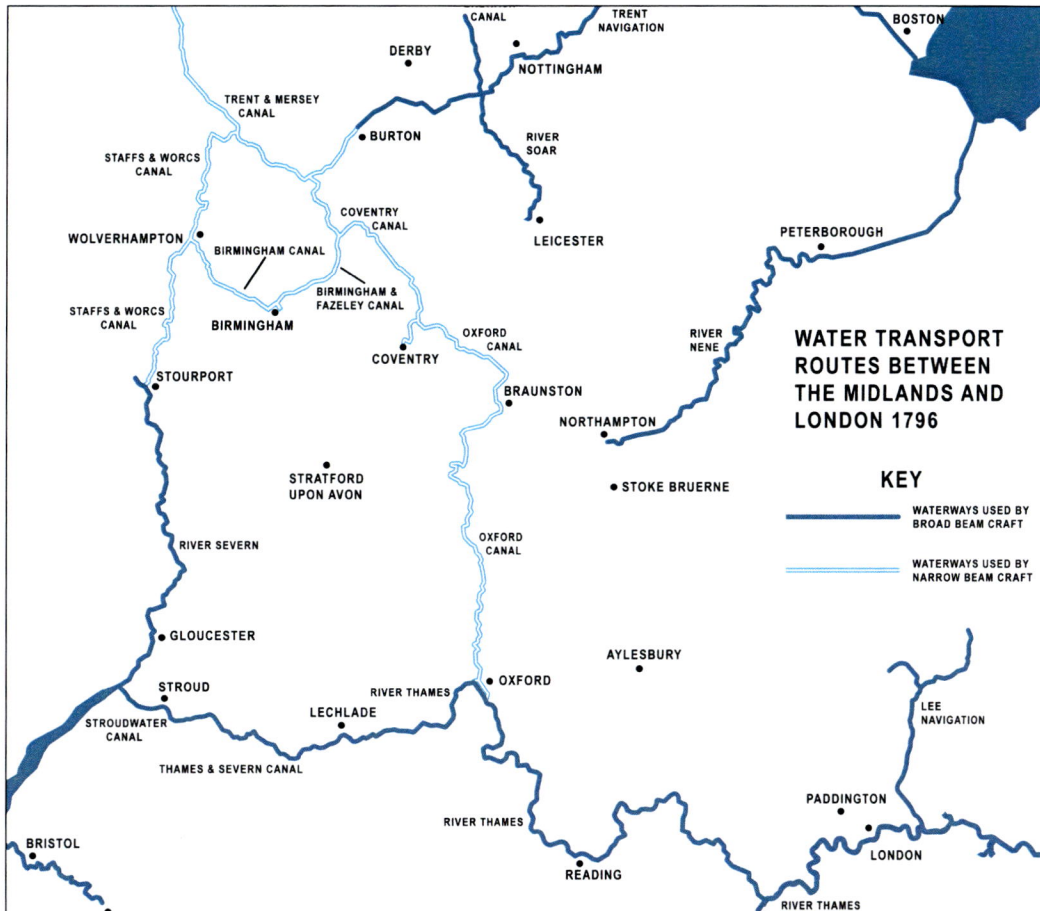

Figure 5 Water transport routes between the Midlands and London 1796
(Christopher M Jones)

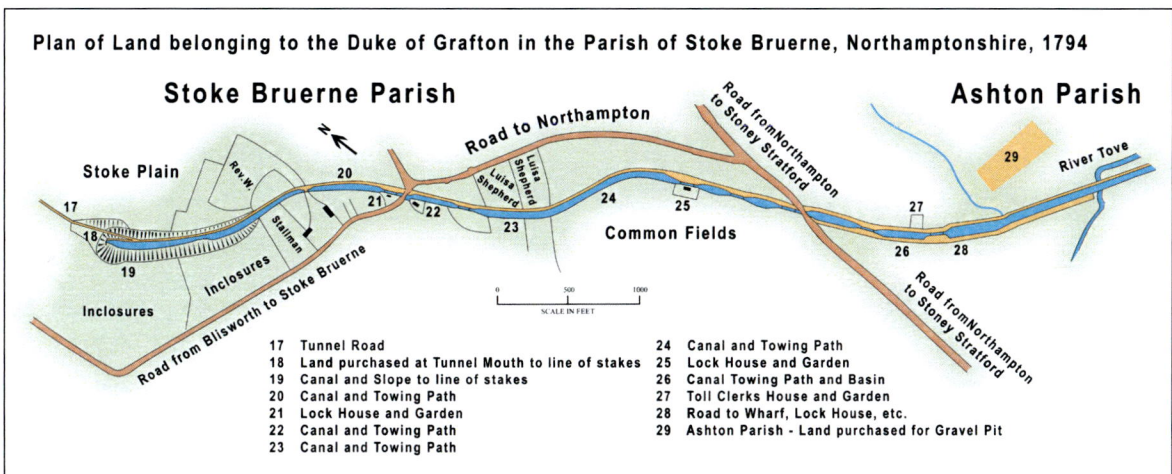

Figure 6 Duke of Grafton land sold to the Company of Proprietors of the Grand Junction Canal 1794
(Christopher M Jones)

19

Table 1: Conveyancing of the Duke of Grafton's plots of land in Stoke Bruerne

Plot	Distance	Name	Details
17	3 Roods, 8 Perches	Stoke Plain	Part of certain Common Land in the parish of Stoke Bruerne … and taken for making the said road …
18	3 Roods	Stoke Plain	Part of the said Common Land … and cut and taken for making the said road and other conveniences at the South westwardly entrance into the tunnel
19	3 Acres, 2 Roods, 36 perches	Well's Home Close	Part of a certain enclosure in Stoke and cut and taken for making the said canal and the towing path thereto and the deep cuttings on the sides thereof
20	1 Acre, 21 Perches	Tite's Home Close	Part of a certain enclosure in Stoke and cut and taken for making the said canal and the towing path
21	15 Perches	Tite's Home Close	Taken for the purpose of erecting a Lock House thereon and making a garden
22	1 Rood, 8 Perches		Part of open field land … and cut and taken for making the said canal and the towing path
23	1 Rood, 32 Perches		Part of open field land … and cut and taken for making the said canal and the towing path
24	3 Acres, 1 Rood, 17 Perches		Part of open field land … and cut and taken for making the said canal and the towing path
25	25 Perches		Part of certain open field land … for the purpose of erecting a Lock House … and making a garden
26	2 Acres, 2 Roods, 10 Perches		Part of open field land … and cut and taken for making the said canal and the towing path … and a dock or basin and wharf
27	32 Perches		Part of certain open field land … taken for the purposes of erecting a Toll Clerk's house and making a garden
28	I Acre, I Rood, 36 Perches		Part of certain open field land … taken for making a road to the said wharf and for other purposes of the said canal

The Grand Junction Canal arrived at Blisworth in September 1796, and by 1800 arrived at the lower end of Stoke Bruerne. Between the two villages was Blisworth Hill, the last part of the cutting which would create the *continuous line of water from Brentford to Braunston*. Cutting through Blisworth Hill to construct the tunnel involved major engineering works, with the first attempt having to be abandoned in 1796 due to flooding. To avoid delaying the goods arriving by boat at either end of the newly *in water* canal, the Grand Junction Canal Company negotiated Blisworth Hill in the summer of 1797 with a horse toll road[11]. At one end of the toll road was Blisworth Wharf, owned by Pickford's the largest canal carrying company of the time, at the other end, the Old Stratford Turnpike in Stoke Bruerne. The Blisworth Hill horse toll road followed a three and a half mile route over the hill as illustrated in Figure 7. Goods arrived by boat at either end, cargo was unloaded and placed into carts, the carts were hauled over the hill by horse and on completion of the journey the cargo was re-loaded onto awaiting canal boats.

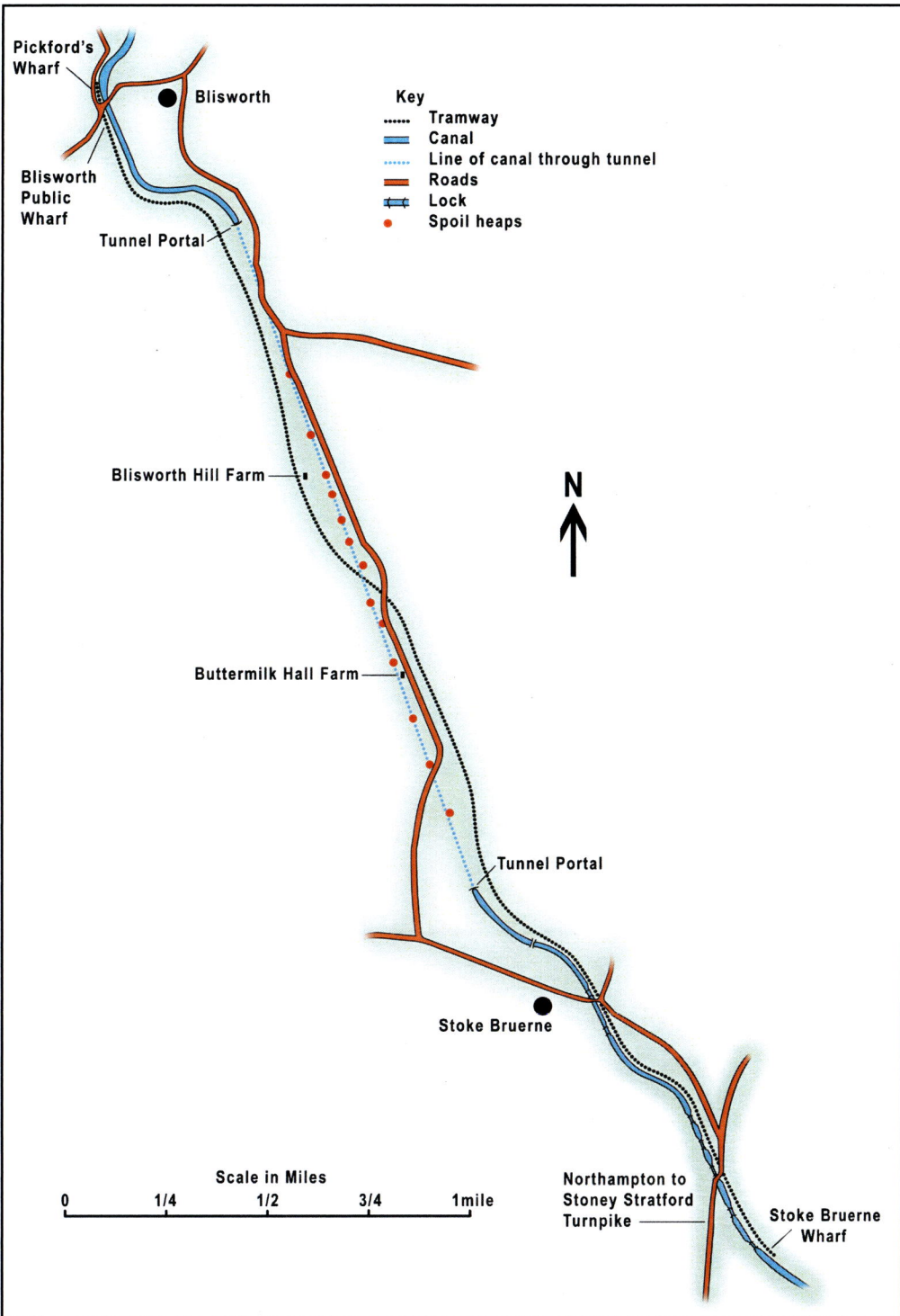

Key
- ······· Tramway
- ▬▬▬ Canal
- ········ Line of canal through tunnel
- ▬▬▬ Roads
- ▭ Lock
- ● Spoil heaps

Pickford's Wharf
Blisworth
Blisworth Public Wharf
Tunnel Portal
Blisworth Hill Farm
Buttermilk Hall Farm
Tunnel Portal
Stoke Bruerne
Northampton to Stoney Stratford Turnpike
Stoke Bruerne Wharf

N

Scale in Miles
0   1/4   1/2   3/4   1mile

Figure   7   Route of Blisworth Hill Road (Christopher M Jones)

21

The Blisworth Hill horse toll road created for the Grand Junction Canal Company *through traffic with punctuation*[12], although it soon became unsatisfactory for the quantity of transhipped goods wanting to use it. The canal company replaced the road with a *double-track tram road*, the first iron (horse) rail-way in Southern England. Images of the rail-way are captured in two paintings by Brian Collings shown in Figure 8 and Figure 9[13]. Completion of the Grand Junction Canal, with the exception of Blisworth Tunnel was announced to the public in June 1801 …

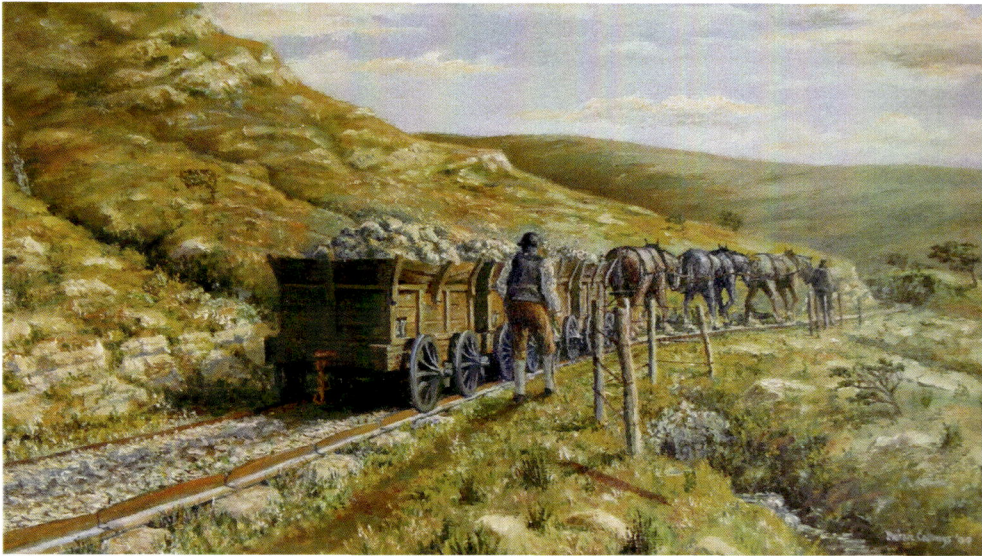

Figure 8   Horse Toll Road in operation over Blisworth Hill (Brian Collings)

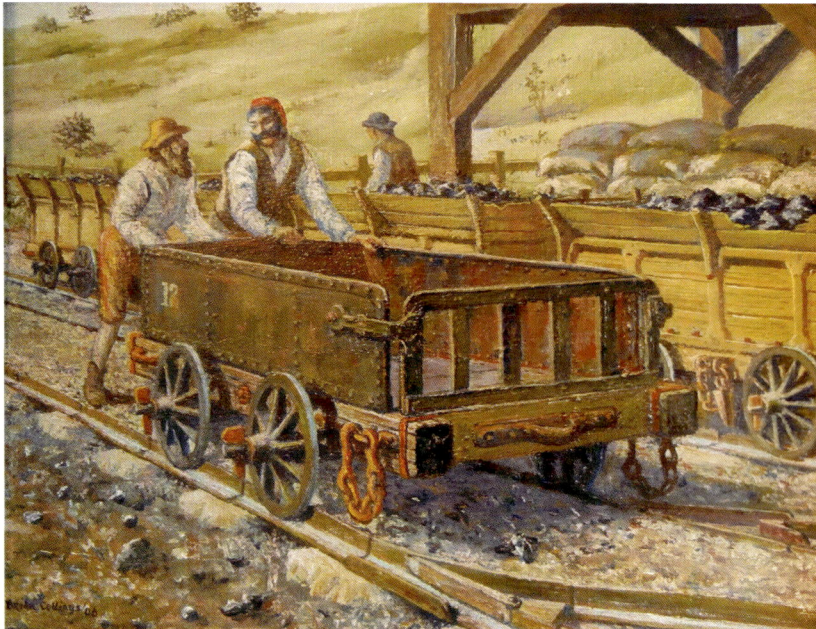

Figure 9   Horse Toll Road in operation over Blisworth Hill (Brian Collings)

The Public are hereby informed, that the whole Line of the Canal, from, the Oxford Canal at Braunston, to the River Thames at Brentford, together with the Branches to Buckingham, Wendover, and Paddington (except the intended Tunnel at Blisworth, where an Iron Railway has been executed for facilitating the conveyance of all articles during the execution of the said Tunnel), are now navigable; but as the Towing-Paths of the New Parts of the Works, and the erection of proper Warehouses, Sheds, Cranes and other conveniences, at Paddington, will not be in a state sufficiently accommodating to receive the General Merchandise before the 10th day of July next, the opening of these New Parts of the undertaking, for the General Trade, will be postponed till the said 18th day of July; when the whole Line is intended to be opened, and a Passage-Boat will immediately after be established to and from Uxbridge.

By Order of the Committee
June 8, 1801[14].

Within two months of opening terminals at both ends of the *Hill Railway* became some of the busiest in England[15], and whilst transhipped goods passed *over the hill* the construction of Blisworth Tunnel recommenced on a new line, but not without tragedy. In 1803 during the sinking of a tunnel ventilation shaft a *melancholy accident* resulted in the loss of life …

… as they were drawing two of the workmen up from the shafts, by a sudden jerk of the horse, the basket in which the men stood flipped off the hook affixed to the rope, by which accident they were both precipitated to the bottom (a depth of fifty yards); one of them was killed on the spot and the other furtive but a few hours[16].

Whilst the tunnel was under construction, in the south of Stoke Bruerne the canal was raised out of the valley by a flight of seven locks with several adjoining lock cottages. As the canal moved nearer to the centre of the village, the existing street was re-aligned and carried over the canal on a single arch brick-built bridge at the tail of the top-lock. During excavation of the tunnel, and as the canal was cut through the village, the Duke of Grafton's tenant farmer George Tite, experienced the lion's share of upheaval. Mr Tite's *Home Close Farm* was on the central line of the canal and because it was near to where the tunnel was being excavated it became a site for the dumping of huge quantities of spoil. After the canal was complete *Home Close Farm* straddled either side of the canal, dividing the village in half, on one side was a barn parallel to the canal, additional barns at angles to the canal and a labourer's cottage, whilst on the other side Mr Tite had a further piece of land[17]. Nearing the mouth of Blisworth Tunnel the Rector also felt the upheaval of the canal as it cut through his glebe land and fish ponds, although the Rector suffered the loss of an orchard and some fish ponds he was compensated by the Canal Company, receiving £300 and a bridge over the new canal to enable him easy access to parsonage land.

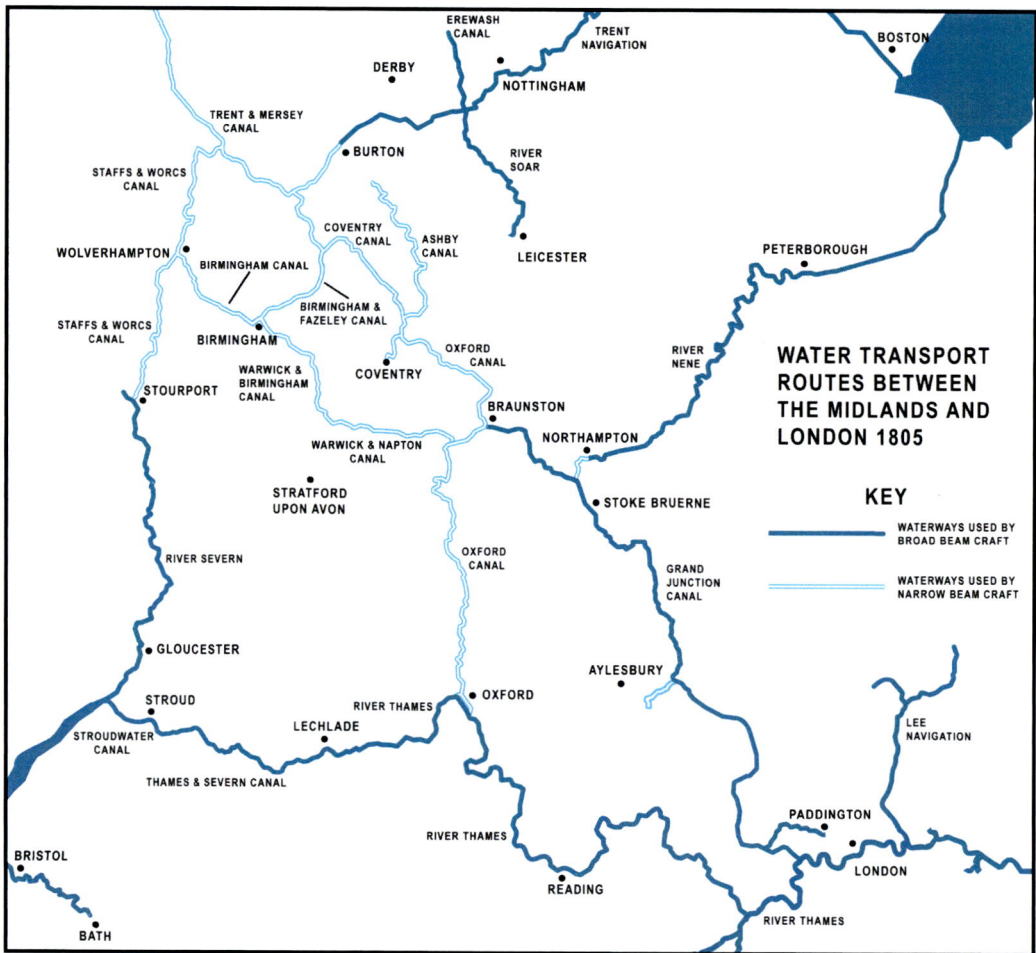

Figure 10   Grand Junction Canal Map 1805 (Christopher M Jones)

The final part of the Grand Junction Canal to be constructed was Blisworth Tunnel, which was completed on February 25th 1805, creating in Stoke Bruerne the *continuous line of inland water communication,* a new route for commercial goods transportation as shown in Figure 10. One month later the Grand Junction Canal was officially opened, the ceremony marking the occasion was by all accounts spectacular …

> That grand line of communication between the metropolis and the most distant parts of the kingdom, which the Grand Junction Canal was to effect, was complete on Monday last, when an amazingly large concourse of people assembled, some of them from considerable distances, to view the stupendous works at Blisworth Tunnel, and to see the grand procession of honour of the opening of it. One of the Paddington packet-boats, called the Marquis of Buckingham, was the first boat which went through the Tunnel, this was early in the morning, in order to join the other boats assembled at the north end of the Tunnel, at Blisworth, to form the grand procession. About 11 o'clock the Committee

of the Canal Company (who had superintended this great work), Messrs, Praed, Mansell, Unwin, Parkinson, Smith, and a great number of others of the principal proprietors, entered the boats: attended by Messrs. Telford, Bevan, and others of the engineers employed on the Canal, and by a band of music, and proceeding into the Tunnel, amidst the loudest acclamations of the spectators. The pitchy darkness of the Tunnel was shortly relived by a number of flambeaux and lights; but the company in general seemed lost in contemplating the stupendous efforts by which the amazing arch of brick-work (about eighteen inches thick in general, fifteen feet wide, and nineteen in height, withinside, being an elliptical form, 3080 yards in length), had been completed between the 10th of August, 1792, and the 26th of February, 1805. The height of the hill, above the Tunnel, being, for a considerable way, full sixty feet, for drawing up the clay and soil which was excavated, and letting down the materials to different parts of the works, nineteen shafts, or wells, were sunk on different parts of the line, and a heading, or small arch, was run or formed the whole length, below the present Tunnel, with numerous cross branches to draw off the springs of water, which would otherwise have impeded the work.

In an hour and two minutes the boats with the company arrived at the south end of the Tunnel, and were greeted by the loud huzzas of at least five thousand persons, who were assembled, and who accompanied the boats with continual cheers[18].

In South Northamptonshire the Grand Junction Canal cut through the centre of Stoke Bruerne and passed by the side of seventeen other places[19] as illustrated in Figure 11, subsequently Stoke Bruerne developed as a canal village, the Parish housing the line of the canal, seven locks and a portion of Blisworth Tunnel. Because the tunnel was constructed without a towing path, as a horse-drawn boat approached the tunnel mouth the horse was detached from the towing line and a member of the crew led the horse over the hill, leaving the remaining crew to perform the strenuous job of *poling* a 70 foot loaded boat through the dark, cold tunnel, the only lighting coming from a tallow candle. During the journey water relentlessly dripped on boaters for two and a half miles, the only break in the monotony being when boats passed in the tunnel, providing an opportunity for boaters to exchange a few words.

After the canal arrived in Stoke Bruerne structures began to evolve alongside the towing path: a Lock House, a Wharfinger House, a Wharf serving the Duke of Grafton's estate and a further Wharf below the bridge. Stoke villagers soon began to experience the consequences of the canal in the Parish, when one native family buried a mother and child following an accident …

Susannah the wife of John Blunt and Mary daughter of John and Susanna Blunt of Stoke … were both drowned in the Grand Junction Canal between three and four o'clock in the morning of the 19th inst, the mother with the child in her arms having fallen into the third lock below stoke bridge and continued in the water at least half an hour before they were taken out[20].

The following December George Wykes was also buried at Saint Mary's following a canal incident …

South Northamptonshire Towns and Villages on or near the Grand Junction Canal

Canals ———

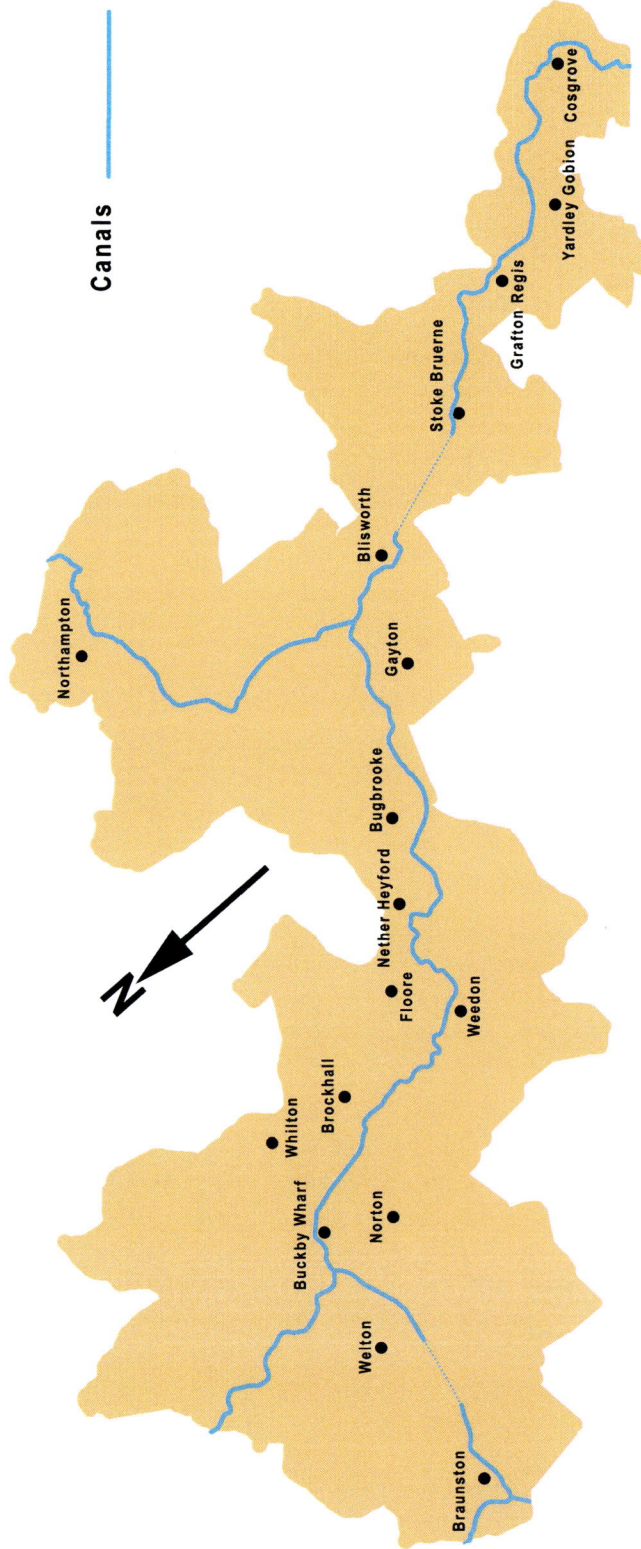

Figure 11   Grand Junction Canal passing through or nearby villages in South Northamptonshire (Christopher M Jones)

… fell into the lock in the middle of stoke field; and altho he was got out of the water almost immediately, yet he had received so much injury on the back part of his neck by the fall that he died in the cart which was carrying him to the general infirmary in Northampton[21].

The canal also brought with it new livelihoods for men residing in Stoke Bruerne and beyond. Immediately after the canal arrived in the village John Child moved to Stoke from Barby, with his wife Jane and their first son John Junior, taking up the position of Grand Junction Canal Company lock-keeper. The Child family had further children over the next few years, as did two of the other young lock-keepers Samuel Dike and Thomas Parish, all three families baptising their children at Saint Mary's[22] as shown in Table 2.

Table 2: Saint Mary the Blessed Virgin. Children of lock-keepers baptised 1813-1817.

Year	Birth date	Child's Name	Parents	Fathers occupation
1813	10th October	Thomas Child	John and Jane Child	Lock-keeper
1814	7th August	Jane Dike	Samuel and Ann Dike	Lock-keeper
1815	25th December	Jane Child	John and Jane Child	Lock-keeper
1816	25th February	John Parish	Thomas and Ann Parish	Lock-keeper
	24th March	Elizabeth Dike	Samuel and Ann Dike	Lock-keeper
1817	11th May	Sarah Child	John and Jane Child	Lock-keeper
	25th May	Joseph Dike	Samuel and Ann Dike	Lock-keeper

The first published account of Stoke Bruerne after the opening of the canal came from journalist John Hassell, written as a result of a horseback tour of the Grand Junction Canal in 1819[23]. On nearing Stoke Bruerne Hassell recounted the scene and illustrated his experience in two published engravings shown in Figure 12 and Figure 13.

Descending the hill we come suddenly upon the seven locks which lift the navigation from the valley to the entrance of the tunnel at Stoke Bruerne (Figure 12[24]). The scenery at the first bridge we pass over is very interesting; the view of that village, and its church on a wooded eminence, with the approach to it by navigation, is singularly beautiful, and has induced us to introduce it in the work (Figure 13[25]). It was harvest time, and the avocations of the farmer appeared on every side. The effects on the landscape was good, and the incidents natural …

Every object that encountered our sight, as we passed to the village, appeared of the picturesque; the team retiring from the glebe had its rustic mate and tired plough boy, with all their paraphernalia, seated on the leading horses; the navigation attendants and their cattle were bustling to pass a lock; the freighted boats presented a motley group of passengers on their decks; while a number of female attendants on the canal horses, reminded me of those hardy Cambrian lasses I have often seen following their laborious avocations.

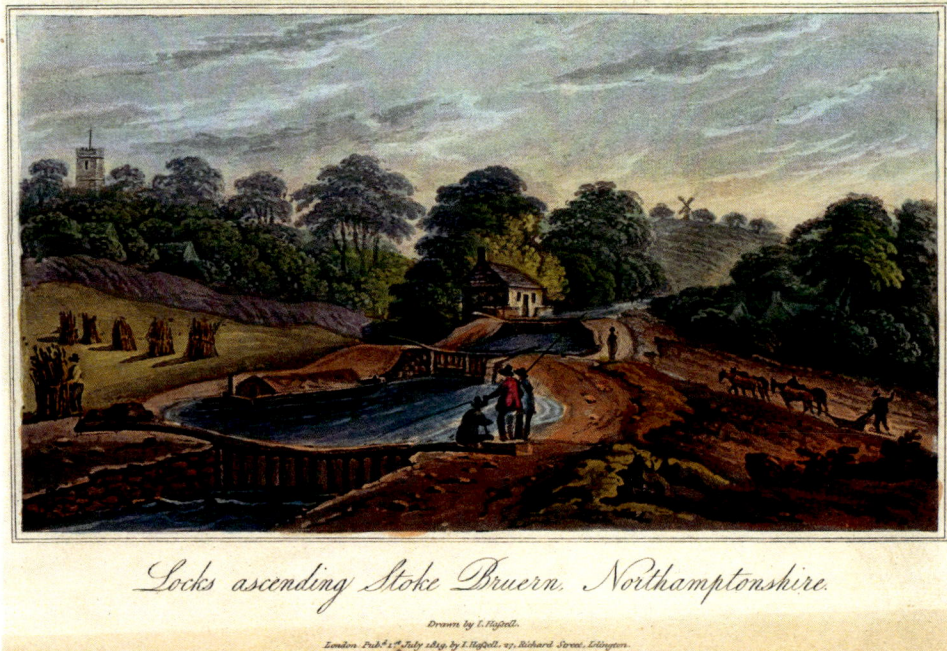

Figure 12   Engraving of Stoke Bruerne from Hassell 1891 (Northampton Central Library)

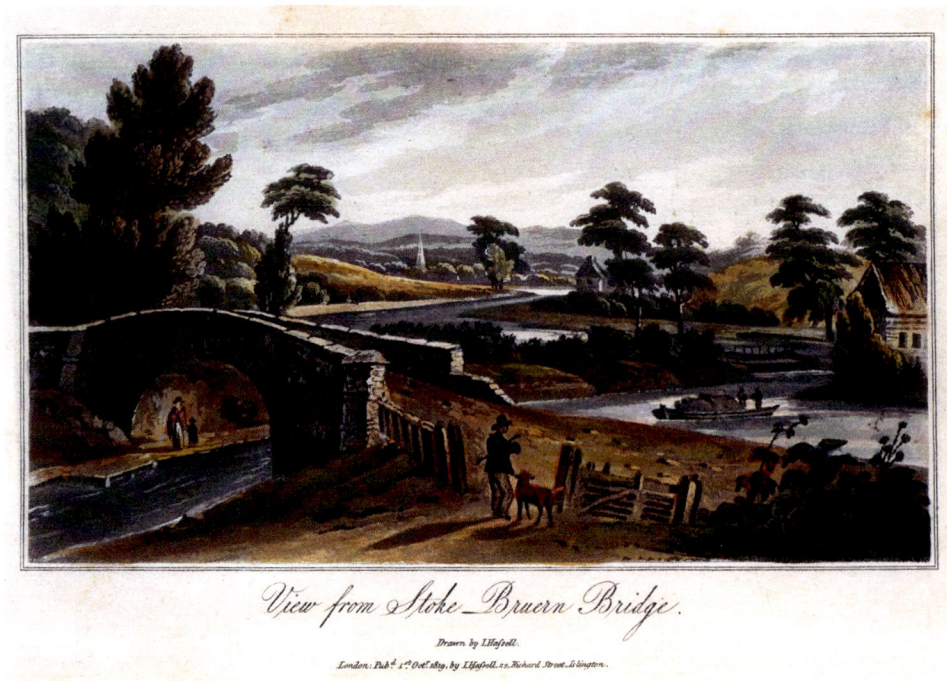

Figure 13   Engraving of Stoke Bruerne from Hassell 1891 (Northampton Central Library)

Stoke Bruerne village has a great affinity in appearance to the Welsh villages, the buildings very much resemble them in their make … The church, which is in an old gothic building, is situated on the highest part of the hill on which the village stands; and there is an extensive prospect from the extremity of the churchyard, overlooking the country and the valley we have just passed. The same view presents itself from the bridge … At the entrance of the celebrated tunnel, a succession of moving objects occur, and as it is a resting place for the navigation cattle, we anticipated finding some accommodation; our wants being moderate, we felt highly gratified by our good hostess announcing her ability to supply us with an excellent piece of corned beef. The servant being from home, I undertook the nursery department, and to the tune of the Sailor's Lullaby, rocked a sweet little babe to its peaceful slumbers, while she provided vegetables to our repast. The chubby infant reminded me of the substantial comforts of Dulce Domum.

The canal is carried by a level above the tops of those houses which are situated at the lower parts of the village, and appears like a trench cut through a hill, made rather wider at this place than usual. A quarter of a mile brought us to the entrance of the tunnel, which is faced with brick and stone, and assimilates in its appearance with the bridges that are thrown over the stream at the requisite places. The ground above the entrance is very rugged and picturesque from its inequalities, and is topped with wood. Several barges were now preparing to enter the excavation; the men throwing off their upper garments and lighting up their lantern, gave the helm for steerage to the women, one or two females generally attending each boat; when ready they loose the tow rope of the horse, and apply themselves to the poles, with which they sturdily shove the boats through the dark channel. On the top of the hill, just above the navigation, there is a small shed erected for the attendants and the cattle that have come over from Blisworth, and are to await the arrival of their proprietor's barges passing through the tunnel from that village. The distance is about two miles and a half underground, and is usually performed by two men with a loaded boat in two hours and a quarter, but some time less if light or un-laden.

We now rise from the towpath by a considerable ascent, and come in sight of a celebrated sporting country… The whole of the way to Blisworth, where the apertures had been made for boring the tunnel, the excavated earth has been thrown together in large mounds, and resembles the tumuli of the ancients - it appears a very rich fat clay, fit for various purposes.

The strenuous job of *Poling* a narrowboat through Blisworth Tunnel was gradually replaced by a new form of propulsion *Legging*. The precarious nature of legging through a broad gauge tunnel is shown in Figure 14, where two men cling to leggers *wings* suspended over the water, especially tortuous in long canal tunnels such as Braunston and Blisworth, when tiredness and fatigue take there toll. The inset top left shows how the *wings* were attached to the boats fore-deck with iron hooks slotted through eyelets bolted into the deck. As legging became established, at either end of the tunnel mouth men would congregated offering a boater their casual labour to *leg the boat for a price*, an attractive offer for a weary boater needing a rest. The *casual leggers* became so much of a concern to a Northampton trader he wrote to the local newspaper with a detailed account of their improper employment[26].

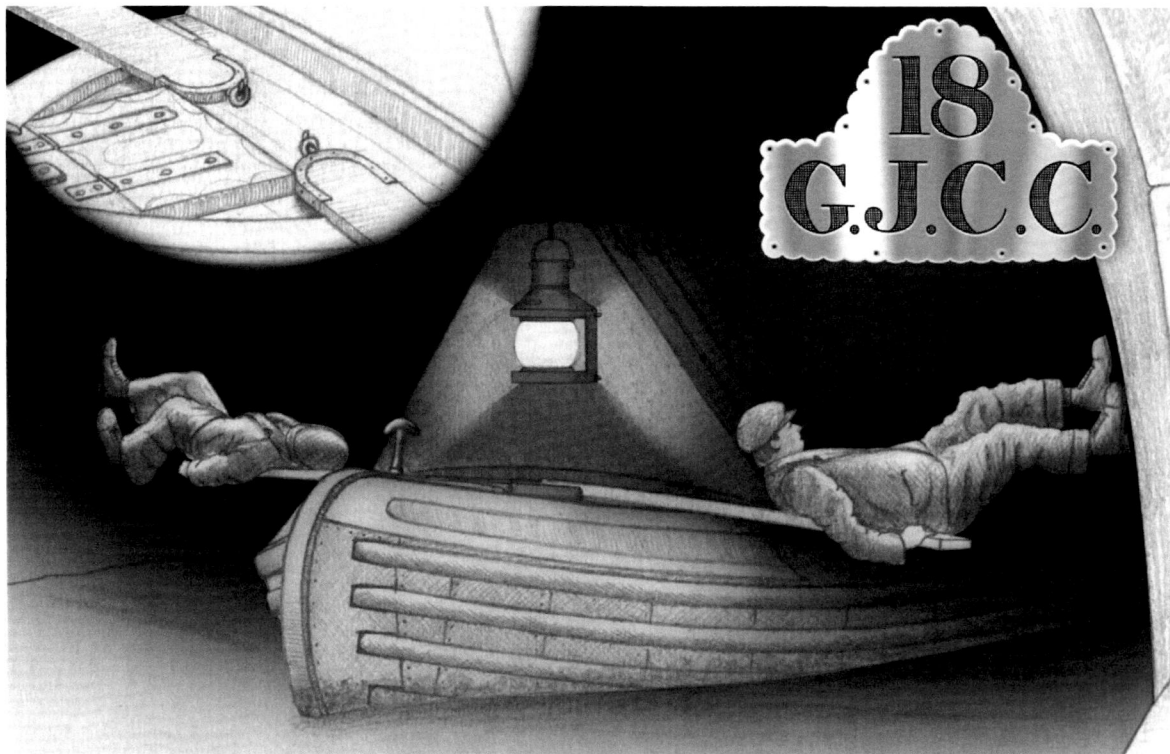

Figure 14   Legging, leggers wings and registered leggers brass arm bands (Christopher M Jones)

To all Traders on the Grand Junction Canal, and more particularly the Traders of the town of Northampton, the following observations are submitted, upon the novel and highly improper employment of men vulgarly called Leggers, to conduct their respective boats through the different tunnels :-

It is a well-known fact, that some few years ago the employment of any men to conduct boats through the tunnels, except the boatmen actually employed by the trade, was unknown. Within these last few years the boatmen, without the consent of their employers, have attracted, by employing them, from 30 to 50 men on the Braunston and Blisworth tunnels, to the annoyance of the neighbourhood, the prejudice of their master's interest, and to the encouragement of idleness in themselves. The general charge is 1s. 6d. through the Blisworth, and 1s. through the Braunston tunnel, thus is a tax of 2s. 6d. per voyage laid upon a pair of boats, supposing they (the boatmen) paid in money. But this is too often not the case: it does not require the calculation even of boatmen to ascertain whether, in paying the leggers with their master's goods and not in money from their own pockets, they do not save the 2s. 6d. It also appears reasonable to conclude, that from the avidity of the leggers to receive goods instead of money (which I am credibly informed is the case), that they are paid better in goods than money; thus the trader is taxed to an extent he is not aware, by a set of men who are only governed by the medium between their rapacity and the boatman's fear of detection. Here then is a wider field; for whether the boatmen endeavour conscientiously to guess at the money's worth, or whether it is given without any idea of quantity or value, I know not; but I must confess the latter case strikes me as the most consistent with their general character.

Numberless are the instances that might be adduced of the evil arising from men partially out of employ, as the leggers are, and particularly so when we regard the degraded state of the morals of these men, being composed of the most idle, disorderly, and unprincipled characters in the neighbourhood. I would therefore propose to the trade to reduce his boatmen to what they originally were, servants, not masters. If they can afford to lose 2s. 6d. per voyage, by keeping in employment men to do their work, they cannot object, as unreasonable, a deduction to that amount as it would only reduce then to the original and proper standard; and if, after notice given, they should give goods instead of money, I would prosecute them for theft; it would be dispersing a worse than useless set of men, and, as it were, forcing honesty upon the boatmen.

The Canal Company are aware of the villainy practiced on the canal by boatmen, as may be proved by the following circumstance:

A friend of mine applied at their office, in London, purposely to state the loss to which he, as a considerable trader, was subjected, by the improper gauges taken by their clerks. Their answer was (and an extremely proper one), "Prove to us satisfactorily that it was our servants, and not yours, and we will attend to it." What could he say, or how could he draw the line between the servants of the Company (whose gauge was, probably, beyond the real weight), and his servants (the boatmen), who had given a part of the goods, in lieu of money, to the leggers? I shall now more particularly address myself to the traders of Northampton, with many of whom I have the honour to be personally acquainted, and trust that they will take it into their mature consideration: there can be no question as to the propriety of it, and an example from so respectable a body of traders, and from a town so well known in the commercial world, could not fail in producing, what the traders generally must see the necessity of, namely, the expulsion of the leggers from the tunnels, and the resumption of the boatmen attending to their business themselves. Thus would the interest of the trader be confirmed, the honesty of the boatmen strengthened, and a horde of vicious, immoral, and unprincipled characters ousted from a situation where they have been enabled in some measure, from the difficulty of obtaining evidence to prosecute, to persist in their conduct with impunity. If we regard public morality, let us endeavour to suppress vice – it is a duty we owe to society, setting aside individual interest. But when we see morality, interst, and the security of the neighbourhood attacked by an idle and useless set of men, we ought not to hesitate, but adopt those measures which would prevent their having the opportunity to be vicious. It is the traders' province, in this instance, to step forward and crush the system at once. Let the cause be taken away, and it is perfectly logical to conclude, that the effect will cease. The cause, in this instance, I conceive, originated in complete indolence on the part of some few of the boatmen; a demand for labour consequently ensued; it appears that the supply, in consequence of the universal want of employment, has exceeded the demand; and the natural consequence is, that there are a great many partially employed, and, in some instances, idle hands, with precarious means of support. The effect is robberies, of various descriptions, from the boats on the canal to the traveller on the highway, - thye encouragement of vice and immorality, from swearing, drunkenness, &c. I anticipate, with pleasure, seeing an example set by the traders of Northampton, which will shew to the world, that amidst the hurry of business they do not neglect the protection of morality.

I am, very respectfully, Gentlemen,

Your obedient Servant.

A TRADER.

The Canal Company responded in 1827 by creating a new occupation *Registered Leggers* to outlaw the casual labourers who bullied and intimidated boaters to employ them to leg their boats through both Blisworth and Braunston tunnels. To distinguish *Company Leggers* from those offering casual labour Grand Junction Canal Company leggers were issued with numbered brass armbands illustrated in Figure 14, where the inset top right is a reproduction of an official leggers brass armlet registration number 18. The Company's legger gangs were provided with a hut in Stoke Bruerne from which they legged in pairs, returning over the hill with their *wings on their backs,* teams being available 24 hours a day, seven days a week.

The landscape changes in Stoke Bruerne.

Passing of the 1833 London and Birmingham Railway Bill posed a threat to the carrying of goods on canals, in response the Grand Junction Canal Company made improvements to speed up canal traffic, made possible in Stoke Bruerne by the Duke of Grafton selling further plots of land to the canal company[27]. In 1835 these improvements altered the village landscape when the company duplicated the seven locks, created a double arch bridge over the canal near top lock, built an additional arch at the turnpike bridge below lock 18, laid a new towing path on the west side of the canal and constructed side ponds on the south west side of the lock-flight.

Although traffic on the Grand Junction Canal was going through a period of change, brought about by the growth of railway companies, for many companies, canals had been the only means by which they could move raw-materials and finished products. Narrow-boat cargo's on the Grand Junction Canal reflected trade of the time: Iron consisted of both manufactured and un-manufactured iron; coal drawn from collieries in Derbyshire, Warwickshire, Staffordshire, Leicestershire, Nottinghamshire and even Lancashire; Grain was a major back-load from London to mills along the Grand Junction and into Oxfordshire, particularly Banbury; Several types of salt, for example fine or table salt for human consumption, and broad salt for agricultural use was carried to London, mainly from Droitwich; Timber and deals were useful back-load for boats returning from London, large quantities coming from the Baltic region. Sand and Bricks were carried due to the numerous brick yards and sand pits along the canal. Lime and limestone was packaged patent or prepared lime, the forerunner of modern cement. General cargo to and from London included sugar, groceries, cloth, wool, boxes or casks of patent [artificial] manure and oilcake, fire-clay products, clay and bricks from Stourbridge, ale from Burton, Cheshire cheese, various types of earthenware and pottery from the Potteries including bricks and drain-pipes, stone bottle ware, Yorkshire paving stone, flour, hides, cullet (broken glass), zinc, flints, tallow, marble, Portland stone, spelter and soaper, and ironstone (quarried in Northampton and taken to the Black Country)[28]. Boaters passing through Stoke Bruerne were the labouring classes whose livelihoods were obtained through being employed by canal carrying companies who transported these cargoes for merchants, traders and manufacturers in their own fleets of boats, or by boats owned by merchants, traders and manufacturers themselves. To a lesser extent some boatmen owned or hired crafts, working for carriers or merchants as independent contractors plying for hire.

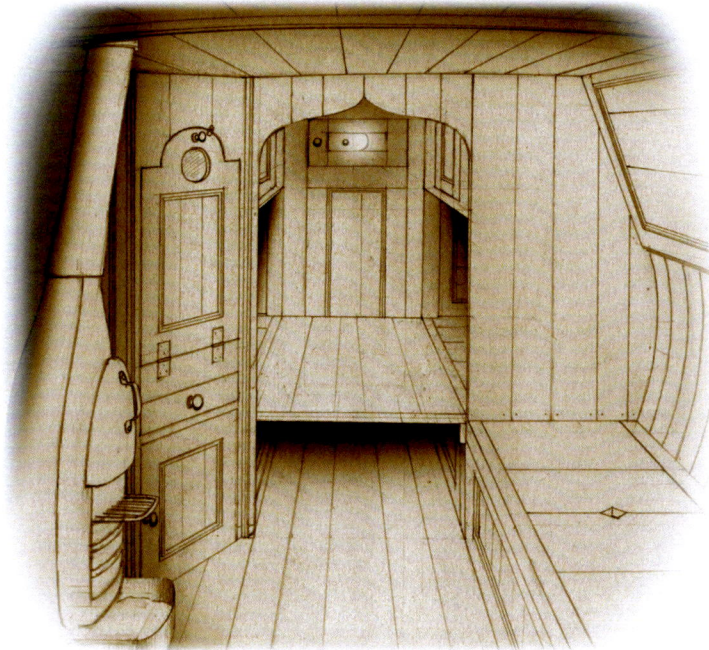

Figure 15   Back cabin layout before the Canal Boats
Act 1877 (Christopher M Jones)

For live-aboard boating families the *back cabin* of the narrow boat provided them with limited accommodation as they were *fitted out* with only the essentials. Figure 15 shows an impression of the basic cabin furniture built into many narrow boats prior to the regulations introduced in the Canal Boats Act of 1877[29], the main points to note from the illustration is the wooden bulkhead on the right with enclosed cupboards behind and above the main bed. A drop down table and side bed, and a stove (the original design being *bottle nosed*). Boat families equipped

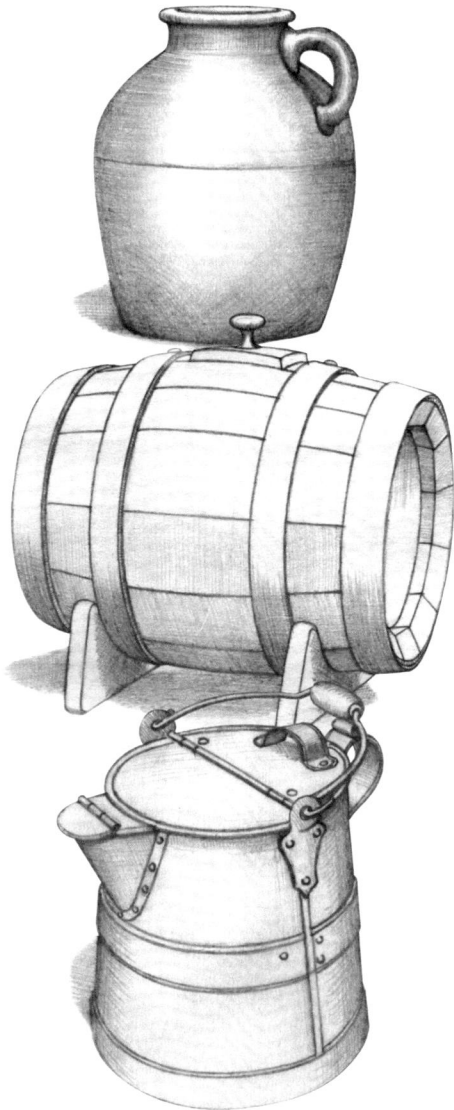

Figure 16   Vessels boaters used for fresh water (Christopher M Jones)

the back cabin with only day to day necessities; a kettle, cooking pots and crockery, kept to a minimum to meet their needs. Clean water was stored in cans, stone jars or barrels as illustrated in Figure 16, boaters filling these at natural streams en route[30]. For boat families their work was fraught with a persistent risk of accident and injury, risks which were exacerbated by the constantly changing weather, and towpaths *filthy with horse muck*. Deaths related to the canal in the early years of the Grand Junction Canal in Stoke Bruerne can be seen from the burial records of Saint Mary's church shown in Table 3, from the records it can be seen children were residing on canal boats as early as the 1820's.

As the community expanded in Stoke Bruerne Rev Lee, Rector of Saint Mary's approached the Parish Council regarding the building of a school-room. Although the initial request was refused, after revising his plans the Sheppard's[31] a local farming family, conveyed in trust a piece of land to the Rector. With a grant from the Anglican National School Society Rev Lee erected a 42 feet by 20 feet schoolroom on the road leading to the church, opening it's doors in 1838.

Lock keeper John Child raised five children following the family's arrival at Lock 15, in the late 1830's the second generation of the Child family began to marry, eldest son John Junior marrying farmers daughter Sarah Ann Sheppard in 1837. After the sudden death of John Child Senior, John Child Junior *followed in his father's footsteps* becoming both head of the Child family and lock keeper. In 1841 John and Sarah Child were living at lock cottage with their daughters Mary and Jane, John's widowed mother Jane, younger brother and boatman Thomas, and younger sister Jane. John Junior's other brother William also lived in Stoke Bruerne with his wife Esther Elizabeth[32].

Table 3: Saint Mary the Blessed Virgin. Canal related burials 1819-1830.

Burial date	Name	Age	Parents	Description
20th Nov 1819	Thomas Lloyd	30		Boatman drowned in Canal at Lock (from or about Bedworth)
16th Jan 1822	Henry Carter	10	Joseph and Elizabeth	Drowned
29th Aug 1822	Eleanor Travis	1	William and Mary	Died on boat 28th August
16th Aug 1823	Unknown female	20 - 30		Found drowned in lock
3rd Nov 1823	George Shaw	Abt 21		Drowned in lock near Turn pike
29th Sept 1826	Mary Hannah Brentnele	4 months	John and Marie	Died on canal boat
3rd Aug 1829	Thomas Harris	38		Drowned at Islington. Transported back to Stoke Bruerne
11th Mar 1830	John Hall	1yr 11 months		Drowned in canal

The first modern census enumerated 435 inhabitants in the Parish of Stoke Bruerne, men of the village being most commonly employed as agricultural labourer, although eleven worked for the Grand Junction Canal Company as labourers[33]. The canal labourer's worked and lived alongside rural tradesmen in the village including: masons, carriers, carpenters, tailors, butchers, a blacksmith, a postman, a shopkeeper, a coal merchant and a miller. Also residing in the village were a number of shoe and lace makers traditional trades in Northamptonshire. Not long after the 1841 census the Duke of Grafton was awarded a Royal Assent for *An Act for inclosing Lands in the Parish of Stoke Bruerne*. On commencing the *inclosing of his land*, the Duke was required to abide by a clause in the statute schedule specific to the Grand Junction Canal which passed through his land in the Parish of Stoke Bruerne.

> LXXVI. Provided always, and be it further enacted. That it shall not be lawful for the said Commissioner to divert, turn, widen, or alter ant Brooks, Streams, Ditches, Drains, Watercourses, Tunnels, Watergates, Banks, or Bridges within the said parish … Now running into or forming part of the Works of the Grand Junction Canal, or to order a new Bridge or Bridges to be made over and across the said Canal by virtue of the said recited Act or of this Act, without the consent of the Company of Proprietors of the said Canal in Writing under their Common Seal first had and obtained; and that nothing herein contained shall extend or be constructed to extend or enable the said Commissioner to do, or order or cause to be done, any Act, Matter, or Thing which shall alter or prejudice the Navigation or Works of the Canal, or the Towing Horse Road over the tunnel of the said canal …[34]

Around the time of inclosure an accident in Saint Mary's resulted in the *death by peculiar circumstances* of twenty-two year old George Pettifer, a member of the local blacksmith's family …

The bell-ropes of the church had been under repair, and on Monday, in consequence of the village feast, four or five persons went into the Church-loft to ring the bells, but the deceased imprudently went unknown to his companions into the place above, where the bells were hung; shortly afterwards, at a time when the bells were ringing, a heavy fall was heard, and blood flowed through the ceiling upon the ringers; it was ascertained that deceased was dead and bleeding profusely in the head, having evidently been struck by the bell, which weighed 12 cwt. It is supposed that he must have walked on a plank which the labourers had placed for their convenience when repairing the ropes[35].

Two businessmen moved to Stoke Bruerne in the 1840's, both played a part in changing the village landscape. Joseph Ebbern[36] [c.1841] acquired the under-developed land on the east side of the canal next to top-lock, originally part of George Tite's Home Close Farm. Mr Ebbern most probably purchased the land from the Duke of Grafton during the Inclosure activities, funding the purchase through a loan from his ageing father[37]. After obtaining permission from the Grand Junction Canal Company Joseph Ebbern built a canal-side warehouse, a canal arm and a dock for loading and unloading boats. To maintain the continuity of the Grand Junction Canal Company towing path he also built a steep bridge in the towing path over the canal arm leading to the warehouse arm. On completion of the building work

EBBERN's WHARF, STOKE BRUERNE.
J.EBBERN
Begs leave to inform his friends and the public that he has constantly on sale at the above wharf, COALS, COKE, LIME, SALT, BRICKS, DRAINING TILES, and SLATES, on the most reasonable terms.

N.B. Goods forwarded by Fly Boats to all parts of the Kingdom.
Stoke Bruerne, Sept. 24, 1844

Figure 17   Joseph Ebbern advertisement (Northampton Mercury)

Ebbern's Wharf commenced trading, with Mr Ebbern regularly advertising his wares in the local newspaper[38] as shown in Figure 17. Details of the Duke of Grafton's Inclosure Award were published on April 9th 1844 with an associated map[39], as illustrated in Figure 18, at the time Joseph Ebbern occupied Plot 32, a cottage and gardens (0 acres, 3 roods, 4 perches). In December 1846 Joseph Ebbern married Caroline Bailey from Kislingbury, on the marriage certificate his occupation is given as Boatmaster, Stoke Bruerne[40].

Mr George Savage with his young family[41] also moved to Stoke Bruerne, initially leasing The Navigation Inn as the family home. Soon after arriving Mr Savage erected Stoke Brick and Tile Works, with a canal arm, a dock on the east side of the canal below Lock 15 and a bridge in the towing path over the canal arm leading to the brick works, on land owned by the Duke of Grafton, the works being located in an ideal position to receive clay from pits on the Grafton estate[42] and opposite the Savage's home. In the late 1840's Mr Savage worked as contractor

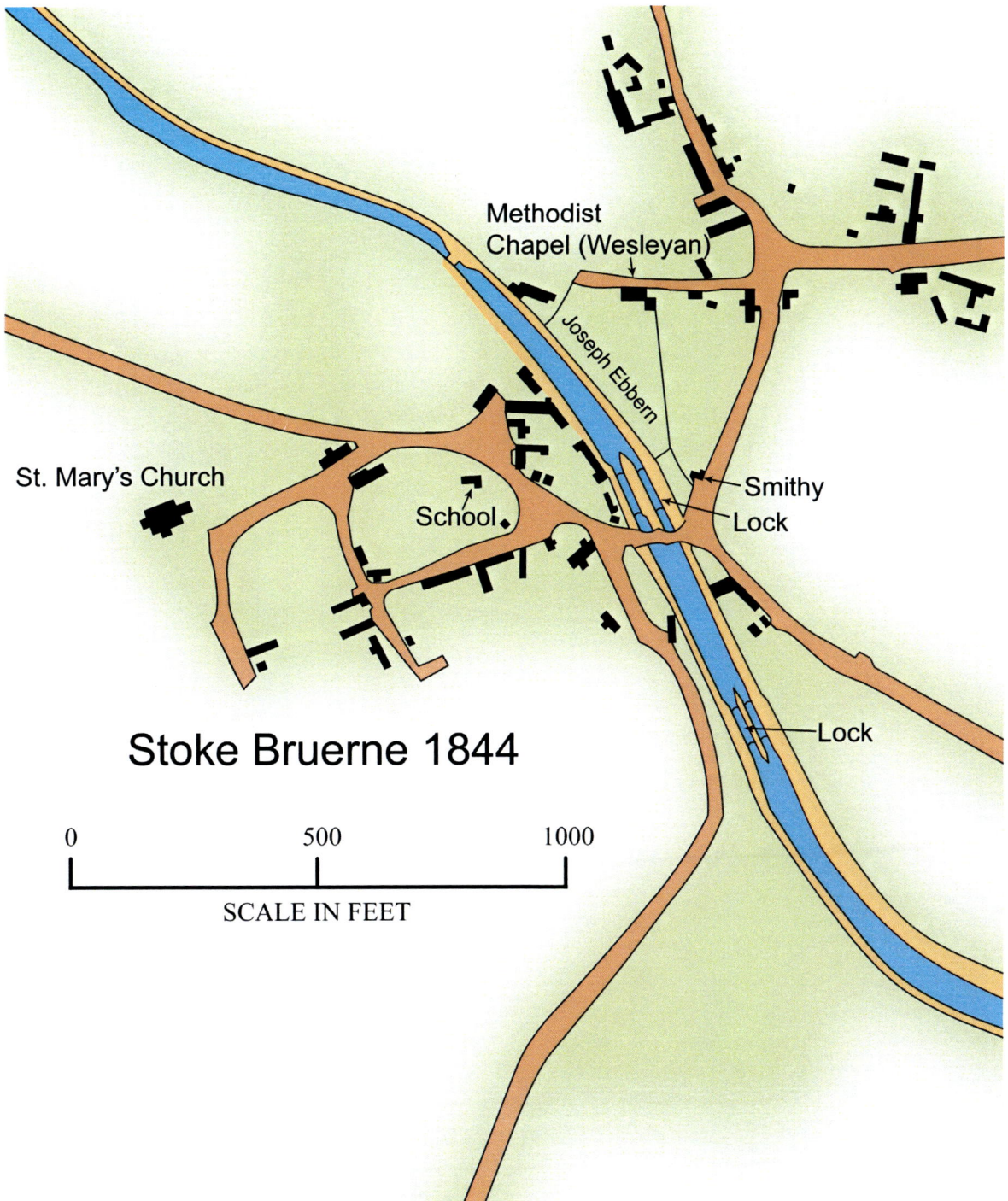

Methodist Chapel (Wesleyan)

Joseph Ebbern

St. Mary's Church

School

Smithy

Lock

Lock

Stoke Bruerne 1844

0   500   1000

SCALE IN FEET

Figure 18   Duke of Grafton Inclosure Map 1844 (Christopher M Jones)

to the Grand Junction Canal Company converting a hut to a semi-detached pair of cottages adjacent to bottom lock for housing the canal company stable keeper. Georgina Jane and Alfred Henry Savage were born after George and Elizabeth arrived in the village, both children were baptised at Saint Mary's[43].

Family boaters caught in the middle.

The industrial revolution saw mass migration from rural to urban settings as a result by the mid nineteenth century half of England's labouring population were living in cheap, overcrowded, insanitary city housing. These squalid living conditions led to the proliferation of diseases' such as Cholera, which caused thousands of deaths before reaching epidemic levels in the 1830's. Typhus, an acute infectious and epidemic disease was also rife in the labouring population, which was believed by Edwin Chadwick[44] to be *fatal to male breadwinners leaving families dependent on relief,* Chadwick insisting epidemics were due to poor urban drainage resulting in towns being covered in a *residue of filth* which contaminated the air [The Miasma Theory]. Government responded to Chadwick by charging him to report on *The Sanitary Conditions of the Labouring Population of Great Britain.* The report published in 1842 gave explicit descriptions of the *grossly insanitary conditions in which the labouring population lived,* conditions Chadwick related to the high incidence of disease (morbidity) and death (mortality) in this class. An illustration of the cause and effect chain is depicted in Figure 19.

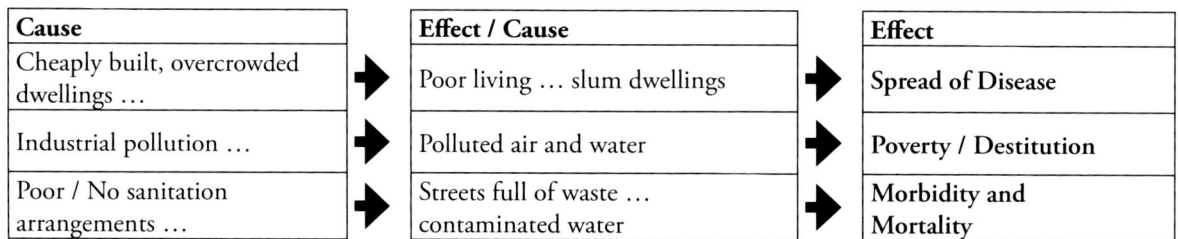

Cause		Effect / Cause		Effect
Cheaply built, overcrowded dwellings …	➡	Poor living … slum dwellings	➡	Spread of Disease
Industrial pollution …	➡	Polluted air and water	➡	Poverty / Destitution
Poor / No sanitation arrangements …	➡	Streets full of waste … contaminated water	➡	Morbidity and Mortality

Figure 19   Cause and effect of poor health in the urban labouring population (Della Sadler-Moore)

Chadwick's report led to a Royal Commission on *the state of large towns and populous districts,* after the report was published *The Health of the Towns Association* was established with responsibility for the diffusion of information on the physical and moral evils arising from insanitary conditions, their mission being …

> … to substitute Health for disease, Cleanliness for filth, Order for disorder, Economy for waste, Prevention for palliation, Justice for charity, Enlightened self-interest for ignorant selfishness and to bring to the poorest and meanest – Air, Water, Light.

Whilst the *Sanitary Movement* was underway, the first parliamentary lens to cast it's eyes on *itinerant live-aboard boaters* was a House of Lord's Select Committee appointed to *inquire into the expediency of Restraining the practice of carrying Goods and Merchandisze on Canals, Navigable Rivers, and Railways on Sundays*[45]. The Select Committee having been appointed as a result of Lord Hatherton and the Marquess of Normanby speaking out in the House of Lord's on behalf of *boatmen on canals*. Lord Hatherton presented to his learned colleagues a petition *against the prevailing system of traffic on canals on Sundays,* signed by boatmen from Penn in Staffordshire, in his speech he outlined his concerns regarding the neglect of boatmen as a class of people …

> The present system was totally unnecessary, and unproductive of good to any class, either to the merchant, the labourer, or the public. With regard to one class, and one especially, deserving the kindest consideration of the House. He should, in a few days, present a petition universally signed by those boatmen who justly complained that they alone of all the labourers in her Majesty's kingdom, were restrained to work on a Sunday. They thought, and he agreed with them, that all considerations, moral, religious, and political-combined to render an abolition of this system in every way expedient. The petitioners, whose petitions he now presented, entertained the same views and made the same prayer, and with that prayer he begged to express his entire concurrence[46].

After the weekend break the Marquess of Normanby rose to bring forward a motion before his honourable colleagues *that a select committee be appointed to consider the present system of Trafficking On Canals on Sunday's*[47], which in his opinion was required for one reason only …

> … an inquiry should be instituted to decide whether the present state of things ought to be allowed to exist. It was the first duty of a moral and religious community-when, at any rate, it could be accomplished without injury to any class, and unless some strong reason were opposed to it-to keep the strictest observance of the seventh day. Now, he believed that in the present system of Sunday trafficking on canals little benefit was derived by anyone.

The motion was agreed, the Select Committee was appointed and a range of people associated with canal and river navigations were called to give evidence as listed in Table 4, not one boater was called to speak for themselves or for their class. The evidence received by the committee gives an insight into a range of *officials* perspectives on boaters and boating work during the early 1840's.

Table 4   Stakeholders giving evidence to the Select Committee on Sunday Trafficking 1841

Name	Position
Sir George Chetwynd	Connected in property with Trent and Mersey Canal Company … acquainted with Boatmen's habits
Alexander Hordern	Shareholder Staffs and Worcs and Birmingham canals
Josiah Anthony Hayes	General Agent and receiving clerk for the Staffs and Worcs canal
John Wheeley Lea	Worcs and B'ham canal … lives near Salt at Droitwich
Thomas Bagnall	Coal and Iron Master – West Bromwich

Thomas Harrison	Superintendent of shipping company – Droitwich and Worcester … Patent Salt Company
Francis Twemlow	Chair of the Quarter sessions for the County of Stafford
John Crowley	Partnership at Wolverhampton
Richard Heath	Carrier owner at Stourport
Benjamin Devey	Carrier on the Severn
John Whitehouse	Carrier at Dudley … Tipton to London
Lord Francis Egerton	Sole interest in the Bridgewater Canal
John Davies	Rector at Worcester
Edward Atherton Lingard	Agent: Old quay company proprietors of Mersey and Irwell Navigation, Runcorn.
William Ward	The Oxford Canal, Carrying Company owner with father
John Moss	Chairman re railways: G J Railway. Deputy Liverpool and Manchester Regs re railway
Rev Frederick Wade	Resident Trent & Mersey / Harecastle Tunnel (legging) p88 sick boatmen
Charles Inman	Previously junior partner at Pickford's now merchant at Liverpool
Philip Pleydell Bouverie	Connected with GJCCCo Member of Select Committee Ceased to be chairman in June
Richard Cowlishaw Sale	Clerk and solicitor to GJCCCo since 1805
Joseph Baxindale	Pickford's representative

Canal company representatives unanimously agreed *transportation by canal was governed by law* and applied in the same manner as to road transport as *both were the queens highways.* As proprietors the canal companies felt they had no power to stop traffic on a Sunday because *anyone has the right to navigate a boat on a canal on payment of tolls.* The canal companies agreed the passage of boats on a Sunday *had increased considerably over the last 20-30 years,* the evils of which they *laid at the doors of factories and merchants who press for quick delivery due to the urgency of traders' to see their loads delivered on time.* The companies viewing the prevailing climate as one of *competition for carrying contracts,* with carriers who delivered *even just a few hours earlier than another* being favoured, whilst *slower carriers lost contracts.*

Carriers reported operating different practices regarding Sunday working, for example Thomas Bagnall a coal and iron master from West Bromwich *never carried materials by canal on a Sunday and prohibits any boatman travelling on a Sunday, wherever they might be on the canal.* Similarly John Whitehouses' company had not *let boats travel on a Sunday for five years,* to which he added *we not suffered at all.* In contrast to the smaller carriers Joseph Baxendale, representative for Pickford's the largest carrying company of the time painted a very different picture when he informed the committee of the regular practice of *prepping cargos on a Saturday night for departure on a Sunday* which resulted in *boaters feeling under pressure to commence their journey once loading was complete.*

The committee were informed of a number of petitions submitted in recent years to government, *which indicated the strong feelings of boatmen wanting a day of rest.* Rev. Davies, Rector of Worcester talked about the petition he submitted, commencing his account with a quote from a boatman who on making his mark on the petition said *I wish I could sign it with both of my hands,* a comment Rev. Davies felt *summed up the feelings of this class of people.* The committee then invited Rev. Davies to give an account of his *connexion and interest with boatmen*, to which he recalled being *asked to visit a demoralised dying boatman*, the experience of which stimulated him to enquire into *the state of this class of men in general, and to trace the source of their demoralised condition*[18]. From his investigations Rev. Davies came to the conclusion *boaters whole lives were detached from those around them as they associate together, they are quite a class of men* sui generis, more specifically he informed the committee he knew of *Four Classes of boatmen …*

The First Class - those who are apparently lost to all right feeling. Men given to profligate and abandonment habits, who, if they think they can escape Human Detention, will be guilty of any of those crimes which are ascribed to them …

The Second Class - who appear to be very well-disposed men, anxious to obtain the Rest of the Sabbath, that they might improve it to the high and holy purpose for which it was originally appointed.

Of this class of men many are really depressed in their minds; they feel themselves aggrieved in two points of view; as British Subjects, that they are deprived of those Rights to which they are entitled, for they consider that every British Subject is entitled to the Rest of the Sabbath; they also have a still higher motive, many of them,- they are anxious to spend it, as I have said, aright. But I think that the First Class oftentimes receives an Accession from this Second Class, from those who have stood out against Temptation for a Time, but ultimately, being cut off from all Religious Instruction, they have yielded to those bad Habits of Drinking and Profligacy to which they have been tempted; and they have filled up those ranks in the First Class which have been thinned by Transportation and other Punishments.

The Third Class – are few in number; but I have met with no Persons in any Situation who surpass the reformed Bargemen or Boatmen in all that constitutes Excellency of Character; kind Fathers, affectionate Husbands, honest Servants, and really Ornaments to their Station in Society. I have been gratified in visiting some of these Men.

The Fourth Class – is a very important Class, to which those who are anxious to benefit these Men should particularly direct their Attention, I humbly conceive. It is the Boys; Lads from Twelve to Sixteen Years of Age. Your Lordships must probably have noticed in the Constabulary Report that one of the Police Officers stated that he found Lads of Twelve or Fourteen as impervious to any Attempts to ascertain the State of Crime that existed as the most hardened Men in advanced years … Although Pains may have been taken by Clergymen in instructing these poor Lads, even the most promising are too often led astray … There have been found in these Men, both individually and collectively, Proofs of the Advantage of Instruction… some of my Brother Clergymen who have visited this Class during Illness have had Reason to believe there has been a salutary Effect produced on their Minds by the Instruction they have received. Upon their recovery they have shed Tears when they have left their Homes to resume their Labours saying, "Now I must go back, and must be obliged to profane the Sabbath". These poor Men are in a peculiar Situation, that if they do not violate the Law of God and their Country thay are liable to be turned out of their Situation and lose their Bread … A Man came to me on Monday Morning, and said "Sir, I worked Four Hours Yesterday Morning, against my Conscience, and because I would not go on a second Time I am turned out of employment."

Two senior officials from the Grand Junction Canal Company gave evidence. Chairman, the Honourable P. P. Bouverie began by informing the committee *the number of boats on the Grand Junction was greater than any other canal,* after which he emphasised *use of the term Sunday Trading was wrong as there was no buying or selling on a Sunday, only liberty of passage.* Bouverie's main concern was with regard to *any future Bill being introduced which would prohibit traffic on a Sunday,* asserting this approach would *lead traders to choose a different mode of conveyance.* A concern to which he suggested an alternative to a whole day's stoppage … *if stoppage enforced on the grounds of observance of the Sabbath it should be limited to the hours of divine service*[49].

Also from the Grand Junction Canal Company was R. C. Sale who reported *his company had on numerous occasions discussed Sunday Trading,* and they were in agreement that any *stoppages should also apply to road and rail transport and not just boaters.* From his position as a Solicitor Mr Sale advised *no changes were needed to the law by introducing a new act as the issue would be better addressed by empowering canal companies to make bye-laws.* Before withdrawing Mr Sale was asked *Do boatmen [on the Grand Junction] have a strong desire for a day of rest in the week?,* he replied …

> Yes, many have, the mass is careless about it. Last 30 years – number ameliorated in their habits, they bear a very indifferent character in the scale of society. No class of society so neglected as these men …

The committee ordered the *report of the evidence* to be printed on May 4th 1841, then forwarded to the House of Lords. In September the Boatmen's Pastoral Instruction Society[50] wrote extensively in support of an Act of Parliament with regard to *the prohibition of Sunday traffic on canals and railways,* having received the evidence Parliament went silent.

The final *Health of Towns* report was published in 1845, in which it highlighted *the continued and deplorable extent of urban overcrowding,* their solution was to recommend the creation of a *Central Inspectorate of Housing* and a new government department to administer; drainage, paving, cleansing and water supply in each locality. The following year the *Removal of Nuisances and Prevention of Epidemic Diseases Act* passed into law, including procedures for the *speedy removal of nuisances,* with powers given to the Privy Council to regulate on *the prevention of contagious diseases.*

The new legislative machinery was a step in the right direction, but it did not go far enough, because in 1848 the measures proved ineffective when Cholera claimed the lives of 60,000 and Influenza the lives of 50,000 in London. Parliament responded by passing the *Public Health Act for England and Wales (1848)[51]*, the Act marked the beginning of a commitment to a proactive (as opposed to a reactive) approach to Public Health[52]. The Act created a central government department, the *General Board of Health* with powers to set up *Local Government Boards (LGB's)* where death rates were high, or where a tenth of poor law rate payers petitioned for one.

Whilst the public health agenda percolated through urban and rural England slowly effecting improvements in living conditions for the *settled* labouring classes, no one thought to focus attention on the health and wellbeing of the itinerant inland waterway's population. Itinerant live-aboard family boaters during this first sixty years of working on the Grand Junction Canal survived in an *era of no work no pay*, there was no *employer provided* compensation for injuries acquired in the course of boating work, and no sick-pay for boaters laid up as a result of illness or injury. Although there is some evidence of the opportunity for boaters to join a Boat Society which would *pay out in times of need*. An example of a Boat Society being started in Long Buckby is seen in an advert below[53] …

TO CARRIERS, BOATMEN, AND OTHERS.

A BOAT SOCIETY will commence on Monday March the 2nd, 1840. At Mrs. BUNTING's, New Inn. BUCKBY TOP LOCK, when the first monthly dues will be received.

Any person desirous of becoming a member,

Will oblige their obedient servant,

John Watson

If a boat family were *laid up* as a result of illness or injury it meant tapping into their savings, if they had any. Because live-aboard boaters were not part of a Parish, it was unlikely they were eligible for Poor Relief unless they had a home or a family on the bank they could return to in times of need, although there was always the possibility of removal from the boat to the workhouse. Boating life was hard, working through all seasons, and for many the pressure of delivering on time meant a relentless seven day working week.

The scene is set in Brick and Stone.

During this first sixty years Stoke Bruerne developed its infrastructure as a direct result of the canal *cutting through the village.* Joseph Ebbern at sometime between his marriage in 1846 and the end of this half century erected properties on his land next to the warehouse and dock: four three storey tenement cottages facing the line of the Grand Junction Canal, a pair of cottages next to top-lock, and a number of tenements in Chapel Lane, despite his financial situation being under question as his canal carrying partnership with his brother was dissolved in 1847 due to bankruptcy[54]. For the Child family who had been living at the lock-keepers cottage since the canal opened, tragedy befell them in the 1840's, when the head of the family John Child, and his wife Sarah passed away leaving two daughters. Only a few years later John Junior's brother William lost his wife Elizabeth and their third child (age 28 and 6 months respectively)[55].

From the mid 1830's deaths related to the canal in Stoke Bruerne continued, as seen from the parish burial register transcribed in Table 5[56], although the records show it was not only boaters' who succumbed to the dangers of the canal, as shown by a local family the Dimpsey's who lost two children due to drowning. At the inquest of eight year old Fanny Dimpsey[57] it was ascertained Frances was playing with other children when she fell in the canal and drowned. Hannah Wickens[58] was also a local child, at Hannah's inquest it was heard she was playing with two friends only minutes before her body was found in the canal … *it appeared that in walking on a board in the canal she fell into the water and was drowned before assistance could be procured.* A number of Stoke men also drowned due to drunkenness. Further deaths in Stoke Bruerne occurred due to the canal, which are unreported in Saint Mary's burial records because these victims were returned to their own Parish, as was the case of William Irons from the nearby village Roade. William went to The Boat public-house after work where he *drank half-a-pint of ale,* on leaving the pub it was an *intensely dark night,* William slipped into the lock and although assistance was instantly procured *he was quite dead when taken out.*[59]

Table 5: Saint Mary the Blessed Virgin. Canal related burials 1835-1848

Burial date	Name	Age	Description
22nd July 1835	Fanny Dimpsey	8	Drowned in canal – accident
23rd Feb 1837	Thomas Wood	6	Died of smallpox
22nd April 1837	Anthony Garratt	70	Drowned in the lock – drunk
5th Nov 1837	Thomas Harris	37	Drowned in canal – drunk
25th Sept 1839	Joseph Scaldwell	6 ½	Drowned in canal – Stoke Wharf
9th May 1843	Hannah Wickens	6	Drowned in canal
7th Feb 1845	Unknown man	27/28	Drowned in canal
1st Feb 1847	Ann Stevens (from the Midlands)	45	Boatman's wife drowned accidentally Stoke Bruerne
2nd Mar 1848	George Dimpsey	10	Drowned

On a more positive note, and just a few miles along the Grand Junction Canal at Long Buckby Wharf lived lock-keeper Thomas Amos, his wife Mary and their nine children[60]. The Amos's youngest son John being a rope-maker having served his apprenticeship at the rope-walk near the family home. John Amos married Elizabeth Ireson[61] from the nearby village of Naseby in 1849, the following year their first child William was born. After the birth of their son the Amos family (John, Elizabeth and William) moved from Lock 7 (Long Buckby) to near Lock 14 (Stoke Bruerne), approximately fifteen and a half Grand Junction Canal miles, on their arrival in the village the landscape along the line of the canal was set in brick and stone.

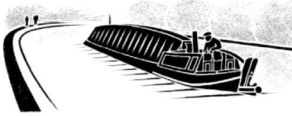

The Amos family arrive in Stoke Bruerne

John and Elizabeth Amos, with son William moved into one of Joseph Ebbern's rented cottages in Chapel Lane. Although John was a new edition to the Parish, he would be familiar with boaters due to his upbringing as a lock keeper's son, and from his own craftsmanship as a rope maker in Long Buckby[62]. On moving to the village John set up his first rope making business, the equipment needed would be fashioned by the local carpenter and blacksmith, because apart from the rope turning machinery and a straight length of ground for the rope-walk, the only other requirement would be hemp or cotton yarn from which the rope would be made[63]. Rope was an essential part of canal boats, and for John the move to Stoke Bruerne would be an ideal position for his business, as it was close to the canal. Carriers with fleets of boats, or canal companies with their own maintenance or carrying boats would purchase rope in bulk from a suitable rope supplier, whereas individual boaters and smaller carriers would usually choose local rope-makers who could supply individual lengths of rope at the required size and weight. Different sizes of ropes were used on the canal for towing boats and mooring lines, as well as straps for stopping the boat at locks, with smaller sizes being used as strings for sheeting up the boats *side cloths* and tying down *top cloths*, whilst old ropes were used for fender making[64].

At the time of the Amos's arrival widowed lock keeper William Child was raising his orphaned nieces Mary (12) and Jane (10), alongside his own children Esther Elizabeth (9) and William (7), in 1853 William re-married Hannah Grisbrook, eldest daughter of John Grisbrook, toll collector. Blacksmith Robert Pettifer was doing well in the village as he had in his employment both sons, as well as two apprentices, between them they were shoeing a large number of Grand Junction Canal Company horses, averaging 75 horses per month[65]. Other tradesmen in the village at the time included[66]; two carriers, two butchers, two bakers, two stonemasons, three beer retailers, three coal dealers / merchant, two boot and shoe manufacturers, a dairyman, a miller, a saddler and a wharfinger. The parish had fifteen people *in receipt of relief,* two males and thirteen females their ages ranging from late 50's to early 90's, there was also a 29 year old woman *not of sound mind* living with her parents and siblings. Fourteen men from the village were in the employment of the Grand Junction Canal Company, named in Table 6.

Table 6: Canal related occupations of men in Stoke Bruerne (1851 Census)

Name	Occupation	Age
William Child	Lock Keeper	40
Thomas Dimsey	Lock Keeper	63
Nathaniel Carter	Lock Keeper	43
Joseph Dyke	Lock Keeper	33
Daniel Dimsey	Labourer on Canal	36
Neal Jeffreys	Labourer on Canal	35
Robert Parkinson	Labourer on Canal	55
Philip Simpson	Labourer on Canal	47
Thomas Williams	Labourer on Canal	46
William Peasland	Labourer on Canal	62
Richard Macdonald	Labourer on Canal	25
Thomas Webb	Labourer on Canal	26
George Smith	Labourer on Canal	55
William Gardner	Labourer on Canal	46

The two businessmen who made Stoke Bruerne their home in the 1840's remained in the village. George Savage now 37, was living at The Navigation Inn with his wife and young family, George being the licensed victualer, as well as farming the 168 acre *Home Close Farm*, employing five men and two boys[67]. George was also operating the brick works opposite his home, and a further brick works in Blisworth, regularly advertising the goods on sale at his brick yards in the local paper[68] shown in Figure 20. Mr Savage's business interests continued to expand, when in 1856 he obtained a contract in association with construction of L.N.W Railway branch from Northampton to Market Harborough[69].

To Land Proprietors, Farmers, Builders, and others.
STOKE BRUERNE AND BLISWORTH BRICK YARDS

George Savage begs to inform the public that he has on hand at the above Yards 1,000,000 well burnt and good Building BRICKS, and 800,000 to 1,000,000 Draining PIPES, of various sizes, from two to nine inches in bore, thoroughly well burnt, and good quality.

Parties requiring, will be liberally treated with, and as the Grand Junction Canal runs alongside the said yards, the carriage to a considerable distance is but trifling, which George Savage would undertake.

Stoke Bruerne, November 2nd, 1854.

Figure 20   George Savage Brick Yards advertisement (Northampton Mercury)

Joseph Ebbern with his wife Caroline and their seven year old adopted son Peter Tite were also in the village, by now Mr Ebbern was a property owner, landlord, coal merchant and a farmer employing several men. In May 1853 it transpired all was not going as well as neighbours might have thought for the Ebbern family, as was revealed when Mr Ebbern was summoned to appear in court by a Northampton linen-draper on account of a debt of £21.8s.8d. incurred by his wife[70]. Mr Ebbern did not attend the hearing, but was represented by Mr Becke who opened the defense by informing the judge *Mr Ebbern was living apart from his wife under a deed of separation.* The proceedings revealed Joseph's estranged wife's spending habits, Caroline having run up a number of debts for *goods of a similar character without the defendant's authority or knowledge;* Mr. West of Towcester £13.16s.6d; Mrs Roby of Towcester £5; Mrs. Randall of Northampton £6; Mr. Whiting of Towcester £6 and finally Mr. Jenkinson of Towcester, £29.10s. The judge declared *it was his job to ascertain whether the debt was of a nature to come within the implied authority given to a wife by the law to pledge her husband's credit for necessities,* Mr Becke responded by pointed out his *client had not been aware of the dealings of his wife until application was made for payment of the balance.* Having heard the claims the judge acknowledged Mr Ebbern's position to be a hard one, but concluded …

> … he did not see how [Ebbern] could escape the claim … If the whole of the goods supplied to the wife had been had from defendant, he might well have suspected that she was exceeding the authority of her husband. But all he knew about was the £20 worth supplied by himself, and he dare say there were many coal-merchants besides Mr. Ebbern whose wives spend £20 a year in dress… He had a right, therefore, to give judgement for plaintiff, debt and costs.

The plaintiff applied for immediate payment, Mr Becke requesting the period be extended over twelve months, His Honour agreeing to this set a fixed payment of £2 each month until the debts were cleared. The year after the court hearing Joseph Ebbern placed his property portfolio of nine properties and stabling for 15 horses in Stoke Bruerne up for auction, the stabling was most probably used for his business interests in relation to fly-boats and what was thought to be *a single-house outside top lock,* was in fact two tenements, one housing the village butcher. Details of Ebbern's properties were placed in an advert in the Northampton Mercury[71] transcribed in Figure 21, the sale drew to a close the family's association with Stoke Bruerne[72].

The rural community of Stoke Bruerne did not escape the ills of infectious disease in the early 1850's when a spate of fatalities struck. Typhus claimed the lives of five women and one man in 1850/51, two years later was particularly tragic when in March 1853 four babies aged three weeks to one year died from Influenza, and the following year Cholera claimed the lives of five people[73]. A particularly tragic loss of life also occurred in 1854 at top-lock when 13 year old John Henoth a lad employed on a boat going to Leicester *endeavoured to jump from the towing path into the boat … he alighted onto some chains, and, his heels tripping up, he fell backwards into the lock. The rush of water carried him under the boats, and before he could be got out life was extinct.* The inquest held at The Boat Inn returned a verdict of accidental death[74].

STOKE BRUERN, Northamptonshire
THE NINE FREHOLD MESSUAGES
WAREHOUSES, BUTCHER'S SHOP,
CANAL-BASIN, WHARFS AND LIME-KILNS
Hereinafter described; unless previously disposed of by private contract
WILL BE OFFERED
FOR SALE BY PUBLIC AUCTION,
By Mr. JOHN MACQUIRE

At the Railway Hotel, Blisworth, on Friday the 17th day of March, at Five o'clock in the afternoon, by order of the proprietor, and in one lot or more, so may be agreed upon at the time of sale.

ALL that brick-built and slated MESSUAGE (now occupied as two tenements), with the Butcher's Shop, extensive Warehousing, Stabling for 15 horses; Canal-basin, Coal Wharf and Yard, Lime-Kilns, Garden Ground, piggeries, hovels, and other outbuildings, situate in the village of STOKE BRUERN aforesaid, now in the occupation of Mr. Joseph Ebbern, the proprietor, and Mr Benjamin Cook; and of the yearly value of £50.

And also all those FOUR brick-built and tiled MESSUAGES or Tenements, adjoining the above property, with store-rooms underneath, having a frontage to the Grand Junction Canal, and a communication at the back with the premises above described, and let to respectable tenants, at a rental of £22. 4s. per annum.

And also all those FOUR stone-built and thatched COTTAGES or Tenaments, standing at the back of the above property, and producing a rental of £17. 11s. per annum. And all that piece of Garden Ground, adjoining the said cottages, containing One Rood or thereabouts, and in the occupation of Mr Ebbern

The whole of the buildings, except the last-mentioned cottage have been recently erected, and are most substantial, and no expense has been spared to make them complete for business purposes, and the warehouse may be converted into mills at a moderate expense by the introduction of steam power.

The property is desirable for occupation or investment, and is still adapted for trade, having a frontage to the canal of 340 feet.

A fair proportion of the purchase money may remain on mortgage, if required.

Stoke Bruern is distant from the Roade station of the London and North-Western Railway, one mile, from Towcester and Blisworth three miles, and from Northampton six miles.

To view the property, apply to Mr Ebbern; and for further particulars to the Auctioneer, Northampton; or to Messrs. R.F, and C. Welchman, Solicitors, Southam and Daventry.

Figure 21 Sale of property by Joseph Ebbern. Stoke Bruerne. Auction advertisement (Northampton Mercury)

Mr Savage purchased a number of Joseph Ebbern's auctioned properties, including the canal-side warehouse which he converted in 1857 to a steam powered corn mill[75]. John Amos at some point moved to a canal-side house adjacent to top-lock, as to whether he purchased the two tenements during Ebbern's auction or whether he rented remains unknown, although he did expand his business interests by opening a grocer's shop, at a time when his wife Elizabeth gave birth in quick succession to five children; Mary Ann (b.1853), Thomas (b.1854), John Henry (b.1856), Elizabeth (b.1857) and Charles (b.1859).

In 1858 writer John Hollingshead, with his friend *Cuddy* travelled the Grand Junction Canal on Captain Randle's fly boat *Stourport* owned by the Grand Junction Canal Company[76], for the duration of their journey John and Cuddy were accommodated on a straw bed in the sheeted hold. *Stourport* departed from City Road in the dead of night, soon after the passengers experienced their first lock, tunnel and gauging procedures. As the journey proceeded John and Cuddy's main concern was their diminishing food supplies, to remedy this as they neared Stoke Brewin (Sic) they decided to walk in search of a *fresh fowl [chicken]* …

> On again we walked, with increasing appetites and decreasing hopes, until we come upon the village of Stoke Brewin … a one small cottage street, with many outlying barns:- a village that does not covet patronage of strangers. The first inquiry we made respecting this phantom fowl, was addressed to an old woman standing at the door of a thatched hut. "A vowl, measter" she asked, in astonishment. "What, a live vowl?" "No, ma'am," I said; "a dead fowl, for cooking. "Dead or alive", said Cuddy, who was more desperate. "I'm sure I don't know, measter," returned the old woman; I doan't think onybody be havin' such a thing in Stoke. Ye cen try Must'r Edwards, at the corner."

> The corner alluded to was only a few yards off, and we made rapidly towards Mr. Edwards cottage. There was Mr. Edwards, a fat man, standing in the low door-way, shaking his head at us as if we had been vagrant tramps, or he had never heard of such a bird as a fowl during the whole of his village existence. Turning our backs very quickly upon Mr. Edwards, we strode along the short street until we came to the village butcher's, whose shop was a little larger than the Stourport cabin, and would not have contained much animal food if it had been filled to overflowing. It was as clean as the cage of a wild beast an hour after feeding-time. Not a scrap of anything was visible but a piece of suet the size of a nut, upon which a dozen ravenous flies and a blue-bottle had settled. This was a state of things that required explanation, and proceeded through the shop and tapped at the half-curtained door-window of the back parlour. This was at once opened, and we saw the master of the shop devouring the only leg of mutton upon the premises.

> "Teo shillings a pound for that leg of mutton," said Cuddy, without the slightest hesitation. "Noa,'', said the man sulkily, seeming to understand the eccentric but very natural offer; "there beant too much 'ere fur my fam'ly, an' I wun't sell to ony mun"

> Further haggling was useless, and we left this mockery of a shop, with the highway-robber part of our character again strongly developed. "I tell you what Cuddy," I said "a

twenty pound note in one's pocket at Stoke Brewin is not of so much use as a pipe-light. We'd better declare on the parish."

A few more steps brought us to the canal bank, where we found another foodless tavern stocked with the thin, sour ale; and as the Stourport and it's butty –barge had not yet arrived, we entered the pale of mild dissipation to drink ourselves into a better humour.

"I suppose Lundun be very cool, now?" inquired the young lady who served us with beer. "Dull!" almost shouted Cuddy, whose gallantry was quite good; "the dullest street, in the dullest party of the city, at the dullest time of the day, and the dullest part of the year, is a beer garden compared with Stoke Brewin!". I started from the house upon hearing this speech, and was soon followed by Cuddy …

After John and Cuddy's rather interesting experiences in Stoke Bruerne they headed for the canal and found *Stourport* in top-lock, the crew preparing for the passage through the tunnel. After getting on-board the journey re-commenced, Hollingshead giving a vivid description of the passage through the tunnel …

The horses were unhooked, and while standing in a group upon the towing-path, one of the child-drivers, a girl about six years of age, got in between them with a whip, driving them, like a young Amazon, right and left; utterly disregarding the frantic yells of a dozen boatmen, and nearly half a dozen family-boatmen's wives. At the mouth of the tunnel were a number of leggers, waiting to be employed; their charge being one shilling to leg the boat through. We engaged one of these labourers for our boat to divide the duty with one of our boatmen; while the youth went over with the horse. A lantern was put at the head of the boat; the narrow boards, like tailors' sleeve-boards, were hooked on like projecting oars near the head; the two legging men took their places upon these slender platforms, lying upon their backs; and with their feet placed horizontally against the wall, they proceeded to shove us with measured tread through the long, dark tunnel.

The place felt delightfully cool, going in out of the full glare of a fierce noon-day sun; and this effect was increased by the dripping of water from the roof, and the noise caused by springs which broke in at various parts of the tunnel. The cooking on board the boats went on as usual, and our spaces being confined, and our air limited, we were regaled with several flavours springing from meat, amongst which the smell of hashed mutton certainly predominated. To beguile the tedium of the slow, dark journey-to amuse the leggers whose work is fearfully hard, and acts upon the breath after the first quarter of a mile, and above all to avail themselves of the atmospheric effects of the tunnel; the boatmen at the tillers nearly all sing, and our vocalist was the captains straw-haired son.

If any observer will take the trouble to examine the character of the songs that obtain the greatest popularity amongst men and women engaged in heavy and laborious employments, he will find that the ruling favourite is the plaintive ballad. Comic songs are hardly known. The main secret of the wide popularity of the ballads lies in the fact, that it generally contains a story, and is written in a measure that fits easily into a slow, drawling, breath-taking tune which all the lower orders know; and which-as far as I can find – has never been written or printed upon paper; but has been handed down from father or mother to son and daughter, from generation to generation, from the remotest times. The plots of these ballad stories are generally based upon the passion of love; love of the most hopeless and melancholic kind; and the suicide of the heroine, by drowning in a river is a poetical occurrence as jealousy.

There may have been a dozen of these ballads chanted in the Blisworth tunnel at the same time. The wail of our straw-haired singer rising, to our ears, above the rest. They came upon our ears, mixed with the splashing of water, in drowsy cadences, and at long intervals, like the moaning of a maniac chained to a wall. The effect upon the mind was, in this dark passage, to create a wholesome belief in the existence of large masses of misery, and the utter nothingness of the things of the upper world.

We were appraised of the approach of another barge, by the strange figure of another boatman, who stood at the head with a light. It was necessary to leave off legging for the boats to pass each other, and the leggers waited until the last moment when a concession seemed inevitable, and then sprang instantaneously, with singular dexterity, on the sides of their boats, pulling their narrow platforms up immediately after them. The action of the light in front of our boat, produced a very fantastic shadow of our recumbent boatman-legger upon the side wall of the tunnel. As his two legs struck out horizontally from the edge of the legging-board, treading, one over the other, against the wall, they threw a shadow of two arms, which seemed to be held by a thin old man-another shadow of the same substance, bent nearly double at the stomach, who worked them over and over, as if turning two great mangle-handles with both hands at the same time …

Throughout the 1850's the rector of Saint Mary's was kept busy baptising children from families associated with the canal as shown in Table 7, which includes two new additions to the Child family following William's second marriage. In the late 1850's the Amos's eldest son William, with four other lads from Stoke Bruerne joined Courteenhall Grammar School[77] shown in Table 8, William, the youngest of the boys was the first to leave after less than a year the reason given being *too far to walk*. His friend William Woodward, son of the village carrier Joseph Woodward, left after just two months to join his father's business, as did Charles Tew who joined his fathers masonry business The two other boys relocated to Stoke Bruerne School; Philip Simpson youngest son of a canal labourer and William Peasland, eldest son of the village baker. These two boys may well have returned to Stoke school due to the recent recruitment of a new School Master and School Mistress, Mr and Mrs William Pink from Chichester. The infants school had its own teacher, 59 year old Martha Shears. The village school was thriving in 1861 as shown in the census return[78], 85 scholars were residing in the village, including the majority of the Amos's young family. The number of villagers working for the Grand Junction Canal Company continued to rise as shown in Table 9, the company having promoted William Child to Canal Agent.

Table 7   **Saint Mary the Blessed Virgin. Canal related baptisms 1850-1859**

Baptism Date	Birth date	Child's Name	Parents	Father occupation
January 1850	16th Dec	James	William and Sophia Gardner	Legger SB
August 1850		Prudence C	Thomas and Elizabeth Webb	Legger
October 1850	Twins 1st October	Samuel	Joseph and Keziah Dyke	Lock Keeper
		Joseph		
November 1851	27th April	Ann Marie	Richard and Katharine Woodward	Legger
November 1851	12th Oct	Henry	Philip and Parthenia Simpson	Legger
January 1852	30th Dec	Harriett	William and Sophia Gardner	Legger
November 1852	15th Aug	John	Joseph Manoah and Louisa Jeffery	Legger
January 1853	19th Nov	Richard	Joseph and Keziah Dyke	Lock Keeper
February 1853		Frederick	William and Sophia Gardner	Legger
March 1853	11th Mar	Henry	Daniel and Elizabeth Dimpsey	Legger
September 1853		Ellen	Richard and Katharine Woodward	Legger
July 1854	25th June	James	Joseph and Keziah Dyke	Lock Keeper
February 1855	27th Jan	Joseph	Philip and Parthenia Simpson	Legger
March 1855		John G	William and Hannah Child	Lock Keeper
April 1855	26th Feb	Prudence S	William and Sophia Gardner	Legger
June 1855		Martha	Thomas and Mary Peasland	Boatman
May 1856	19th Feb '55	Elizabeth Jan	Thomas and Mary Webb	Legger
May 1856	6th April	Alfred	Thomas and Mary Peasland	Legger
September 1856	13th Aug	Annie Grisbrook	Joseph and Priscilla Putman	Ostler to GJCCo Fenny Stratford
April 1857	5th Mar	Sarah	Joseph and Keziah Dyke	Lock Keeper
April 1857	15th Mar	Thomas Henry	William and Hannah Child	Lock Keeper
July 1857		Francis	Richard and Katharine Woodward	Legger
April 1858	28th Feb	Sarah Phebe	Philip and Parthenia Simpson	Legger
January 1859	22nd Dec	Alice	William and Hannah Child	Lock Keeper

Table 8　　　**Attendance at Courteenhall Grammar School 1859-1860**

Reg No	Name	Age	Baptised	Entered	Left	Reason for leaving
90	William Peasland	14	Yes	26th January 1859	Midsummer 1860	To be under the new master at Stoke
91	William Ireson Amos	9	No	26th January 1859	Xmas 1859	Too far to walk
92	Charles Tew	10	Yes	7th February 1859	Midsummer 1859	Work
108	William Woodward	14	Yes	3rd October 1859	Xmas 1859	Work
113	Peter Simpson	10	Yes	17th October 1859	Lady day 1860	Stoke School

Table 9　　　**Canal related occupations of men in Stoke Bruerne. Census 1861**

Name	Occupation	Age
Thomas Frost	Lock Keeper	55
Richard Woodward	Legger	33
Joseph Wickens	Legger	29
Samuel Doughty	Lock Keeper	45
Benjamin West	Lock Keeper	48
Joseph Dike	Lock Keeper	43
William Gortness	Legger	58
George Smith	Legger	70
Samuel Harris	Legger	39
William Child	Canal Agent	50
Thomas Webb	Legger	34
George Warren	Legger	31
William Peasland	Legger	71
Philip Simpson	Legger	54
Thomas Williams	Legger	60
John Nicklin	Legger	23

Catastrophy and new communications come to the village.

The children and no doubt everyone else in Stoke Bruerne were excited when the Grand Junction Canal Company introduced coal burning steamers to their fleet of canal boats in 1860, excitement which was sadly short lived. On Friday 6th September 1861 an incident in Blisworth Tunnel resulted in two fatalities (William Webb and Edward Broadbent) and three men injured (William Gower, Joseph Jones and John Chalmers)[79], at the time of the incident five boats were in or passing through the tunnel …

1. A boat with two men (Stoke Bruerne carpenter **William Webb** and an unnamed boatman) employed by the Grand Junction Canal Company to do tunnel repairs.

2. The Grand Junction Canal Company steamer *Bee* with two engineers (**William Gower** and **Joseph Jones**) and two boatmen (**Edward Broadbent** and **John Chambers**)

3. A haul boat towed by the steamer *Bee* (with a crew of three un-named boatmen)

4. A Mr Fellows boat, legged by **Joseph Wickens and an unnamed legger** (Grand Junction Canal Company employees)

5. A further Grand Junction Canal Company steamer *Wasp*

Late on the Friday afternoon the steamer *Bee*, steered by Joseph Jones with a crew of three and a tow boat were on a return journey from Birmingham to London. The two boats entered the tunnel at Blisworth, at which time the wind was blowing in the same direction as the steamer was proceeding. On approaching *stanks* recently married Stoke Bruerne carpenter William Webb was doing repairs, Steerer Joseph Jones cut the steam on *Bee* to collect Webb who wanted a lift to the village to sharpen his tools. After Webb alighted *Bee* it moved off and continued the journey with the haul boat, soon after they met a boat being legged by Joseph Wickens (and an unnamed legger). *The steamer passed [Wicken's] boat on one side, and the haul boat passed on the other* at which point the tunnel was *very smoky [and] their towing lines became entangled.* The three boats were caught up for about ten minutes, until one of the haul boat crew let go of the ropes. Meanwhile Joseph Wickens and the other legger *lay down to recover till wind blew through tunnel,* Wickens recalling he shouted to *Bee but received no response.* After ten minutes the boats moved on in either direction, around the same time a second steamer *Wasp* passed Wickens's boat causing a further accumulation of smoke in the tunnel.

On *Bee* carpenter William Webb keeled over, falling onto John Chambers who was sleeping in the cabin, this caused Chambers to wake, on which he heard Webb say *one engine driver down and other taken the same.* Chambers went to the boiler room where he *became overwhelmed and fell in the water,* the shock of entering the water woke him and he swam and caught hold of the back of the boat, shouting to Broadbent to pull him in. As there was no reply Chambers raised himself onto the boat as it was exiting the tunnel in Stoke Bruerne, after turning off the engine Chamber's went into the cabin and fell asleep. On exiting the tunnel mouth *Bee* was seen heading *into the mud and reeds* by agricultural labourer John Sturgess who was leading cows by the towing path. At the hearing Sturgess recalled the incident …

> … the boat was so full of smoke I couldn't see anyone, I called out as I ran towards the tunnel when I saw a man hanging over the side, I shouted to him but there was no answer, I shouted again and a man came from under the cloth [he told me] two men were nearly dead inside, near the bed I saw a man's face. I then ran to get my master Mr Phipps. I turned back and saw a man fall in the canal, he scrabbled about and got out.

Men from Stoke Bruerne alighted *Bee* and removed William Gower and Joseph Jones to The Boat Inn, both men having been badly burnt. Later on they found out Edward Broadbent had fallen from *Bee* into the canal whilst in the tunnel, the body was recovered later that evening.

The following Monday the inquest was held at the Boat Inn, local businessman George Savage was foreman of the jury. After the jury were sworn in the proceedings were moved to the village Schoolroom due to the number of people in attendance, including Chairman of the Grand Junction Canal Company, Mr Anderson and other company members, witnesses called to give evidence are listed in Figure 22.

Joseph Wickens (Legger)

William Gower (2nd engine driver) and Joseph Jones (Engine Driver) lain on beds on the floor of the Boat Inn due to extensive burns

John Chambers (Steerer 'Bee')

John Sturgess (Labourer Shutlanger)

Samuel Harris (Legger)

William Tew (Shoemaker)

Mr Robert William Parsons Knott (Apprentice surgeon)

Mr Robert Webb Watkins (Surgeon Towcester)

Figure 22   Witness's called to give evidence at Blisworth Tunnel accident inquest 1861

The inquest opened with an account of Blisworth Tunnel, indicating it's length as 1½ miles, with one ventilation shaft ¾ mile inside the tunnel from Blisworth, the surface of which was covered with a *wooden hut like structure*. The initial lines of enquiry were directed at factors which could have led to an increased amount of smoke in the tunnel, including the type of coal used on the steamer (as to whether it had a high sulphur content) and when *Bee's* engine was last cleaned. The final question was about the fire, as to whether sufficient time had passed for it to settle before entering the tunnel. Having heard the evidence the coroner summed up …

> The facts are few and simple … medical evidence is very strong as to the real cause of death; could be no doubt it arose from asphyxia, of suffocation as it is more commonly

termed …. If they believed the death arose from suffocation, there was an end of the question. So far as the company was concerned they would, no doubt take eminent engineering opinion as to whether the smoke could be condensed or got rid of in any way, but with that the jury had nothing to do.

Of course, had there been any blame attached to the company, had the engine not been properly cleaned, that would be a question as to their liability, but not in this court. The captain of the boat, however had distinctly told them that he had examined the engine at London and Birmingham and that they in clean and good order.

All they had to do in this inquiry was to ascertain whether, as to the origin of the incident, there was any blame attached to any persons. It did not appear that there was, but this would seem to be one of those unfortunate occurrences which took place without there being able to account for them. Many other men had passed through the tunnel without meeting with such an unfortunate result.

There might have been something in the coal, as the chairman of the company had told them that a description of the coal had been complained of in the Regent's canal tunnel and consequently they immediately ceased using it … if it had not proved that sulphur did arise from the coals that would not have materially affected this inquiry, as all these had to decide on was the cause of death, in which they must be guided by the medical testimony.

The jury found the deceased men met with *accidental death by suffocation in Blisworth Tunnel.* In summing up it was strongly recommended the canal company *give more ventilation to the tunnel by sinking additional shafts in the shallowest places,* at which point the company Chairman confirmed the instructions had already been given to the engineer, he also reassured those in attendance *the widow and children of the deceased [Broadbent, who had a wife and eight children, the youngest born that month] would be taken care of by the company.*

George Savage at the time of the tunnel incident was in his mid 40's and a successful businessman, having increased the size of his farm to 400 acres and expanded the number of employees in his brick-works at Stoke, Blisworth and Towcester[80], his ninth and last child Herbert Augustus was born in 1861. The Savage family were active in village life, as was evident at the second Stoke Bruerne *Floral Fete and Harvest Festival* held in the village school-room in 1863. The Savage's children were awarded numerous prizes, although these were honorary *as the money prizes were for the labourers only.* Miss Savage came first in the model garden category, with a facsimile of her fathers garden. In the under 12's flat race Master C Savage won first prize and Master W Savage won the pole jump at a height of 7ft 2 inches, their father being awarded an honorary first prize for 12 pods of kidney Beans[81]. Mr Savage was the owner of the canal-side steam mill where a further tragedy occurred. 54 year old miller John Turner died in Northampton Infirmary from injuries sustained at the steam mill. At the inquest the receiving surgeon from the Infirmary confirmed Mr Turner arrived suffering from a compound fracture of the skull and bones of the face, John died that morning from inflammation of the brain. The surgeon told the coroner

John spoke to him before his death … *he told [me] the accident was caused by his falling down a trap door, and being caught by a hook which was attached to the end of a chain. Did not blame anyone, and said he was quite alone at the time the accident occurred*[82]. At the inquest Adam Wilcox, the mill engine driver also gave witness …

> … on the 20th, inst, the deceased was on the top floor of the mill by himself and [I] was on the bottom floor sending up wheat by way of a chain and windlass worked by an engine. The duty of [John] was to receive the wheat, and for this purpose he was standing by the trap door. [I] did not see the accident, but … heard something fall, and after waiting about a minute … went to see for the deceased. [I] found him lying at the bottom of the steps, with his head on a hook. [I] immediately lifted his head off the hook. He was soon afterwards taken home, when he spoke, but he did not tell [me]. [I] was of opinion the deceased was coming down the ladder when his foot slipped, and he consequently fell down. [I] had finished sending up wheat to [John], and imagined he was coming down the steps …

The jury returned a verdict of *accidental death*, after which a juryman suggested Mr. Savage be asked to *place a railing by the side of the steps to prevent future accidents*, although the coroner reminded jurors *they could not make a recommendation of that kind, as they had not seen the mill,* but he went on to ask Mr Wilcox to inform his employer of the opinion of the jury. Another tradesman in Stoke Bruerne who wasn't doing so well was the village blacksmith Robert Pettifer, who was declared bankrupt in the County Court of Northamptonshire towards the end of 1861[83].

Two of the deceased men from the tunnel incident were buried at Saint Mary's shown in Table 10. The burial records also show the death of an un-named 13 year old in December 1865, a lad employed only a week earlier in London by Boatman Burton, who knew the boy only by the name Thomas. Burton's boat was propelled by steam, he also had a horse which he directed the boy to ride over the hill to the tunnel mouth in Stoke Bruerne. At the inquest in the Boat Inn a witness gave an account of the incident …

> As the boat neared the bridge [I was] in the cabin, heard the deceased and the horse plunging in the water. It was then a little after six, and was quite dark, and it was quite half an hour before the body could be got out of the water. A legger, named Warren, said a few minutes before six he saw the deceased riding a horse under Stoke Bridge, and all at once, without the horse being frightened, it slipped into the canal. Witness caught hold of deceased's hair whilst he was in the water, but it slipped through his hands, and it was quite 25 minutes before he could be taken out. When he was brought to the public-house restoratives were applied without success[84].

Table 10   Saint Mary the Blessed Virgin. Canal related burials 1858-1865

Burial date	Name	Age	Parents	Description
26th July 1858	William Whitlock	7	Benjamin	Drowned
9th September 1861	William Webb			Blisworth Tunnel Incident
9th September 1861	Edward Broadbent			Blisworth Tunnel Incident
26th December 1865	Unknown	13		Drowned in canal

By the early 1870's John and Elizabeth Amos were living with their teenage children, oldest son William was in Buckingham working as a grocer's assistant[85]. Thomas and John Henry were working for their father as rope-makers, the family rope-walk being behind their home and running in a straight line to Chapel Lane shown in an artists impression in Figure 23. John Amos was doing well, employing three boys in addition to his two sons, as well as expanding his business interests to include the village post-office. When the telegraph line was laid in the village it was connected to the Amos's post-office and became an important communication point for boaters, carriers and canal companies. Because for canal transport to function effectively the two main centres of communication were *canal company toll offices and post offices*, the latter particularly if they were near the canal side.

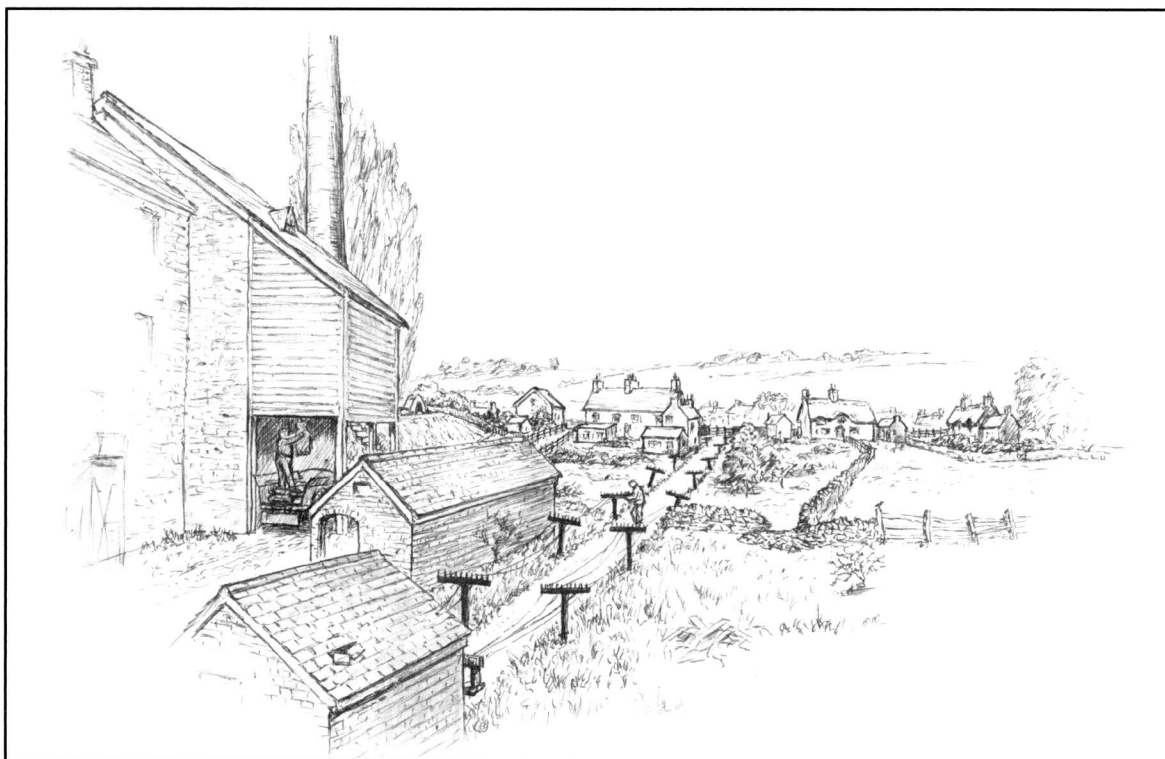

Figure 23   The Amos family *Rope-Walk* (Brian Collings)

Certain toll offices such as Braunston or Hawkesbury Junction (which were at some distance from actual post offices), acted as unofficial post offices, both for carriers and their boatmen. Money was sent to boaters by their employers, including; the balance of their outstanding pay, an advance on their future earnings, or money to pay tolls, usually by postal orders which the toll clerk had the authority to cash, (the same as post masters/mistress's), with many carriers having toll credit accounts with canal companies or sometimes individual toll clerks. Canal companies preferring this arrangement as clerks acted as local agents for the companies, collecting rents and managing other financial matters, and held a bank book for a local bank account to deposit tolls and other income on behalf of the canal company. Clerks were also insured against theft and other financial problems. Letters for boaters were also sent to toll offices so the boatmen could collect them when next passing[86].

During this decade Rev. Lee continued to baptise the children of workers in the canal industry shown in Table 11, from the records it is worth noting one boating family, the Whitlock's showed a preference for baptising their children over a number of years in Stoke Bruerne. Leggers continued to be employed by the Grand Junction Canal Company until the introduction of steam tugs, tug drivers being recruited locally (Benjamin Wood age 36 and his 13 year old son John). The canal company by now had reduced the number of lock keepers to two; Benjamin West age 53 and Richard White age 34, but continued to employ 60 year old William Child as Canal Agent. In 1871 two boats moored in Stoke Bruerne on census day shown in Table 12. In fact Captain Joseph Hollis, who was born in Netherton, Worcestershire[87] appears on the census twice as he is also enumerated at his home address, Miles Street, Deritend, Birmingham with his family, which is not unusual for boatmen as they may have filled in the census form (or more than likely, someone else would have filled it in for them) before they left on a journey[88]. Looking at the census entry, you would think this family had no connections with Stoke Bruerne, that they were just passing through, and had moored up that night, but on closer examination of Joseph's family history, his son William Adam Hollis married Esther Hood (from Tipton) by licence on January 23rd 1872 at Saint Mary's, Stoke Bruerne, their son Joseph William was also baptised here on September 5th 1875[89].

Table 11   Saint Mary the Blessed Virgin. Canal related baptisms 1860-1874

Baptism Date	Birth date	Child's Name	Parents	Father Occupation
May 1860	16th May	James	Thomas and Mary Peasland	Legger
June 1860	4th Aug	Susannah	Joseph and Keziah Dyke	Lock Keeper
November 1861	11th Nov	Alice	William and Hannah Child	Lock Keeper
December 1861	19th Oct	John Charles	John Gill and Ann Diane Wickens	Legger
May 1863	5th Nov '58	Eliza Jane	Thomas and Mary Webb	Legger
June 1864	5th March	Emma	William and Mary Whitlock	Boatman
	15th Jan '62	William		
	21st April '60	Hannah		
October 1864		Mary Jane Peasland	William Carter & Ann Pettifer	Legger
May 1865	2nd April	Faith	Joseph and Keziah Dyke	Lock Keeper
May 1865	6th June '64	Joseph William	Richard and Katharine Woodward	Legger
July 1865		Alice	Joseph and Keziah Dyke	Lock Keeper
		Ann		
April 1866	21st Feb	Linda Marie	Thomas and Marie Willby	Legger
June 1866	20th April	William E	John Gill and Ann Diane Wickens	Legger
September 1866	10th Aug	Rosa Eleanor	William and Mary Whitlock	Boatman
February 1867	29th Oct	Emily	William and Ann Peasland	Legger
June 1867	15th Oct	Kate	Joseph Eyden and Sarah Jackson	Lock keeper Hardingstone
March 1868		William James	Thomas and Marie Willby	Legger
May 1868	Jan 1868	John Thomas	John and Hanah Jackson	Lock Keeper: Stow Nine Churches
October 1868	May 21st	Alice Selina	William and Mary Whitlock	Boatman SB
December 1868	27th June	Ann Selina	John Gill and Ann Diane Wickens	Legger
February 1869	11th Nov	Agnes	William Carter and Ann Pettifer	Legger
September 1869		Mary Alice	William Taylor and Elizabeth Jeffery	Legger SB
May 1870		Annie Frances	John and Rosanna Linnell	Lock keeper SB

Table 12   Boats moored in Stoke Bruerne on census night 1871

Boat / place	Occupants	Age	Occupation	Birthplace
Stoke Lock	Emmanuel Chambers	61	Master	Oldbury. Staffordshire
	Sarah Chambers	59	Wife	Oldbury. Staffordshire
	Elizza Chambers	31	Daughter	Leicester
Stoke Tunnel	Joseph Hollis	55	Captain of boat	Netherton. Worcestershire
	George Perrett	39	Mate	Tewkesbury. Gloucestershire

Sanitary reform and the floating population[90]

The itinerant lifestyle of *family boaters*, unless loading and unloading in major ports or townships, meant they were traversing the canals, shielded from the many problems associated with urban squalor and disease, evading the gaze of the Local Government Board's newly appointed sanitary inspectors, and the self-appointed sanitary reformers. This was true with the exception of one non-conformist Wesleyan Methodist whose gaze was firmly fixed on *family boater's*. Mr George Smith of Coalville had for a number of years fought vehemently for improvements in brickyard children's lives, after the somewhat tortuous and lengthy campaign Smith was instrumental in obtaining amendments to the Factory and Workshop Acts with regard to the employment of children, although not without a toll on himself and his family.

George Smith was raised in the Potteries (near the Trent and Mersey Canal), from the age seven he worked as a brick maker, during which he gained personal experience of the conditions under which boaters lived and worked, gleaned from helping load hundreds of narrow boats, experiences he later reported *opened his eyes to the sad conditions of the poor canal children*. In October 1873 Smith publicly inaugurated a second campaign in a letter published in a number of London and provincial papers[91] titled *Boatmen and their children – an appeal,* Smith's aim being to *improve the situation of boat children …*

BOATMEN AND THEIR CHILDREN. - AN APPEAL.

I have now very respectfully to claim the attention of the public, through the press, to a much too long neglected department of our sailor-population—if sailor be the proper word, when not the sea but our canals are the scenes of their occupations. As the heading of my letter indicates, I refer to the boatmen and their children. At rough estimate there are 11,000 of canal boatmen with the women and children in active employment in England alone, so that it will be seen in a glance that it is no trivial or small interest that I am now concerned about. Well, sir, it will probably be news to 99 out of 100 readers, that these boatmen, their wives and families, in a very large proportion, have no home on land, but pass their lives habitually on board their boats. By an accepted phraseology the boat-home is called a cabin (as is poor Paddy's), but practically it is a miserable hole, averaging 6 feet by 7 feet 6; or in other words, the cabin contains about 202 cubic feet of space; and in such places will be found from four to seven persons, over and above fire-stove, seats, beds, pots, and other necessities. So they are stowed together from year's beginning to year's end. I may be permitted to give actual examples, as (1) J. K., of Stoke Golding, with wife and five children, live constantly in the boat, having no other home. (2) W. G., Cropredy, near Banbury, with wife and six children, the same. (3) J. O., of Stockton Wharf, with wife and seven children. So throughout.

Of the children of these 100,000 boatmen, not more probably than 2,000 will be found to attend either day-school or Sunday-school. Of the boatmen themselves, 2 per cent. As able to read and write will be a full proportion.

I do not enter at present on the condition either physically or morally of this population. Very appalling are the facts within my knowledge, and these must sooner or later come out. Neither do I just now enter on the question of wages and earnings. But even these few data must prove, I humbly think, that there is a loud call for legislative inquiry, legislative supervision, and legislative redress. On the face of it, it seems monstrous that with the Factory and Workshop Act of 1871, passed and in activity, it should be possible to have women and children herding together and employed as in these boats, so that the Education Act should be inoperative in relation to these boatmen's children.

Trusting that the whole subject of our boatmen and coasting coal-boat families will secure the powerful advocacy of the press, so as to command legislation.

In response to the letter *London Figaro* published *Our Floating Population* which reiterated Smith's key points and offered support to his campaign, afterwards the article was widely quoted in the press. Smith's employer saw the letters and he was called to a meeting and given an ultimatum, *give up the campaign or leave*. George Smith chose the latter, he was now unemployed with a wife, five children and another on the way, fortunately Smith was made a partner in a firm, and for a short while all went well, until in his partners eyes he failed to fulfil his contractual arrangements, his contract was terminated and as a consequence the family were evicted from their home, forced into poor housing and lived in poverty[92].

With the support of his wife the campaign continued, Smith walking scores of miles along the towing path to gather first hand evidence regarding the boat people. During Smiths' travels the *Potteries Examiner* published a powerful article titled *Life on the canals* flagging up Smith's *appeal for legislative inquiry, legislative supervision, and legislative redress* on behalf of the boatmen and their families[93]…

Mr. Smith has hit another blot in our social system, for the floating population of our canals have had as little care bestowed upon them in regard to moral and intellectual training as if they were a pariah race. We have no doubt but that Mr. Smith's estimate that there are 10,000 boaters in active employment in this country, is a fairly accurate approximation, and our readers will agree with him that it is no small matter for us to have in our midst a population so large as this, that is almost totally neglected educationally. Moving about from place to place in the 'slow barge' they have no settled home, but pass their lives in 'cabins', not much too large for dog-kennels, which serve as kitchen, parlour, and bedroom. We well remember, many years ago, having our attention called to the condition of these gipsies of our canal system, by a young man who had become interested in their welfare by observing their habits, and that they neither attended chapels nor churches themselves, nor as a rule sent their children to school. Actuated by an earnest desire to see more of the life in their cabin homes, and to carry an influence for good there, he commenced to visit the boatmen on the Sunday evenings …. We went with him on one occasion … in the first boat that we applied for admittance, we were told that a little girl lay dangerously ill, by the mother, the father having just run for the Doctor. There were several other children in the cabin, and it appeared to us that such a small crib was not the best place in which the battle against disease and death could be fought, or in which infection could be prevented …

Smith did not respond in the press because of his continued excursions, although his friends from *Figaro* again drew to the attention of the country the case of the canal population (April 1874) in the article *The Boatmen's Friend*. The same month Smith gave a speech at a Sunday School anniversary at Moira, Leicestershire, which was fully reported in the *Leicester Daily Post*, after which the press did not leave the subject alone[94]. The year concluded with the article *Modern Mermen* appearing in the satirical journal *The Hornet*, which focused on the conditions of the labouring population and working class progress …

There is plenty of work for a Government determined to deal with the social conditions of the labouring population, although the unhappy tendency of our working men to go on strike has caused some persons, very unwisely, to hesitate in lending their support to schemes of working-class progress. Among the subjects imperatively calling for legislative attention is the condition of the immense floating population to be found on our rivers and canals. It may astonish most people to learn that we have thousands of men, women, and children who do not know what it is to sleep in a dwelling-house. Such, however, is the fact. The men who are employed in canal navigation reside almost exclusively in the tiny cabins on board the barges of which they have charge. Were they the only occupants of these floating dens perhaps it would be difficult to get up a feeling of sympathy on their behalf, but when we find that they have as companions their wives and children, we begin to perceive the real evil of the matter.

Mr George Smith, of Coalville, who so gallantly fought the battle of the brickyard children, and who has now become the champion of our water babies, mentions the case of a boat-woman who had not slept in a dwelling-house for the last twenty years. This woman, to whom the domestic comforts of life were little more than a name, had actually reared no less than eight children in a cabin, containing not more than 202 cubic feet of space, in which must be included stove, seats, beds, pots, &c. Fancy living in a room little larger than an ordinary wardrobe ! Of course, families thus circumstanced cannot practise the common decencies of life. One of this woman's children slept at the head of herself and husband, another at their feet, two in a tiny cupboard, and the other four wherever they could be packed.

Such a state of things ought to be impossible. Were the case related by Mr. George Smith in any was exceptional, we might shudder for a moment and then forget it. But it is only one instance out of hundreds-nay, thousands; and we cannot afford, either as Englishmen or Christians, to stand idly by in the face of such evils. Are we to let these remain in this fearfully degraded condition? Are we to allow their children to grow up in that unhappy state of ignorance which has rendered the name of 'bargee' synonymous blackguardism and filthy slang? Certainly not. It is our duty to put an end to this crying scandal, that it may no longer remain our reproach and shame. But the Government will not or cannot interfere, unless compelled to do so by the force of public opinion. As of old, they attempt to shirk the responsibility. 'Am I my brother's keeper?' they cry. But we must have no excuses. When Parliament again meets, the subject must be persistently forced upon its attention, until it earnestly sets about redressing an evil which ought never to have been allowed to exist in a civilised country[95].

Smith received a raft of letters in response to the campaign and numerous articles appeared in the press, including the poem *The Children's Friend* by a Cornish poet the papers also carried a portrait of Smith reproduced in Figure 24. When Smith's campaign was gaining public support disaster struck on the Regents Canal when a Grand Junction Canal Company boat carrying explosives blew up, resulting in three deaths and comprehensive damage to local structures. The incident was reported in the Northampton Mercury because boatman Edward Thomas survived although his boat was blown to pieces and sunk[96]. The outcome of the disaster caused the company to sell their canal carrying department.

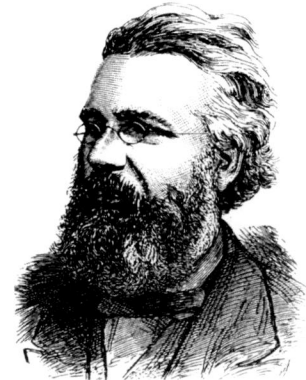

Figure 24   Portrait of Mr George Smith of Coalville

By now Smith was campaigning for a Royal Commission, the difficulty being knowing which government department to appeal to, as each department dealt with different legislation [Education Act, Sanitary Act or Factory and Workshop Act]. Smith was invited to deliver a paper on *Church Work among boatmen* at an event which was widely promoted in the press, Smith wrote the paper but to his surprise the Church Congress Secretary announced in The Standard *Smith had been substituted*. Not deterred Smith wrote to editors enclosing a copy of the paper and they responded by publishing it, from which a number of extracts are reported …

Many of the boaters and their families have but one home, little more than one bed, and one suit of clothes, and these filthy, and not much better than rags. Taking all in all, or canal population is in a worse condition than it was 25 years ago, Their "cabin home" of about 200 cubic feet of space, scarcely the size of an ashpit belonging to a town house. This is not the place to bring up a large family, have confinements, and grapple with disease and death; but these things are taking place daily under our own eyes and nose.

They have been lying at the foot of the ladder all these long years, and no one has cared to help them to take the first step … We can no more better the condition of our boatmen and their families … by simply throwing into the canal a bottle of scented rose-water. Desperate diseases require desperate remedies. The boatman, their wives, and their little ones are in the mud and mire, mixing up with everything that is abominable and filthy, and instead of getting out of it they are deeper in it than they were 25 years since …

England, professing as she does to have the wisest and most Christian-like statesmen, the best laws, and most liberal form of government in the world, is sadly neglecting her duty in quietly standing by with folded hands while the seeds of immorality, disease and death are being scattered broadcast along our canals. The law must go first, and I am thankful to say the wheels are set in motion. A Royal Commission is sitting at the present time taking evidence … and very likely before another year is over an Act will be passed having for it's object the bettering of the conditions of our "canal population"…

The boaters are somewhat like the Ishmaelites of old, everybody seems against them and they seem to be against everybody. They are treated as the bastards of society, and the water tramps of the community. Even the children out of the gutters get upon the bridges to throw all manner of filth at them as they pass along[97]…

William and Thomas Amos.

On a backdrop of urban and rural sanitary reform and an increasing interest in George Smith's campaign *family boaters* continued to ply the Grand Junction Canal uninterrupted. The 1870's canal scene at Stoke Bruerne was probably at its most bustling, with staff at Stoke Bruerne Primary School continuing to caution pupils on the dangers of the canal as extracts from the school log book show [98]…

June 20th 1873: Cautioned the lads to keep away from the Canal, in the dinner time; as some had been fishing, I was afraid it might encourage others to go …

Monday August 4th 1873: A very hot day. Cautioned the scholar's against bathing in the canal in the dinner time. School work today was satisfactory …

John and Elizabeth Amos's second son Thomas was a member of Roade Baptist Chapel, the second oldest Chapel in Northamptonshire[99] and just over a mile from Stoke Bruerne. The Chapel's congregation had for a number of years experienced difficulties retaining a minister, after appointing Rev. How in 1866 the congregation significantly increasing[100], Rev. How announcing major re-developments for the chapel, including re-seating, enlargement of the burial ground and the building of a new schoolroom at an estimated cost of £600. Part of the development money was raised by a bazaar[101] in Miss Lalor's schoolroom opposite the chapel. On the day of the bazaar …

> … a large Union Jack waved in the breeze on the chapel entrance, over which an arch formed of evergreen and flowers had been erected. From the windows of the school-room floated the French tricolour, and a flag which was a combination of the English and Danish national standards, whilst two standards representing England and Denmark separately were placed on either side of the gateway leading to the school. The passage through the front garden, too, was rendered attractive by stands bearing beautiful plants in pots and choice bouquets of cut roses, geraniums … In the school-room the most tempting array of articles was displayed, including most of the things which came within the definition of the term "useful and fancy", from a baby's shoe to a musical portrait album … a well patronised refreshment stall … The weather, which during the morning had been very wet, cleared up at noon, and the change brought a larger than anticipated number of visitors. Arrangements had been made with the London and North Western Company to convey passengers at cheap fares, and almost 80 persons from that town availed themselves of the opportunity afforded … A tea meeting was held in the chapel after the children's treat, at which about 300 members and friends sat down. The bazaar was thronged during the whole afternoon and evening, its success being beyond the most sanguine of its promoters …

At around 8 o'clock young Thomas Amos assembled the children close to the chapel where he conducted the closing hymns which the children sang the previous Sunday *in a very pleasing manner*. A few years later Rev. How announced the whole amount for the chapel developments were *in hand*, the same year Thomas Amos with his two sisters Annie and Elizabeth were baptised by immersion in the brook at Hyde Farm, the home of Steven Warwick the eminent Northamptonshire Baptist[102]. For Thomas Amos his baptism marked the start of a long relationship with Roade Baptist church. In the 1870's boaters' continued to baptise their children in Stoke Bruerne shown in Table 13. Although on examining the records more closely Barnabus Alderman and William Bustin were in fact tunnel tug drivers employed by the Grand Junction Canal Company, two pictures of tunnel tug *Pilot* near the mouth of Blisworth Tunnel are shown in Figure 25a, with smoke and in Figure 25b without smoke.

Table 13   Saint Mary the Blessed Virgin. Canal related baptisms 1870's

Baptism Date	Birth date	Childs Name	Parents	Father Occupation
October 1871	29th July	Keziah Ann	George and Sarah Inns	Boatman SB
August 1873	15th April '63	Harry	Benjamin and Eliza Wood	Boatman SB
	14th June '69	William		
	15th Nov '72	George		
August 1873	10th Dec	John Thomas	Barnabus and Mary Alderman	Boatman SB
January 1874	31st Oct	John Henry	William and Harriet Bustin	Boatman SB

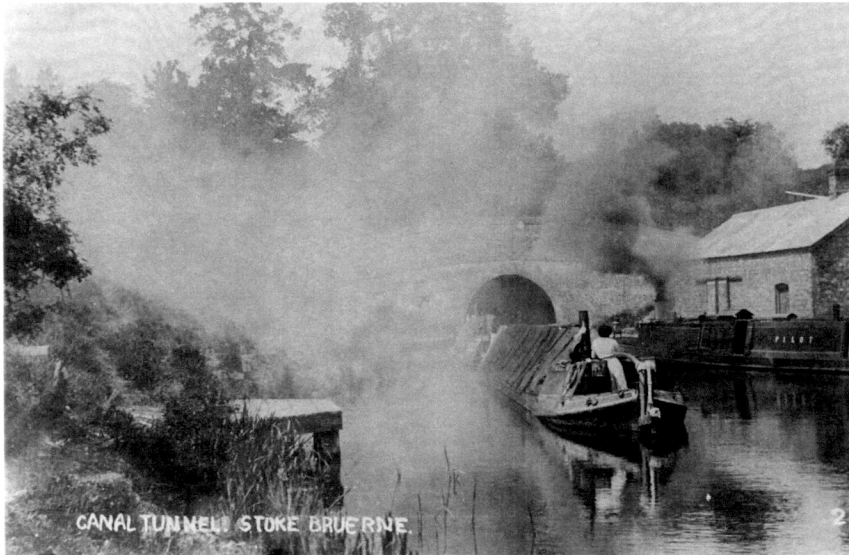

Figure 25a   Grand Junction Canal Company tunnel tug Pilot with smoke
(Waterway's Archive)

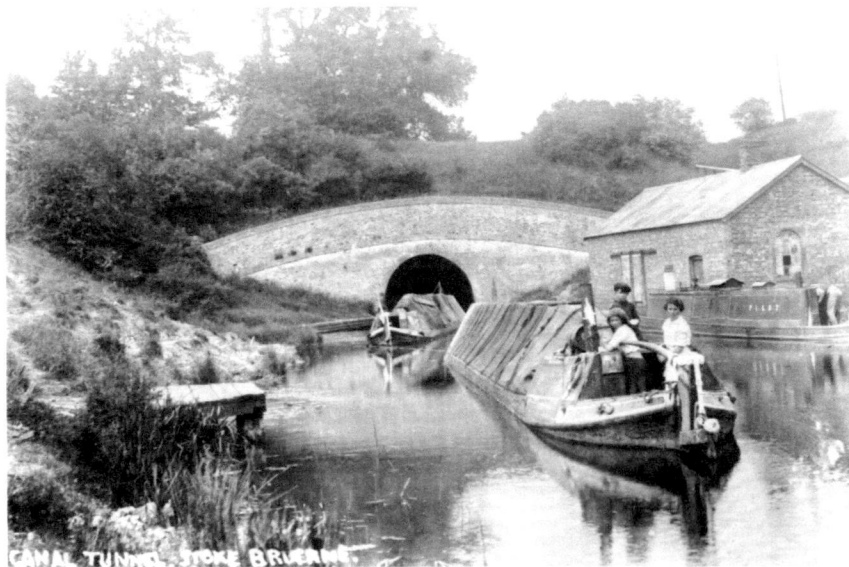

Figure 25b   Grand Junction Canal Company tunnel tug Pilot without smoke
(Della Sadler-Moore)

Between 1850 and 1875 John and Elizabeth raised the second generation of the Amos family in Stoke Bruerne, alongside increasing the family's business interests as a result of John's entrepreneurial and steadfast work ethic, John also got the right to vote in 1870[103]. Sadly this happy and productive period was brought to a close when eldest son William Ireson Amos passed away in the family's canal-side home as a result of complications associated with Rheumatic Fever[104].

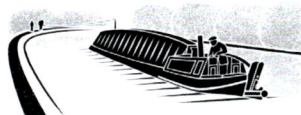

Thomas Amos following in fathers' footsteps

After the death of eldest son William, John and Elizabeth with their son Thomas continued to run the rope business, the shop and the post office in Stoke Bruerne. John Amos being appointed rate collector and census enumerator at a time when his children were coming of age. Thomas Amos continued to develop his interests outside of Stoke Bruerne, initially as a member of the Northampton *Band of Hope* temperance association. At temperance events across the county he regularly performed his musical talents …

> … 1000 people assembled in the Corn Exchange to listen to the Annual Concert, between the verses of the piece "Whistle and hoe", a novel effect was produced by interludes of lively airs whistled by a number of the orchestra, led by Mr Amos of Stoke Bruerne on the flute[105] (shown with his flute in Figure 26).

Figure 26   Thomas Amos with flute (Waterway's Archive)

Thomas was the first of John and Elizabeth's children to tie-the-knot when he married Sarah Ellen (Nellie) Hollowell[106] in 1878, a member of the *Hollowell* family from Brafield-on-the-green, Nellie's family being *influential* in non-conformist and temperance circles in Northamptonshire and beyond. Her brother Rev. James Hirst Hollowell *being one of the most prominent non-conformist leaders of the day*, a second brother Mr William-Cromwell Hollowell was *chiefly instrumental in promoting the scheme which resulted in the building of the Temperance Hall in Northampton* with her other brother Richard Hollowell being *the first chief of the Good Templar organisation in Northamptonshire*[107]. In 1879 two of Thomas' sister's married scotsmen; Mary Ann married William Wilson Mitchell at Saint Mary's in Stoke Bruerne[108], and Elizabeth married George Chalmers at Roade Baptist Church[109]. The most likely reason for the Amos girls marrying Scotsmen was because both men were building contractors working on construction of the railway at Roade.

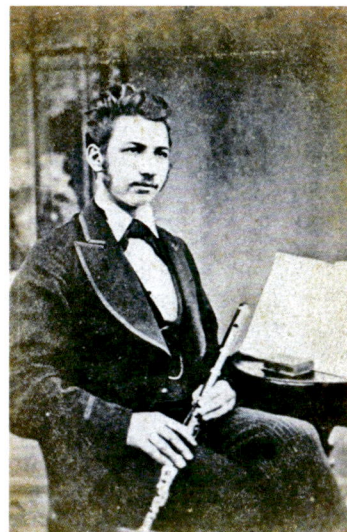

John Amos enumerated his first census in 1881, at the time the Amos family were living at the canalside cottage next to top-lock, their neighbours in the adjacent terraced cottages included;

brickyard labourer Adam Wilcox and his family, engine fitter William Valentine, servant Benjamin Palmer and his family and, engine fitter Barnabus Alderman with his young family. On census day John recorded six boats moored in the village as listed in Table 14. Two boats *Blue Lias* and *The Warwick* have on board the Woodfield family. On *Blue Lias* are John and Mary Ann with children Frederick Samuel and Thomas, whilst on *The Warwick* are James, Edward and Albert, the sons being stated as in the employment of their father, which was not unusual at this time. Fourteen year old James Woodfield went on to become the first captain of Fellows, Morton and Clayton steamer *President*[110].

Table 14   Boats moored in Stoke Bruerne on census night 1881

Boat	Occupants	Age	Occupation	Birthplace
The William	William Smith (Head)	49	Captain of Boat	Birmingham
	Sarah Smith (Wife)	45	Wife	Ludlow
The Thames	William Smith (Son)	16	Boatman	Birmingham
	James Johnson	18	Boatman	Eilstree
Blue Lias	John Woodfield (Head)	46	Captain or Steerer	Warwick
	Mary Ann Woodfield (Wife)	45		Warwick
	Frederick Woodfield (Son)	7		Braunston
	Samuel Woodfield (Son)	5		Braunston
	Thomas Woodfield (Son)	2		Braunston
The Warwick	James Woodfield (Son)	14	All employed by father	Tamworth
	Edward Woodfield (Son)	13		Stockton
	Albert Woodfield (Son)	9		Birmingham
The Moon	Frank Roadhouse (Head)	48	Captain or Steerer	Longford
	Mary Ann Roadhouse (Daughter)	15		
Employed on canal boat	Bedworth Hill			
	Suzanne Roadhouse (Daughter)	12		Bedworth Hill
The Nebold	Henry Berry (Head)	41	Captain or Steerer	Warwick
	Jane Berry (Wife)			Knowle

The youngest of the Amos children Charles initially worked as a letter carrier[111], later becoming a miller and corn dealer in Stoke Bruerne[112]. On his marriage to Emma Ayres (Figure 27), a draper's assistant from Stony Stratford the newly-weds moved to Roade to run a grocery and drapery shop. At the age of 35 John Henry was the last of the Amos children to marry, after which John and Georgina left the village[113]. The landscape in Stoke Bruerne at the time of the Amos children's marriages is shown in Figure 28.

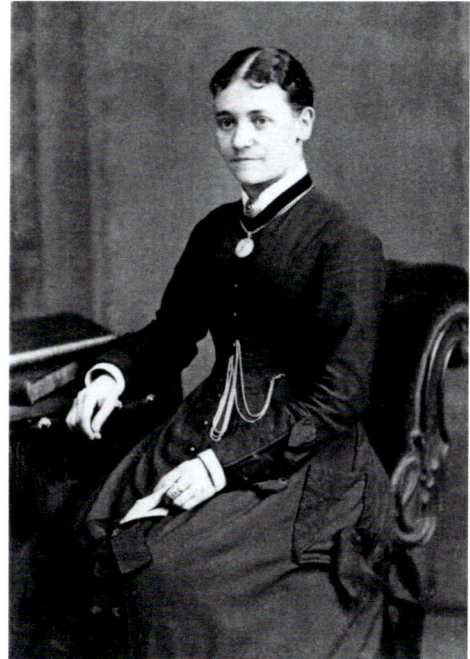

Figure 27   Emma Amos
(Waterway's Archive)

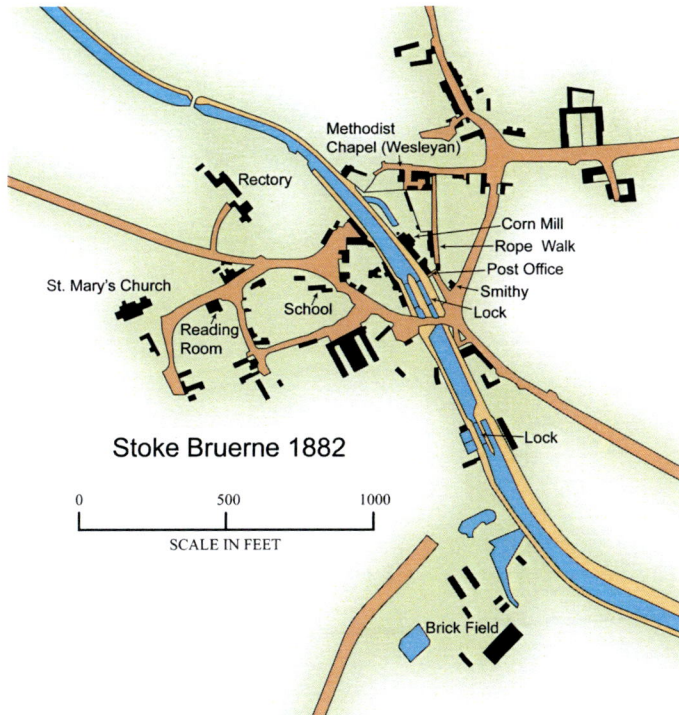

Figure 28   Stoke Bruerne map 1882 (Christopher M Jones)

Thomas and Nellie Amos's first home was in Mill Lane, Stoke Bruerne, Nellie at the time was committed to the Temperance Movement, an interest she derived from her relative William Hollowell. Nellie was the twentieth member of the first Good Templar Lodge in Northampton, the *Pioneer Lodge of the Independent Order of Good Templars (IOGT)*, Nellie having been initiated shortly after the Order was granted the Charter. It therefore came as no surprise that on her marriage to Thomas she opened a *Pride of the Valley Lodge* in their new home, Sister Amos holding weekly sessions on a Friday evening[114]. Thomas Amos and local businessman George Savage were also members of a number of temperance movements[115], including the *South*

Northamptonshire District Lodge of the Good Templars who held regular quarterly meetings in the *comfortable reading room in Stoke Bruerne*[116], after meetings members were provided with *Tea* by Mr and Mrs Amos. In 1885 Mr Savage and Mr Amos Junior were appointed to serve on the lodge committee[117].

Thomas and Nellie's first child Ethel Margaret was born a year after their marriage, Ethel being the first grandchild for John and Elizabeth and the first of the third generation Amos family to reside in the village. Thomas and Sarah's second child Ernest was born in 1882, shown in Figure 29 is Ernest with his mother sitting in the garden of their home, two years later Sarah gave birth to twin girls: Mary Hollowell and Ellen Hollowell[118] (Sister Mary).

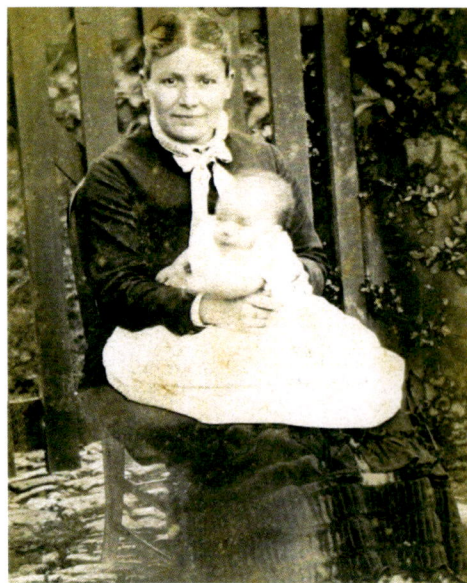

Figure 29   Nellie Amos with son Ernest
(Waterway's Archive)

George Smith's campaign comes into fruition

After George Smith published *Church work among boatmen* considerable correspondence came forward in support of his campaign. At the end of 1875, and at a cost to himself Smith published *Our Canal population: The Sad condition of women and children – with remedy, an appeal to my fellow country men and women,*[119] the book being an amalgamation into one volume a large amount of published correspondence with an extended set of arguments in support of *the legislative requirements of parliament to improve the conditions of the boating population.* Smith dedicated the book to Richard Cross. M.P. Her Majesty's Secretary of State for the Home Department in which he stated *Sir, I have taken the liberty of dedicating this little work to you, having observed with satisfaction during the time you have been in office your honourable and successful attempt to grapple with some of the difficult problems which affect our national and social life, and the well-being of the working and other classes of this country.*

In response to the book the Local Government Board (LGB) received a flood of letters in support of Smith's proposals[120], after which he presented at the *Council of Social Science Association Congress* a set of proposals on *canal boat inspection and enforcement* as a way to achieve improvements for the floating population. A year later the Home Secretary invited Smith to discuss a draft Canal Boat Bill which provided for *the registration and regulation of canal boats used as dwellings,* although the bill did not include all the requirements Smith wanted he endorsed it because *he was keen to see it on the statute books*[121]. At the first reading the *Canal Association*[122] pushed for a Select Committee, who, after several hours of debate passed it. After further opposition from the Canal Association and a further Select Committee lasting 26 hours, the Bill was moved to a third reading then passed for Royal Assent.

The Canal Boats Act came into force on January 1ˢᵗ 1878, enacting the following legislative mechanisms; All canal boats to be registered. Registration authorities empowered to fix the number; Age and sex of persons allowed to live on boat; Local sanitary authorities to inspect boats for infectious diseases; Elementary education for boat children (responsibility assumed by school attendance committee in registration area); Empowerment of canal companies to set up schools for children of employees; Registration authorities given powers to initiate inspection to the enforcement of the Acts provisions via sanitary authorities. Under the Canal Boats Act 1877, the Local Government Board issued regulations to the Registration Authorities on May 17ᵗʰ 1878, appended to these were copies of the Act, a set of forms (A-C) for conducting inspections and registrations, and the first *Schedule of Canals, with their nominated Registration Authorities*. The Grand Junction Canal in this first wave of canal boat legislation had five registration authorities[123] listed in Figure 30.

> **The vestry of the Parish of Paddington**
> **The Brentford Urban Sanitary Authority**
> **The Tring Urban Sanitary Authority**
> **The Aylesbury Urban Sanitary Authority**
> **The Buckingham Urban Sanitary Authority**

Figure 30   Initial Sanitary Districts / Registration Authorities. Grand Junction Canal (Christopher M Jones)

One *crucial measurement* under the Canal Boats Act of 1877 was for the cubic air space allowed for each person living in any cabin intended for use as a dwelling. This should be *no less than 180 cubic feet of free air space in the after cabin, and no less than 80 cubic feet of free air space in a fore-cabin*. This figure was arrived at by measuring the maximum interior length, width and height of any cabin to calculate the gross cubic air space, then subtract a portion of this figure for space occupied by cupboards, lockers, etc., to calculate the net cubic air space or free air space. The number of people allowed in any particular cabin depended on this amount of free air space; 60 cubic feet for all persons over 12 years of age, and 40 cubic feet for all persons under 12 years of age. Initially there was some flexibility in the figures due to boats that were built before the Act, but any old craft having its cabin rebuilt or a new boat constructed after the Act, had to have sufficient cabin interior free air space to conform with the Act[124].

After the Act came into force George Smith was disappointed at the speed and quality of its enforcement, so on December 28ᵗʰ 1878 he left home to walk the towpaths *to visit the principle wharves on the Grand Junction Canal looking for evidence of the Act's enforcement*. Smith arrived at Braunston locks to find *fifteen to twenty un-registered boats frozen up, in which there were men, women and children huddling together*. In Braunston Smith met a boatwoman following a terrible accident …

In one of the boat cabins I came across a most heart-rending and pitiful sight; ... A poor boatwoman, named Phipps, known among the boatmen as "Banbury Bess" lay in the cabin with her jaw almost broken by the kick of their horse as she was "doing him up" the previous day … Her head was knocked and her face lacerated by the shoe of the horse to such a degree as to render her insensible and unrecognisable … the Doctor would not call to see to her, nor do anything towards dressing her wounds, unless the good Rector would guarantee the expenses. This poor [woman] lay in this wretched state from ten o'clock in the morning till ten o'clock at night before the Rector's guarantee was given to the doctor that he would be responsible for the expenses incurred. The woman could have been sent to the Northampton Infirmary, but 15s, the amount required for conveying her, could not be raised among the number of boats tied up[125].

Smith continued to Blisworth and on arriving declared *no steps had been taken … for putting the Act into force.* Un-be-known to George Smith, and almost a year after the Canal Boat Regulations were formulated the Towcester Sanitary Committee (November 1879) clerk was informed members of his receipt of the *LGB regulations on the Canal Boats Act (1877)* and the *need to appoint a Canal Boat Inspector.* At which Stoke Bruerne farmer, property owner and member of the sanitary committee Mr George Savage declared he would find an inspector for the area[126], and true to his word at the following meeting he proposed Stoke Bruerne lock-keeper Mr William Child. The nomination was accepted, and the salary agreed at 5/- per boat plus a nominal sum in addition[127], Mr Child's appointment commenced a new canal related occupation for a villager in Stoke Bruerne.

In September 1880 George Smith commenced his *canal wanderings … to obtain first-hand about how the Act was being implemented,* on this occasion he toured the Grand Junction Canal for *six days on a Monkey Boat.* On nearing Blisworth Tunnel on a hot day and having just had dinner, Smith observed .the crew washing the dinner pans *in the cut* and two of the crew *enjoying a swim,* after which he vividly recounts the passage through the tunnel …

I crept upon "all fours" along the top plank to a little space in the centre of the boat to get "forty winks", when I heard something like a thundering monster issuing from the mouth of this dark abyss. As the author and source of this thundering voice kept coming nearer and nearer to daylight, with its trail of boats, the various discordant dismal noises, which had lost their distinctive features through the distance and gloom, could now be faintly heard – the whistles of the steam-tug, the shouts of the men, the chattering of the women, and the cries of the children, the creaking, crushing noises of the boats, the escape of the steam, and the motion of the screw, till at last the whole appeared in view…

Our iron canal-horse had fastened the end of his tail to our boat, and on we began to move: "puff," "puff," a whistle, screech, and a plunge, and we had entered Blisworth tunnel, about which all sorts of ghost stories, frightful apparitions, dreadful murders, and a thousand other things, enough to make your hair stand on end, have been said, and by the superstitious seen. These occurrences took place during the bygone legging days. Some boatmen of the present day-aye, and women, too-still believe in them. I must confess myself it is not pleasant, at least I should imagine so, to be in the midst of this dark, very dark, terribly dark place for two hours without light, with two or three rough fellows at your elbow not over particular as to what deeds they did, enveloped in the dark sounds of the dismal dripping of water into the canal from the roof and sides of the tunnel, each drop seeming to over-sensitive ears like the popping of children's air pistols. "Pop!" "pop!" "pop!" and then as if a battery of "pops" were at work. A splash would be heard, caused by the "spilching" of a piece of a brick out of the side of the tunnel into the "cut". On we moved. In some parts of the tunnel it sounds to me, while sitting under the tarpaulin covers, as if we were going under a multitude of water-taps turned on at full bore. I tried at times to draw my tarpaulin curtain on one side to see what was the matter. Splashes in my face, as if from a watering can, soon satisfied me that one peer was "quite sufficient for the time being," and I hastily drew my blinds together. A few yards further, and then bang! bang! crush! went our boat at the side of the tunnel, as if my friend the boatman had a grudge against it for some past grievance. I made sure our boat, which was laden "top heavy", was going to "topple" us over and bestow upon us the pleasure of swimming for our lives …

In the midst of these thunderings, groaning, and unearthly sounds, Mrs. ----, of the Birmingham boat, which was still accompanying us, would strike up with a good, clear voice, but with a kind of "tin-can" ring about it, and which would have been vastly improved if she had indulged in singing only, instead of oaths and curses upon the heads of her little ones, the following strange mixture of songs and hymns:- "Home, sweet Home," "Sweet William of Dundee," "The girl I left behind me," "Just as I am, without one plea," "Safe in the arms of Jesus," "Rock of Ages," etc. The latter she could only render very imperfectly, her only tutor being her littler boy, who had learnt them in the Birmingham Hospital …

After our boat had made several other attempts at the foundation of the left side of the tunnel, without any effect on our part except to beat a hasty retreat to the centre of the "cut" again, I could not help wondering, during our passage through this "dreary region of the dead," how many poor women and children have found this to be their death and burying-place. Just as I was rumbling these things over in my mind, the whistle of our steam-tug told us that we were getting towards daylight, and the watery caverns of the dismal-sounding darkness were being left behind[128].

Smith arrived at Buckby wharf in the early hours of Sunday morning, and before sleeping he spent time *thinking about legislation for the country's welfare,* his conclusions being … *now-a-days to have got upon the wrong line. Men seem to be finding their way into Parliament to exhibit themselves and their tomfoolery[129].* Next morning Smith's clothes were wet on account of him leaving open *the slide.*

After the monkey-boat journey Smith concern was how to get Local Authorities to enforce the Canal Boat Act and the LGB regulations, he published his conclusions in a second book *Canal Adventures by Moonlight (1881),* which contains details of the boat journey as well as an account of the problems boaters experience when faced with disease and illness …

> The ignorance displayed in the matter of the boaters' health arises no doubt from an imperfect knowledge of the subject. The fact is, the boatmen are nearly always on the move-at any rate a great part of their time; and instead of going to doctors like town folk, when sickness overtakes any member of the family, the woman or man … runs to the nearest chemist or drug-seller on their route for "powders and a bottle o'physic", and on they go again; and unless the sickness ends in death nothing further is known. Colds, bronchial affections, diseases of the chest, and rheumatic complaints are much more common among boaters …

Smith also included *six measures*[130] by which the Canal Boat Act should be amended. **First** - government should take the matter into their own hands. **Second** - more registration authorities should be established with properly qualified inspectors who have the power to enter a canal boat at any time. **Third** - all boats, barges, etc., used for the conveyance of goods should be registered. **Fourth** - the education of canal boat children living on board to be free, with liberty to attend any day-school conducted by properly qualified masters, which attendance to be facilitated by means of a pass-book furnished by the Government for one shilling, and procurable at any bookseller's. **Fifth** - the expenses attending the education of these travelling children, to be defrayed by the school authorities. **Sixth** - an abstract of regulations issued by the Local Government Board, to be hung in a prominent place in each toll-house on the canal side. Smith concluding with the assertion …

> … The children connected with other working-classes are subject by law to three elevating, educating, and healthy influences-viz., the factory laws, the educational laws, and the sanitary laws. None of these have been extended to the poor boat-children and its floating home".

Because he received no response to the campaign for an Amendment Act Smith came to the conclusion *the Act was becoming a dead letter*. The following year he took it on himself to write a *Draft Canal Boat Amendment Bill*, which he delivered to the House of Commons and the Home Secretary. The Canal Boats Act 1877 Amendment Bill was subsequently introduced into parliament and although the first reading went well, at the second it was referred to a Select Committe[131], where Smith was questioned for 3½ hours, throughout which he insisting *no act would work without central government involvement*[132]. On August 14th 1884 the Amendment Bill received royal assent, on which it created the new post of Chief Inspector of Canal Boats. Clauses related to canal boats were also incorporated into the Public Health (Control of Diseases) Act 1884. The first Chief Inspector of Canal Boats was expected to be George Smith, but the position was awarded to 44 year old manager of Stoke Prior Salt Works [Droitwich] John Brydone, on a starting salary of £500 rising to £900 incrementally (plus expenses). For George Smith passing of the Amendment Act drew to a close his 10 year 10 month (October 1873 - August 1884) campaign.

When the Amendment Act came into force the arrangement of the narrow boat back cabin furniture slightly changed. Figure 31 shows these alterations when compared with Figure 15, the wooden bulkhead on the right hand side has been mostly removed, along with cupboards above the main bed, alterations which increased the cubic air capacity of the back-cabin. In order to separate the main bed from the side bed on the right, a panelled and hinged flap was fixed dividing the two bunks, here shown with a fancy curved top. Its this general layout and cupboards which remained the norm in narrow boat cabins until the end of commercial carrying. Figure 32 shows the basic structural features of a narrow boat cabin interior looking from the 'Bed-ole' to the stern entrance doors, before the boaters personal possessions have been fitted. The cabin stove is a typical 19th century 'Bottle' type, manufactured by Matterson, Huxley and Watson of Lion

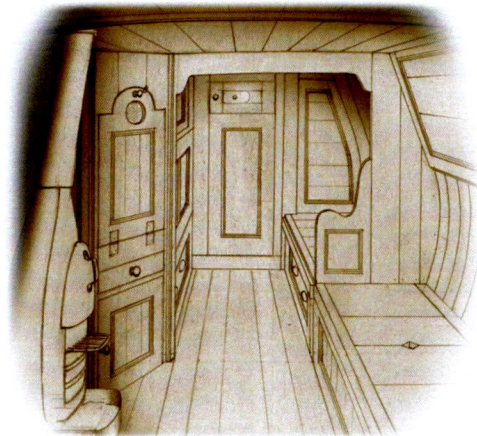

Figure 31   Back cabin furniture after the Canal Boat Act 1877 and Amendment Act 1884 (Christopher M Jones)

Foundry, Coventry. It was supplied with an external chimney, security chain and roof bolt. In between its legs is a removable ash pan. On the left hand bench the sloping lid of a cupboard provides a head rest when used as a bunk. Beneath the steerer's foot board in the cabin entrance lies a coal box with its leading edge making a handy step when entering the cabin. In the corner built beneath the cabin ceiling and stern bulkhead is a narrow drawer which was used for various papers including the boat's Canal Boat Acts 1877-1884 Registration Certificate[133].

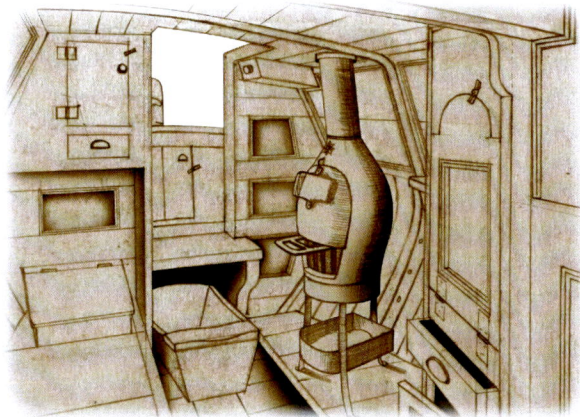

Figure 32   Back cabin furniture after the Canal Boat Act 1877 and Amendment Act 1884 (Christopher M Jones)

Thomas Amos Canal Boat Inspector ...

In Stoke Bruerne Towcester Canal Boat Inspector William Child unexpectedly died in 1884. On looking at his tenure George Smith's observations of poor implementation of the 1877 Canal Boat Act are borne out, as Towcester Sanitary Committee records show no evidence of Mr Childs having registered or inspected any boats during his five years in office. At the meeting after Mr Child's death Mr Savage nominated Mr Thomas Amos as replacement canal boat inspector, the nomination was approved and the salary set at £5 per annum[134]. Mr Amos registered his first boat *Indian Chief* in 1855, owned by his neighbour William Woodward[135], he presented this for approval to the Sanitary committee in February[136]. At the same meeting the clerk reported receiving the new LGB regulations which required canal boat inspectors *to present an annual report on their work and to forward this to the LGB no later than 21 days after the 31ˢᵗ December each year*[137].

John Brydone the first Chief Inspector of Canal Boats started his position in September 1884 after which he spent the first three months travelling over 3,000 miles visiting 94 authorities. In his first annual report Brydone stated *there is no uniformity in application of the acts* even though *a large number of inspectors had been appointed.* In this first year he also began to compile a central register of boats examined and registered, concluding on one hand *his experiences along the canals confirmed the many difficulties of the vice and immorality which pervade this class of people, the one great cause underlying the matter is the old old story, drink* … on the other hand he acknowledged …

> Many of the boat people keep their cabins clean and bright, with here and there some suitable illuminated texts displayed, some have flowers and birds along with them. Some have at their own expense introduced glass into the roofs of their cabins to make them more light and cheerful, and owners would do well to supply these where they are not at present.

> My observation of the canal population by no means leads me to believe that they are a class as to whom one need despair of doing any good. They are amenable to kind influences, and the work of the clergy of different denominations, and of residents in the neighbourhood of the canals, as well as the system established by recent 'legislation', are beginning to bear fruit in raising these people in the social scale, in making them feel they are not regarded as degraded, almost outcast race, but as a useful body of men engaged in an arduous yet honourable calling, helping to carry on with advantage the commerce of the country, and though their conditions of life may not be so fortunate as some other classes, still their usefulness as a class is becoming more apparent to the traders of the country.

Brydone's report appeared optimistic … *I may say that I hope and believe, that in my subsequent reports, I shall be able to recount some rapid strides in the advancement to good citizenship of the floating population*[138], although one fact that came to light which caused him for concern was from the Registrar General who raised the issue of high mortality rates in the floating population …

> The floating population might be expected to be a healthy class, since they live much in the open air, are forced to a reasonable amount of exercise, and earn wages sufficient to procure a proper supply of good food. But … it would appear that the mortality among them is higher than that of all but a very few classes of the community. Among 2 Bargemen, Lightermen, and Watermen", between the ages of 25 and 65, the death rate is nearly twice as high as among agricultural labourers. Probably some part of this excess is to be ascribed to the numerous accidents to which bargemen are liable, but there must be other reasons to account for the great difference between the average duration of their

lives, and that of the lives of the field workers who are presumably exposed to much the same vicissitudes of weather[139]

Brydone worked tirelessly in the background to develop standardised systems to enable local canal boat inspectors to report *inspection outcomes* with greater accurately. In 1886 Mr Brydone issued a circular reminding authorities of the *eight statutory obligations* they were required to enact as listed in Table 15[140], with a request inspectors include data on each points in subsequent annual reports.

Table 15   Eight Statutory Obligations **for annual reporting (Brydone 1886)**

(1)	The arrangements made for the inspection of boats, and the remuneration of the Inspector;
(2)	The number of boats inspected in 1886, and the conditions of the boats and their occupants as regards the matters dealt with in the Acts and Regulations;
(3)	Any infringements of the Acts and Regulations with respect to (a) Registration; (b) Notification of change of master; (c) Absence of certificates; (d) Marking; (e) Overcrowding; (f) Separation of the sexes; (g) Cleanliness and ventilation; (h) Removal of bilge water; (i) Notification of infectious disease; (j)Refusal of admittance to Inspector;
(4)	Legal proceedings taken in respect of any such infringements, and penalties inflicted;
(5)	Cases of infectious disease dealt with, and measures of isolation adopted;
(6)	Detention of boats for cleansing and disinfection; and, in the case of Registration Authorities,
(7)	The number of boats on the register;
(8)	The number registered in 1886, distinguishing the cases in which fresh registration had been rendered necessary by structural alterations in boats previously registered.

After two years as Towcester Canal Boat Inspector, Thomas Amos wrote to the Sanitary Committee requesting an increase in salary from £5 to £10[141]. The request was declined and the committee replied *the appointment would be thrown open unless Mr Amos was willing to continue the duties at the same salary as beforehand.* Mr Amos tendered his resignation with effect from *Lady Day next unless an increase in salary previously asked of by him was granted*[142], the matter was discussed at the January meeting where the committee resolved …

> Messrs Franklin, Savage and George form a committee to wait upon Mr Amos and after making inquiries as to duties and to report thereon to the authority [at the march meeting a decision had been made] Mr George reported regarding committee appointed to consideration of Canal Boat Inspector salary. Considered that the remuneration of the Canal Boat Inspector was insufficient and that £10 per annum was not in their opinion too much. Proposed and seconded that £10 be paid in full – carried[143].

In Northamptonshire Canal Boat inspection was initially performed on behalf of the local Public Health Authority, from 1888 it became the responsibility of the Rural District Council (RDC). In response to these changes a map was produced of the newly created Sanitary districts in Northamptonshire shown in Figure 33[144]. Thomas Amos was working under the revised RDC structures when he presented his first report for the year ending December 31st 1889 …

> I have entered on the inspectors journal 36 boats for the year 1889, of which I find, 5 boats not registered in name of present owner, 8 without certificates of registration, 2 needing painting for cleaning. I have examined boats as follows for registration by your authority:

Date of examination	Name of boat	Owner	Address
January 17th	George	Edward King	Boatman no address
May 9th	Resolute	E J Brown	Gayton
May 13th	Victory	E J Brown	Gayton
July 12th	Liverpool	Greaves, Bull and Lakin	Stockton
August 6th	Lily	Thomas Simpson	Sowe (Coventry)
August 13th	Laura Emma	John Lightbourne	Simpson Wharf
August 13th	Mary Jane	John Lightbourne	Simpson Wharf
October 13th	Two Sisters	Edward King	No address
October 17th	Our Daisy	Alfred Simpson	Berkhamstead

> I met HM Chief Inspector at Towcester 4th July 1889 when he examined the books, forms etc. Have not been refused admittance to any boat.
>
> I remain gentlemen,
> Your obedient servant
> Thomas Amos

Subsequent annual reports by Thomas Amos during his tenure as canal boat inspector are transcribed in Appendix 2. By 1890 Brydone was including statistical data in his annual canal boats report; numbers of boats registered, number inspected and the number of infringements, and he used the data to highlight where improvements could be made when enforcing the Canal Boats Acts. An increasing concern for Brydone related to *overcrowding* on canal boats, which he noted canal companies had responded to *by creating fore-cabins*. Brydone did not approve of fore-cabins as demonstrated by including in his annual report a quote from Doctor Collingridge, Medical Officer of Health for the Port of London who made a recommendation against their use …

> strongly urge upon registration authorities the advisability of putting every possible obstacle in the way of registering fore-cabins, especially to allow of carrying females on board … they are always low and damp and ill-ventilated[145] …

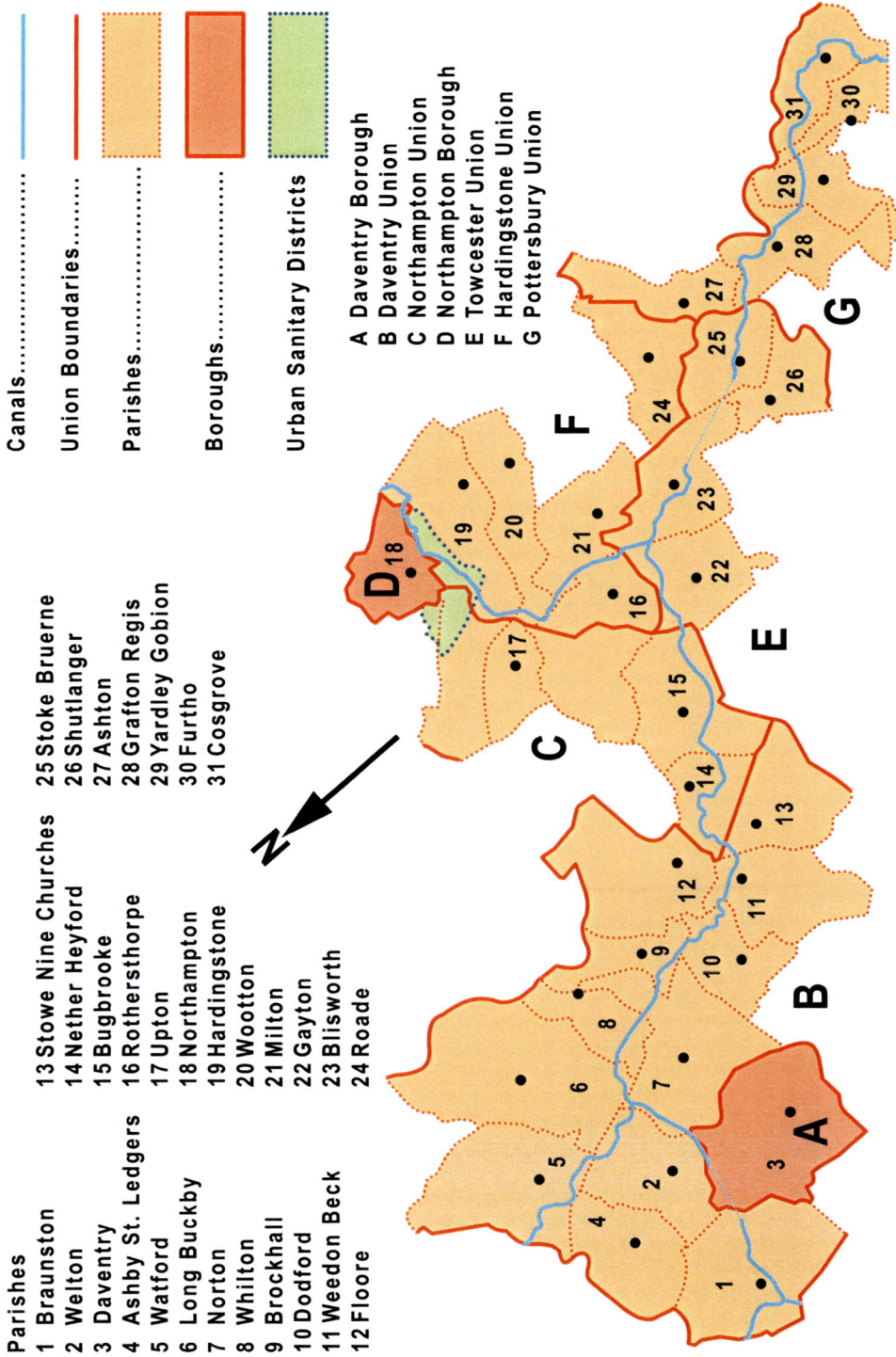

Care on the CUT

Sanitary Districts of Northamptonshire in 1888

Canals..............
Union Boundaries..........
Parishes..............
Boroughs..............
Urban Sanitary Districts

Parishes

1 Braunston
2 Welton
3 Daventry
4 Ashby St. Ledgers
5 Watford
6 Long Buckby
7 Norton
8 Whilton
9 Brockhall
10 Dodford
11 Weedon Beck
12 Floore
13 Stowe Nine Churches
14 Nether Heyford
15 Bugbrooke
16 Rothersthorpe
17 Upton
18 Northampton
19 Hardingstone
20 Wootton
21 Milton
22 Gayton
23 Blisworth
24 Roade
25 Stoke Bruerne
26 Shutlanger
27 Ashton
28 Grafton Regis
29 Yardley Gobion
30 Furtho
31 Cosgrove

A Daventry Borough
B Daventry Union
C Northampton Union
D Northampton Borough
E Towcester Union
F Hardingstone Union
G Pottersbury Union

Figure 33   Northamptonshire Sanitary Districts 1888 (Christopher M Jones)

81

After reminding inspectors of their *eight statutory obligations* Brydone developed an *eighteen point classification of contraventions*[146] listed in Table 16, which he forwarded to local inspectors with a requirement to produce annual data related to each contravention in their district.

Table 16   Eighteen point classification **for reporting canal boat contraventions (Brydone 1891)**

I	Boats not registered
II	Non-notification of change of master
III	Boats without certificate
IV	Certificates not identifying owner with boat
V	Boats not properly marked
VI	Cabins overcrowded
VII	No proper partition separating the sexes
VIII	Females over 12 improperly occupying
IX	Cabins not in a cleanly condition
X	Cabins requiring to be painted
XI	Cabins not sufficiently ventilated
XII	The woodwork of cabins dilapidated
XIII	Removal of bilge water not attended to
XIV	Boats being without pumps
XV	Refusing to admit the local inspector
XVI	Boats being without proper water vessel
XVII	Boats carrying offensive cargoes without the requisite double bulk-heads
XVIII	Non-notification of infectious disease

Growing up in Stoke Bruerne.

Whilst Thomas and Nellie's children were growing up in Stoke Bruerne they experienced a number of local disasters, including the *Sad death of boatman Thomas Smith*[147] in 1885. Thomas Smith had been working with George Varney since Christmas, on the morning of the incident the two men were taking an empty boat from Stoke to Nuneaton, and were in a hurry to catch the 5am tunnel tug. Smith dragged the boat from top-lock to the tunnel mouth, and Varney took the horse over the hill, on arriving in Blisworth Varney was informed *Smith had been found dead in the cabin of the barge*. At the inquest tug driver Richard Dyke gave witness …

> … started 6 or 7 minutes before 5 0'clock … and passed Smith as he was hauling the boat. He asked [me] to wait for him … when he came up he said 'Dick this has given me a "bellowin", he did not say more, and seemed quite exhausted. [Dyke] said he saw him go into the cabin as soon as they got inside the tunnel, although he usually kept outside to help to steer … they reached the mouth … at the end he called to deceased to steer clear

of the head, but he did not respond. [Dyke] turned his tug around … entered the boats cabin, he found Smith inside, with his mouth on his knees. Thinking he was asleep, [Dyke] set him up straight, but on striking a match he found he was quite dead …

On finding the body Dyke gave notice to the village policeman, the body was moved to the Half Moon and Mr W Popplewell, M.R.C.S was called, he reported he found …

> … no signs of violence. A very livid and congested appearance … had no doubt that the cause of death was 'failing of the heart's action, hastened by congestion of the lungs. The exertion he had used drawing the boat, and also the coldness and rawness of the air in the tunnel, would contribute materially to the cause of death[148].

This same year (1885) following a Church of England temperance society meeting held in the village schoolroom an incident occurred which shook both the village and the county as the newspaper headline sums up *Attempted Triple Murder and Suicide Stoke Bruerne*[149]. Thomas Brookes a 44 year old labourer who lived with his father Charles and the housekeeper Mrs Webb. But because Thomas did not get on with his father he regularly spent time with a neighbour Ham Tite, who lived with his 24 year old daughter Mary Ann, whom Thomas Brookes was *keen on* but Mary Ann *did not reciprocated*. On the night of the incident Mary Ann went to the temperance meeting and Thomas followed behind, on looking through the schoolroom window he saw Mary Ann talking with a young man. Thomas then returned to Ham Tites and Mary arrived home at 9.30 at which point Mr Tite went to bed leaving Mary Ann and Thomas in the parlour. On hearing raised voices and a shot fired Ham Tite rushed downstairs to find his daughter bleeding from the head and the door wide open. Brookes had gone to his father's home where he pointed the pistol at the housekeeper, she struggled with him and was shot in the hand, his father then struggled with his son during which he was also shot, Thomas then shot himself in the head and was lying on the floor, Mr Tite and Mrs Webb thought he was dead and ran out of the house.

The police by now had arrived and on entering Mr Tite's home Thomas was gone, a search of the village and surrounding area lasted all night, eventually Thomas was found in Stoke Park Wood. Meanwhile the surgeon attended Mary Ann at her fathers home, although there was very little he could do for her. Thomas Brookes was transferred to Northampton Infirmary on one of George Savage's wagons after which he slowly recovered. Mary Ann passed away at home, after which Brookes was charged with murder at the infirmary. At the inquest George Savage was the foreman of the jury, with John and Thomas Amos and Henry Augustus Savage jurors, the outcome of the coroners case was a verdict of *Wilful Murder*, Brookes was committed for trial before the Duke of Grafton, who after a five hour hearing committed Brookes to a trial[150]. Six weeks later the Grand Jury sat at a summer session, Brookes was indicted and pleaded guilty, although both the defence and the prosecution felt he was *not of fit mind to plead,* on the grounds he had been detained in the Criminal Lunatic Asylum during the weeks since the magistrates hearing. After a review by two doctors and presentation of the findings to the jury the case was concluded *not in fit state of mind to plead – detained in custody*[151].

The Amos family were very active in organisations outside of Stoke Bruerne in the late 1880's, Thomas as a member of the South Northampton Liberals, regularly chairing meetings in the old Wesleyan chapel in Stoke Bruerne[152], he was also a regular delegate at South Northamptonshire branch meetings[153]. Thomas and Nellie regularly attended Roade Baptist Church, which held it's bi-centenary celebrations in 1888[154] . Under the leadership of Rev. Gardiner the congregation went from strength to strength, brothers Charles and Thomas Amos were appointed trustees to the church, and their wives Nellie and Emma were members of the Ladies Committee, their duties included assessing the suitability of women for inclusion or exclusion from the congregation[155]. The Church built a Board School in it's grounds in the mid 1890's and Charles Amos was appointed to the School Committee, later he became Chairman[156]. Thomas Amos also worked with Temperance organisations in Northamptonshire, becoming a speaker on the *Temperance and Band of Hope Union circuit*[157], whilst his wife continued her Pride of the Valley meetings in the family home.

Thomas Amos took over from his father as Stoke Bruerne census enumerator in 1891, on census day he included more detail on the boats and boat families moored on census night than when his father did the job, as shown in Table 17. Of the seven boats moored at Stoke Bruerne on census night, three contain members of the same family travelling in convoy. On the boat *Emscote* is John Powell and two of his sons John and Edward, at this time his wife Jane is residing at their home in Cross Lane, Braunston. On *Banbury* is John's son Thomas, with his wife Elizabeth (nee Kendall) and their two daughters, whilst on their third boat *Economy* is John's other son William and a mate, William's wife Sarah Ann and their son are living with Sarah Ann's mother, Mary Archer at The Wharf, Braunston[158].

Table 17   Boats moored in Stoke Bruerne on census night 1891

Boat	Occupants	Age	Occupation	Birthplace
Alice '459'	William Williams (Captain)	31	Captain	Wolverhampton
	Matilda Williams (Wife)	31		Brierley Hill
	William Williams (Son)	4		Tipton
	Samuel Williams (Son)	6 /12		Tipton
Emscote '100'	John Powell (Captain)	27	Captain	Braunston
	John Powell (Son)	15	Crew	Warwick
	Edward Powell (Son)	13		Braunston
Banbury '22'	Thomas Powell (Captain)	27	Captain	Braunston
	Elizabeth Powell (Wife)	29		Warwick
	Elizabeth Powell (Daughter)	2		Stockton
	Mary Ann Powell (Daughter)	6/12		Braunston

Economy '3'	William Powell (Captain)	24	Captain	Braunston
	Thomas Sparks	10	Helper	Oldbury
Contractor '143'	George Lawton (Capt)	22	Captain	Foleshill
	John Wateley	47 Widow	Crew	Braunston
Monarch '176'	Thomas Lapworth (Capt)	27		Braunston
	Sarah Ann Lapworth (Wife)	23		Wood Lane Staffs
	Bertha Lapworth (Daughter)	3		Braunston
Dundee	Joseph Goddard (Capt)	36 Widow		Tipton
	Joseph Williams	5		Tipton
	Thomas Edwards	15		Tipton

Thomas and Nellie's last child, Olive Eunice was born at Stowe Hill in 1892, around the same time John and Elizabeth Amos moved from Stoke Bruerne near to their son and daughter-in-law and three grand-children in Roade, a year after moving Granny Amos, shown in Figure 34, passed away. After the death of his wife John's health began to fail, he made an application for membership of Roade Baptist Church which was accepted without the need for him to attend the church[159]. Mr Amos Senior passed away in Roade two years after his wife, age 68, his assets of £156 were passed on to his eldest son Thomas.

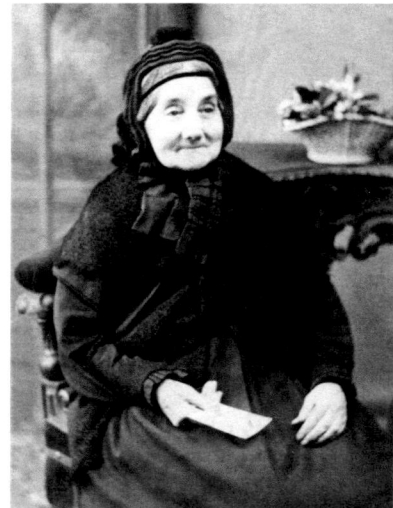

Figure 34   Elizabeth (Nanny) Amos (Waterway's Archive)

In the last decade of the century most canal traffic in Stoke Bruerne was *long distance, through traffic,* passing between the two large centres of population, London and the Midlands. Much traffic also terminated within the line of the Grand Junction Canal such as the Hertfordshire paper mills and at Uxbridge. In Stoke Bruerne there were two boat owners; George Savage and William Woodward. Steam tugs were still operating through Blisworth Tunnel, and when Thomas Amos presented his annual canal boat inspector report in 1894 he drew to the attention of the Sanitary Committee his observations of the dangers associated with these …

> On July 3rd last several children almost suffocated in Blisworth tunnel by the smoke from the steam tug which plys through the tunnel 16 times a day. I made a report to Mr Brydone HM Chief Inspector and received a reply to say the GJCCo engineer had promised to remedy the complaint, but nothing to my knowledge has been done to prevent a similar occurrence.
>
> The same complaint has come under my notice several times during the summer months; if your authority can make any suggestions the company's local engineer informs me he

will lay the matter before the committee and endeavour to carry out the suggestion to remedy the evil[160].

Outside the Amos home on October 1st 1894 the Fellows, Morton and Clayton (FMC) boat *Daisy* arrived crewed by the Humphries family. Mrs Humphries was in the back-cabin with her three day old daughter when Captain Humphries informed Mr Amos that his wife and child were both ill. Mrs Amos after visiting Mrs Humphries immediately took mother and baby into her home and called Mr Ryan the local Doctor, who initially diagnosed *milk fever* but cautioned Mrs Amos *there was a risk of typhoid*. Not deterred Mrs Amos *pluckily resolved to take the risk of infection, and nurse the woman[161]*, soon after Baby Humphries died. Mrs Amos and a trained Nurse provided by the local authorities continued caring for Mrs Humphries during which and to the surprise of everyone the diagnosis was later confirmed as *a virulent case of small pox*. Mrs Humphries died of the disease ten days later and her burial took place the same night[162]. At the time of the tragedy Mr and Mrs Amos and their six children (age 2-15 years) were ordered by the Medical Officer to be vaccinated, and the family furniture and clothing burnt.

Mr Humphries after leaving his wife and child in Stoke Bruerne continued his journey by boat. When Mr Amos was informed of the final diagnosis he made contact with other sanitary authorities so they could stop Mr Humphries and disinfect the boat. Chief Inspector Brydone was on the Birmingham Canal Navigation when he was contacted about Mr Humphries. As Mr Humphries continued to ply the canal Mr Brydone immediately tried to trace the boat by telegraph, the boat was located and precautions taken, Mr Brydone including an account of this in his annual report …

> … The boat was met with on its return journey from London on the Monday morning, before 10 o'clock, at Berkhampstead, by Mr Baines, the Canal Boat Inspector for Tring, who had gone in search of it. The boat tied up on its arrival again at Stoke Bruerne. The woman died on the Thursday (October 11th) and was buried at midnight, the husband being present. On the following Monday (15th) the boat reached the boundary of the borough of Birmingham, where the officer of that authority was waiting for it, and at once stopped it, in order that he might question the master as to what steps had been taken for proper disinfecting of his boat, &c. The master informed him that it had been done twice-the second time at Leighton Buzzard; but, as he was unable to produce, as required by the Statute, and certificate from that authority's medical officer of health, the boat was again disinfected, and a certificate supplied by the medical officer of health of Birmingham, after which the boat was allowed to go on and complete its journey[163]

At the following Towcester Sanitary Authority meeting, on the proposition of Mr Savage the Guardians resolved a vote of thanks be passed to Mr Amos and his wife for *their kind treatment and the manner in which Mrs Amos devoted time to the assistance and treatment of the poor woman Mrs. Humphries[164]*. Subsequently the committee discussed compensation for the Amos family, and the recouping of costs incurred by the Sanitary Authority, although discussion was suspended *to see what the company (Fellows, Morton and Clayton) did[165]*. At the November meeting costs were discussed again[166], Mr Savage reporting *only a little had been collected and that went to pay the doctors account*. Mr. Amos submitted a claim for compensation which the authority scrutinised and *resolved they pay Mr. Amos £29.18.0* made up as follows; Furniture £25.10.0., Mrs. Amos's apparel £3.10.0., charwoman's apparel £0.7.6. and damage to bedstead £0.10.5.

The committee also agreed to pay £3.14.0. to Northamptonshire Nursing Institution, concluding Mr Humphries be called upon to pay the sum of £8.14.9. (the amount expended by the relieving officer and the nurses expenses), the clerk being directed to write to Messrs Fellows, Morton and Co., to inform them[167] *this Authority have resolved to ask the man Humphries to repay the cost incidental to his wife's removal £5.0.7. and the bill from the Nursing Institute Northampton £3.14.0.*[168]. An exchange of letters between the carrying company and the Sanitary Authority subsequently took place[169]. In concluding the event Mrs Amos's caring disposition was later acknowledged …

> … Mrs Amos attributed her safety, and the safety of her family and the village, to the prayers offered in the churches and chapels in the district. … the Deptford Mission which works among boatmen, presented Mrs Amos with a tea and coffee service bearing the simple inscription "Inasmuch"[170]

As the Amos children were growing up Stoke Bruerne was also the site of altercations between steamer Captains, a particularly illustrative case being a difference of agreement which caused a major hold up on the canal outside the Amos home. The incident was anonymously reported in a newspaper far away from Northamptonshire[171], which includes details that could have only been conveyed by a close and knowledgeable observer of the incident …

GREAT BATTLE OF THE BARGEES.

BY AN EYE-WITNESS.

The little village of Stoke Bruerne, near Blisworth, was excited, beyond anything remembered by the oldest inhabitant, one morning this week. A village of fifty houses does not often rise to a climax. But it did so on this occasion. On the whitewashed bridge that spans the Grand Junction Canal might be seen the postman, the policeman, three farmers, nearly all the agricultural labourers–for it was raining pitilessly, and men could not work in the fields-two lads from the ropewalk, the butcher, the squire's gardener, the Northampton carrier, the shoemaker's man, and all the small-fry that could stand the rain. The women were not on the bridge, but they were peeping nervously out of front doors and windows, in the intervals of their early morning work. It was only 7.30 a.m., but a crisis was on the village. Never since the ivy began to grow round the old Stoke church tower had its canal been black with a hundred motionless barges. It looked half like a naval bombardment. And it began to fell remarkably like one towards midnight, when the battle had lasted seventeen hours, and some of us got to know that one of the barges was laden with barrels of gunpowder!

How did the battle begin? Very simply. It was emphatically a row between "Bill" and "Joe." There had been a race in the tunnel soon after daybreak, and, like more splendid racing on the iron roads to the North, the result had not been all glory. The skipper of the Birmingham Canal Co.'s Boat had gained on the river steam-barge of "Fellows, Morton, & Co," and there is said to be a rule that a barge so gaining must be allowed to go ahead of the other. But the rule did not operate that morning. "Bill" played the nasty game of slanting his barge across the track, thereby not only refusing precedence to his rival, but making him push his own boat forward. Emerging from the tunnel, the skippers raced round the curve to the lock. The "Fellows-Morton" man got into the lock first, and his two linked barges were in position to pass out ahead. But the Birmingham "captain" was incensed. They felt they had been "done," and refusing to accept the situation, they rammed the nose of their barge far enough through the gate of the lock to prevent the lock-keeper from shutting it to let out water. Then set in the grim struggle that lasted well-nigh thirty hours, and brought, for Stoke, a vast crowd to the whitewashed bridge near the tiny post-office. At five in the morning, the prolonged hissing of steam betokened something unusual. At five o'clock next morning, the same hissing from the rival engine told that steam was being kept up in readiness for a move forward, if the obance came. About noon of the first day a messenger was despatched by cycle to fetch the engineer of the Canal Company. But it was a long time before he came. A row between bargees is often an ugly affair, and in past years one has rarely been settled without fighting with fists and boots. The engineer perhaps had his reasons for deliberation.

Meanwhile, barges from Blisworth, through the tunnel, stopped short, and formed in the line that way; while barges from the Yardley and Wolverton side were brought up in the net-work of the locks on the lower levels southward. In either direction stretched a long and steadily increasing line of the great barge fleet, "Bill" and "Joe" had the traffic as much under their control as a ten weeks frost, in such a winter as the one before last. The canal banks soon began to look like vast stables, from the number of horses tethered there. No doubt the rest came as a sweet surprise to the weary animals after their long sleepy tramp on muddy towing-paths.

Still no engineer. What was the Company doing, asked more than one bystander, "to let this sort o' thing go on, stopping all the traffic!". "Ah!" said another, "the captains will have to pay smart for it. Every barge stopped will cost these two fellows a pound a-day damages." The "two fellows" aforesaid had not exchanged a word since hostilities began, some said "Bill" was in his bunk fast asleep, and "Joe" was over the "pub" with his mates. Each hero sulked in his tent. I am sorry to say that while there was temper on the canal there was incessant activity at the canal-side "public." "They were drinking all day, and they'll fight at night," said someone. So thought the County Superintendent of Police, for there were soon three policemen in the village, which ordinarily is startled by the sight of one. But, strange to say, the fighting never came off. A lot of drinking no doubt there was. Language of no very choice kind was flying about. Navigation was at a dead stop. The brown water-rat swam from bank to bank without knowing that a foe was at hand. Money and temper were being squandered. But there was no fighting.

At last the engineer came, clothed in the authority of the Grand Junction Company. He at once ordered the Birmingham Barge to be pulled back out of the lock, but before the lock-men could do it, "Bill" had put his engines full steam ahead, and the attempt failed. Once more the lock-keeper made fast a rope to pull her back, but this time Bill's son, more eager for fight than his father, lifted his delicate foot, with the intention of placing it on the lock-keeper's stomach. But the lock-keeper was no baby, and turned to rush on William junior, when the latter ran below, and both saved his skin and put on fresh steam. The engineer at length abandoned his task, declining to rise force. Telegrams now began to fly to London and Birmingham, indicating the serious position of affairs. Drinking continued. The publican, it was shrewdly observed, was the only one that would make a profit out of the bother. Night fell, midnight approached, and few villagers slept very well in their beds. Everybody thought the storm would burst. So few, in particular, knew that one of the barges was laden with gunpowder. It did not carry its red light, as it ought to have done, but it lay right under our windows, and gave us an uneasy night. By this time there were hundreds of bargemen and barge-women about the village, and no one knew what might happen. Almost before the church clock had sounded the hour, the beershop was cleared of its last man, and those guided loose might soon work havoc.

But the gratifying fact has to be recorded that they didn't. Civilisation is advancing among our bargee brothers as elsewhere. Perhaps, too, I ought to mention a local ca… (unreadable), which had its share in preserving the peace. Close to the lock lives a little, kind-hearted woman, whose husband, worthy of her, is a sort of head man of the village. He holds all the offices, save parish clerk, for, as a matter of fact, he leads the singing in a little chapel not far away. A strange, terrible thing occurred at this very lock a few months ago. It happened to a brother of one of the very men who this week raced, fell out, and stopped the traffic for over thirty hours. Nor is it likely to be forgotten, for bargemen have hearts, and tender ones, if we only knew it. One day a bargeman stopped his boat opposite the house of the kind-hearted woman and asked for her. His wife and child were dreadfully ill on board: in fact, the baby had been born on the barge only a few hours before. The woman was delirious. The man begged her to take his wife in. A doctor was fetched, and he certified the poor creature would be dead in an hour if left on the boat. There was no hospital for many miles, and the doctor thought it was not an infectious case. The kind-hearted woman was ready, and soon the sufferer was carried upstairs and put into one of the best rooms. Then began a fearful struggle, for next day the baby died, and the next day the mother's case proved to be a most virulent case of smallpox. Husband and children were sent out of the house and all business stopped, but the brave Christian woman remained beside her poor, distressed sister of the bargee night and day, battling with the disease, and administering Christian sympathy as only a woman can. The poor creature lasted but two days longer, but before her eyes closed on a sorrowful world she breathed devout blessings on the good Samaritan who had taken her in and cared for her at risk to life and no little loss of goods.

Close to where the hundred barges were kept waiting stands the cottage of the bargeman's friend. No one was so grieved as she at the bad spirit and the quarrel. On her sideboard stands a silver tea and coffee service presented to her for loving kindness to the wife of the barge skipper, and subscribed for by some of the men themselves. Sir Walter Foster, then at the Local Government Board, wrote her a letter of highest praise for her humanity and devotion.

Most people wondered why there was no fighting opposite her door, and why in the grey morning light of the next day the Birmingham skipper stole out of his bunk, and by gad to pull his craft back past the lock gates. By noon the canal was again astir, and every water rat ran to its hole. There were various reasons, of course, but I venture to say the presence of the bargee's "Good Samaritan" helped to bring about the pacific solution.- Christian World.

Although the article omitted to name the Captains, these were recorded by Grand Junction Canal Company engineer Mr Milner, in letters arising from his dealings with the incident. Captain W Edwards was in charge of the Fellows, Morton and Clayton Ltd steamer *Phoenix* and Captain A Humphrey the London and Birmingham Canal Carrying Company steamer *Buffalo*. On the morning of the incident Mr Milner was at Braunston, after arriving in Stoke at 3.30pm he *tried both persuasion and force to remove Edwards,* but it was not until the next morning when Mr Milner returned to the scene *that he would give way, which he did by pulling out of the lock*[172]. After the incident Mr Milner sought advice on how to proceed from Mr Thomas at Bulbourne[173] … *whether I am to take out a summons against Edwards or both Captains under Penal Enactment 30 and claim full penalty,* he decided …

I have taken out summonses against the Captains of the Steamers *Buffalo* and *Phoenix* under the 89th section of the Company's act and a third summons on the *Buffalo* for strapping round the lock gate balance on our endeavouring to force the boat out of the lock (under Bye Law 13).

After receiving his summons Captain Humphries saw Mr Milner to inform him of his intent to respect the summons, Mr Milner responding *he could not do anything for him,* although he wrote to his colleague *I do not attach so much blame to him as the lock was his and the stoppage was caused by Edwards. I think a small fine before the magistrates would meet Humphries case but Edwards I should like to make an example of and get off the Canal if possible*[174]. The case was heard at Towcester, Mr Milner conveying the outcome to his colleague …

I beg to report that this case was heard at Towcester today At Lord Euston's suggestion Mr Whitton withdrew the summons against Humphrey and Edwards was fined 20/- for strapping round the lock gate … 20/- for obstructing the traffic with an additional 12/- costs. Our case against Edwards was only partially heard when the Chairman intimated the bench had heard sufficient evidence and had made up their minds. It would be a good thing to get the Edwards family removed from the canal if possible.[175]

Only a few months after the steamer incident trouble occurred inside as opposed to outside the

Amos home when Ernest Amos, Thomas and Nellie's only son brought shame and upset to the family in 1897. Ernest and his friend Herbert Whitlock were arrested, charged and placed on remand for stealing postal orders to the value of £1 17s[176]. The case was brought before the Duke of Grafton at Towcester Petty Session[177] but was immediately adjourned because no evidence had been tendered, both boys were placed on remand for two weeks. On coming before the bench Ernests' case was heard first, with both his parents being summoned to give evidence, for his mother it was noted *Mrs Amos was very much affected in having to give evidence against her son.*

Thomas Amos from his position as Assistant Post-Master was first to give witness, he commenced by producing the postal order registration book, showing the court *postal-order number 784,104 received in the post office on April 9th and issued by S E Amos on April 14th.* Ernest's defence Mr Phipps informed the Duke the Amos boy *had always been a good boy till now* and that his father had *paid cash to Towcester Post Office before receiving the orders,* stressing *neither the post office authorities or the Amos family had suffered through these orders being taken.* Mrs Amos then confirmed *she did not issue order 784,104 to anyone on 14th April,* and after being shown the postal order she confirmed the signature was *not in her handwriting.*

Marian Pike, daughter of the Post-Master confirmed Ernest *brought the order to Blisworth office made payable to Thomas Jones and signed,* and that she gave the prisoner *a sovereign for it.* Supt. Norman who charged Ernest then confirmed the prisoner confessed to the offence on being arrested …

> … 'I took the order for 20s the Thursday before good Friday, I stamped it and cashed it at Blisworth' … the prisoner has been on remand, in custody, three weeks … In view of that fact and what we knew of the lad's circumstances and the respectability of his parents, and the provision likely to be made for the lads future, he was honestly of the opinion that the case could be dealt with under the First Offenders Act (hoping he not prejudicing the case).

Mr Phipps summed up by drawing to the attention of the bench how distressing the occurrence had been for the Amos family and stressed again *the Post Office had not suffered a loss, and he hoped the court would take into consideration the prisoners youth, extreme penitence, previous good character and that he had suffered by being kept on gaol three weeks.* No verdict was made on Ernest until Whitlock's case had been heard.

Mrs Amos also gave evidence at Herbert Whitlock's hearing confirming he was employed by her as an assistant in the post-office, his duties being to deliver letters in Stoke Bruerne. Mrs Amos also confirmed that on *14th April the order for 2s was received into the office, and on 21st the order for 10s was also received … they were never issued from the office, they were not stamped.* Miss Ellen Tew assistant in Roade Post-Office reported receiving a blank postal order from Whitlock which she made payable to T. Jones at the prisoners request, receipted it and *cashed it without noticing it did not bear an issuing stamp.* Finally Marion Pike from Blisworth post-office confirmed Whitlock tried to cash a postal order for 15s which she refused because it was not properly filled in …

> … I asked him how he came about it, he replied that he undertook to get it cashed for a man named John White of Stoke Bruerne. I asked him where White got it from, and he seemed confused, and said he thought it came from White's daughter at Ashton. I went for my father and he subsequently PC Rose was sent for and the order was given to him.

On charging Whitlock Supt. Norman confirmed he pleaded not guilty, stating he *found two postal orders, one for 2s and one for 15s on 27ᵗʰ April, under a truss of hay in Mr Amos's Chaff House at Stoke Bruerne'. I went to Roade and changed one for 2s and tried to change this one for 15s at Blisworth, I told no one I had found them.* Because Whitlock pleaded not guilty he was committed to a future trial but allowed on bail. Ernest Amos was discharged under the order *his father was bound over to be responsible for his son's good behaviour, in the sum of £10 for twelve calendar months.* Whitlock returned to the petty session where his defence opened by announcing *this was a bad case*, as the accused had been committed by the Towcester Magistrate *on the charge of stealing two postal orders,* the property of the Post-master General, his objection being …

> When the prisoner was called upon to plead, that the indictment was had, because under the Vexations Indictment Act it was necessary in a charge of false pretences that prosecutor should be bound over to prosecute on that charge. This had not been done. No proceedings had been taken before the magistrates for false pretences, the prisoner being committed for larceny …

The defence also pointed out *the indictment was bad in itself, and will be bad [if taken to] a next session,* on this point the indictment was quashed and young Herbert Whitlock was discharged[178].

Whilst all the upset was underway regarding Ernest's court case Queen Victoria's diamond jubilee was celebrated in a most spectacular way at Stoke Bruerne Park. The event included the whole of the population of Stoke Bruerne and Shutlanger *not forgetting the sick, the aged and the feeble for whom a special tent and a covered shelter, with comfortable armchairs provided, with carriages to bring them to and fro.* Mr and Mrs Wentworth entertained their guests to a whole day's celebrations including three square meals, music, sport, pastimes and a procession. The weather remained fine and as dusk came the park and the hall were *illuminated with upwards of 12,000 little lamps*, to conclude the day there was a *spectacular display of fireworks*[179].

The Amos's twin girls Mary and Ellen were teenagers at the time of the Jubilee celebrations and Ellen was already showing an interest in becoming a Nurse, as recalled by her childhood friend and neighbour from the Boat Inn Beatrix Woodward[180]… *[Ellen] was too busy being a tomboy, although I do remember that with her dolls, it was always the broken ones she cared for most.* During *This is Your Life* Eamonn Andrews expanded on Ellen's (Sister Mary's) childhood …

> Then, as you grew up, the day came when the broken dolls were fed with 'medicine' and put to bed for the last time. Much more fun, of course, to have a real live patient and so

– no sooner did a barge tie up at the lock – than you were there to hoick some squalling infant from its' mother's arms and carry it home for 'treatment' Nursing care not always popular with your grandfather, I believe … who often had to harness pony and trap and drive to the next lock to return infant to parents[181] …

Deaths related to the canal continued in Stoke Bruerne, although drowning was not exclusive to those working canal boats or those residing in the village as seen from the entries in Table 18. Mr Thomas Jelly, a 77 year old general labourer went for a walk one bright moonlit evening in the direction of Alderton, during which he walked over a brook on an 11 inch plank with a handrail. At the inquest it was reported *the floods had been in* and it was uncertain *as to whether the plank had broken as Mr Jelly passed over it, or whether the floods had washed him away* as the broken plank, part of the handrail and Mr Jelly's body were found ¾ of a mile from *Plank Bridge*, the verdict was returned *found drowned (in the river)*[182]. Three year old Frederick Jeffery was buried in August 1892 after drowning in a lock in the village. Freddie was visiting his grandfather with his mother both lived in London, the child was playing in the garden when his grandfather noticed he was missing. The child's hat was seen near the canal and after seeing bubbles in the water tunnel tug driver Richard Dyke jumped in and recovered the body but *there were no signs of life and attempts to restore animation proved futile*[183]. A death not recorded in Saint Mary's records was that of 62 year old boatman Thomas Simpson from Sowe. Thomas and fellow boatman Amos Barnes tied up in the village just before six o'clock one evening. Amos on giving evidence at the inquest reported *he had never seen Thomas in better health* and confirmed the last time he saw Thomas *he was sober*, at the inquest it was resolved the deceased *probably fell from the lock-gate as he tried to cross over*, the body was transported to his home town where he was buried.[184]

Table 18   Saint Mary the Blessed Virgin. Canal related burials 1875-1899

Burial date	Name	Age	Description
12th August 1880			A woman found dead in the canal
1st November 1882	Thomas Jelley		Found Drowned
7th March 1888	Elizabeth Ann Creswell	5 weeks	Stoke Bruerne canal barge
12th September 1891	Alfred James Peasland	14 years	Drowned from Barge
21st August 1892	Frederick Jeffery	3 years	Drowned in canal lock
4th May 1896	Clara Fenton	11 years	Died on barge
28th February 1899	Eliza Creswell	8 years	Drowned in canal lock

A significant number of men were employed in jobs related to the canal in Stoke Bruerne; Engine drivers, lock-keepers, canal labourers who together with the boaters continued to baptised their children at Saint Mary's Church[185] shown in Table 19. Between 1875-1899 there were 20 canal related baptisms at St Mary's, of these Dyke, Johnson, Inns, Gibbon and Wood worked for either the Grand Junction Canal Company or local businesses. The rest were long distance boatmen; Vaughan from Birmingham; Hollis and Stokes from Brierley Hill Staffordshire; Stevens from Tipton Staffordshire; Bond from Leicestershire; Simpson from Foleshill Warwickshire and Harrison from Droitwich Worcestershire. You may have noticed that on 25th December there are five baptisms all of them are long distance boat families. Christmas day was the only guaranteed day boatmen would not be working[186].

Table 19   Saint Mary the Blessed Virgin. Canal related baptisms 1875-1899

Baptism Date	Birth date	Child's Name	Parents	Fathers occupation
6th June 1875	May 4th 1874	Martha Edith	Benjamin and Eliza Wood	Boatman Stoke Bruerne
5th September 1875	February 10th	Joseph William	Adam and Esther Hollis	Steam Boatman Stoke Bruerne
16th March 1878		William	Jonah and Eleanor Stokes	Bargee Stoke Bruerne
25th December 1878	26th October 1877	George	Henry and Ann Harrison	Boatman. Droitwich.
25th December 1878	About 4 years	Samuel	Emmanuel and Mary Ann Steven	Boatman Stockton.
	About 2 years	Hannah		
	About 1 month	Emmanuel		
25th December 1878	23rd July 1878	Sarah Ann	James and Phoebe Vaughan	Boatman Birmingham.
15th December 1880	2nd January	Alice Louisa	Richard and Annie Dyke	Boatman Stoke Bruerne
6th June 1880	2nd March	William T. A.,	Thomas and Mary Gibbon	Engine Driver Stoke Bruerne
25th December 1883	10h August	Lilian	Richard and Annie Dyke	Boatman Stoke Bruerne
5th October 1884	7th July	Charles William	Henry Walter and Alice Johnson	Lock Keeper Stoke Bruerne
24th March 1889		Frank	Henry Walter and Alice Johnson	Lock Keeper Stoke Bruerne
13th March 1891		Matilda	Samuel and Sarah Bond	Canal Boatman Stoke Bruerne
14th April 1895		Doris Annie L	George and Louisa Sophia Inns	Canal Labourer
7th July 1895	16th April	John Henry	Richard and Annie Dyke	Lock Keeper
9th April 1897		Henry	Henry and Anna Simpson	Bargeman on Barge
8th July 1897	26th August 1896	Beatrice N	Samuel and Sarah Bond	Canal Boatman Stoke Bruerne
10th October 1897	1st September	George Thomas	George and Louisa Sophia Inns	Canal Labourer
12th February 1899	8th January 1899	George Henry	Samuel and Sarah Bond	Bargeman Stoke Bruerne
18th June 1899		Dorothy L	George and Louisa Sophia Inns	Canal Labourer
8th September 1899	25th June 1899	Richard S	Richard and Annie Dyke	Lock Keeper

The Watershed.

The final year of the millennium began with the sudden death of John Brydone the first chief inspector of canal boats, who died *due to overwork and illness at the age of fifty-eight*[187]. Before his death Brydone delivered fourteen annual canal boat reports, from these it can be seen there was progressive development in relation to the duties of local inspectors, the culture of boat families and, the increasing responsibilities of employers (carrying companies) to their employees. In what was un-be-known to Brydone his final annual report, he poignantly commented on the success of the Canal Boat's Act(s) …

> It is now twenty years since the passing of the first Canal Boats Act, and I think the legislation on the subject has produced great and beneficial results, and with very little friction. For the comfort and cleanliness of the cabins little more can now be done than to keep up the surveillance which is at present exercised. The men and women engaged in boating contrast favourably with any of the working classes. The one regrettable incident, however, in connection with the carrying out of the Canal Boats Acts, is the difficulty of securing the education of the children of boatmen. This question does not, however, come within the purview of the duties imposed on the Local Government Board by the Canal Boats Acts.
>
> I have the honour to be, Sir,
>> Your most obedient servant,
>
>> JOHN BRYDONE,
>> Inspector under the Canal Boats Acts[188].

The same month as Brydone passed away, Thomas Amos resigned as Canal Boat Inspector after two decades of service[189], during his tenure Thomas registered 125 boats. Mr Amos was replaced by another resident of Stoke Bruerne Mr George R Phipps whose starting pay was £10 per annum[190]. Not long after taking up his post as Canal Boat Inspector Mr Phipps's father in law, farmer and businessman Mr George Savage passed away age 84[191]. From humble beginnings as a butcher Mr Savage astutely built up his business interests, including the Brick and Tile Works, which his family continued to run after George's death, some of the men employed at the brick-works are shown in Figure 35. In September 1899 Annie Woodward of the Boat Inn acquired her first boat in her own name *Industrious,* an old boat dating back to 1872[192].

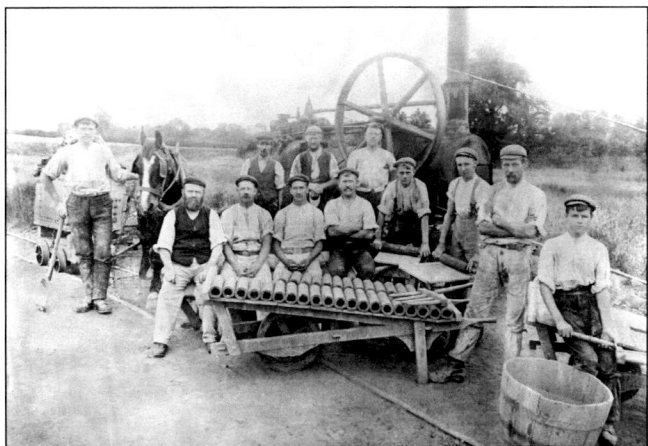

Figure 35   Men working at George Savage's brick works Stoke Bruerne (Northampton Central Library)

Nellie Amos's brother (Sister Mary's uncle) Rev. James Hirst Hollowell was an outspoken advocate for non-sectarian education and had for a number of years written books in his own name[193], in 1899 and under the non de plume Katherine Ireton Rev. Hirst Hollowell published *Ritualism Abandoned*[194], which had incorporated into it an account of the smallpox incident his sister managed in her home in Stoke Bruerne. The account paints a dismal picture of the fear engendered in the village in response to the very first *variola confluens* (small-pox) case …

> … nothing but absolute necessity, and considerations of extreme personal inconvenience, prevented the whole population from simultaneously migrating to another country. They felt that the disease was in the air; it was in the pebbles of the […] yard; it was in the ivy of the […] house; it was in the spouting, and the old bird's-nests; it was in the […] books and cushions …; it was in the gown of the woman that cleaned … ; it was in the smoke from the […] kitchen; it was in every vegetable in the garden, and in every egg laid, at this most inopportune moment, by the reckless poultry in the […] back-yard[195].

The new Chief Inspector of Canal Boats, Mr Owen John Llewellyn[196] started work in April 1899 the same year of the London dock strike, which was particularly significant at Brentford (and Limehouse) where canal boat workers came into contact with lightermen, rivermen and other dock workers during loading and un-loading[197]. Owen Llewellyn in his first annual report paid tribute to the work of his predecessor …

> I cannot conclude this, my first report as Inspector, without paying tribute to the memory of the late Mr. John Brydone. I never had the pleasure of meeting him, but it is my lot to follow directly in his steps, and to visit in all parts of the country the officials of sanitary authorities to whom he was well known. He was a man of whom one hears, without exception, nothing but good. In the words of one inspector: "To few men is it given the chance by his own efforts to raise, as Mr. Brydone has done, a whole class of fellow-creatures from a low and debased standard to becoming honest useful members of society;" and from my own experience I can vouch for the success that has attended his unceasing toil on behalf of the canal boat men, women, and children of England and Wales[198].

Following the passing of the Canal Boats Amendment Act (1884) canal boats and their occupants, the *family boaters* were more regulated than those living on the land due to the requirement for *registration as a dwelling and regular inspection by public officials*, the latter having powers to summons and prosecute. Without a doubt the Act brought many benefits to boaters, some of which were

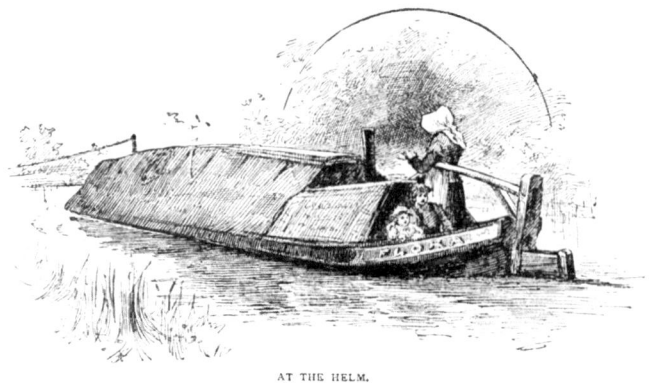

Figure 36   At the Helm (The Penny Magazine 1899)

reported in *The Penny Magazine* accompanied by two pictures. The first is an engraving shown in Figure 36, which depicts a typical horse drawn slow boat of the period with a boatwoman and her children in the hatches. Although some details are suspect the overall depiction is very accurate, including the curving top plank over the hold. This distinctive profile was mainly a 19th century feature; in the 20th century the planks were straight, showing the boats were continually evolving despite canal boats being regarded by some as an outmoded form of transport. The second engraving shown in Figure 37 is of a humorous domestic scene inside the back cabin of a narrow boat. Points to note are the bottle stove with boiling kettle surrounded by various utensils and a pair of boots behind drying in the heat. Attached to the table cupboard wall next to the stove is an oil or paraffin lamp with umbrella shade above to protect the ceiling from heat and soot. Hanging from the lamp bracket appears to be a horn which was blown to warn oncoming boats at blind bends and bridge holes. The cabin furniture is the same as most other boats conforming to the requirements of the Canal Boats Acts of 1877 and 1884 (see figures 30 and 31). Events outside the Amos home continued right up to the turn of the century when two boats sunk in top-lock …

> It appears that the boats, one of which contained powder, was towed into the locks in the usual manner, and the water was then let in. Owing to a defect, however, in the gate, the boat, which had caught against it, could not rise with the water, and the consequence was both boats were swamped. It is stated that other boats have been similarly sunk[199].

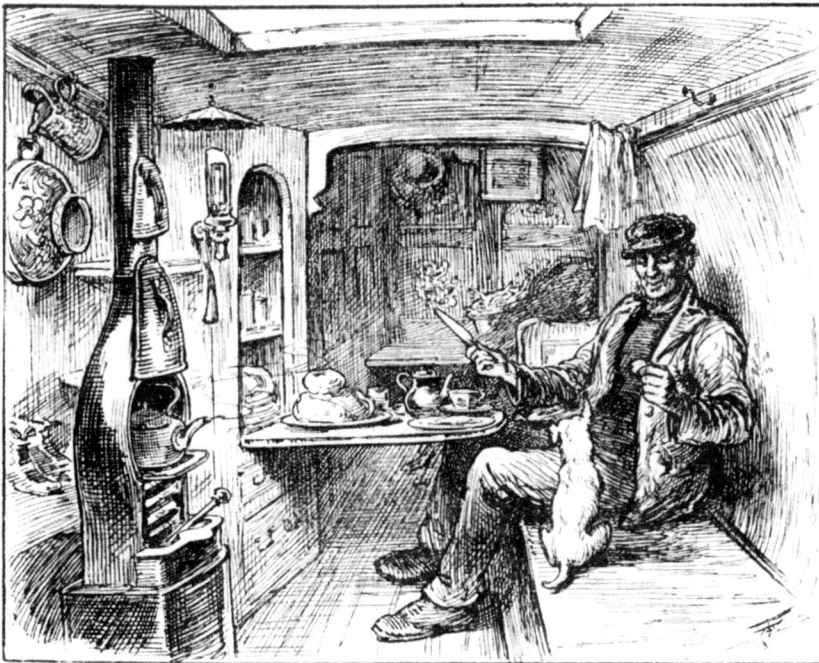

A BARGEMAN'S CABIN.

Figure 37   The Back Cabin (The Penny Magazine 1899)

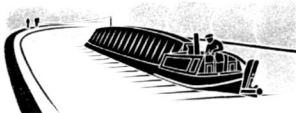

The watershed continues for the Amos family ...

At the beginning of the twentieth century the only members of the *second generation* of the Amos family in Stoke Bruerne were Thomas and Nellie, who together ran the rope business, shop and post-office from their home beside top-lock. Figure 38 shows a regular scene outside the Amos home, where a pair of horse drawn boats enter Top Lock laden with small coal, most likely for some canal side industrial concern. To make life easier for both steerer and horse, the tow line has been attached to a point on the lock side by the photographer, run through a pulley block attached to the towing mast, then back to the horse out of view on the right. This significantly reduces the effort needed to pull the boats into the lock. In the distance is the mill and engine house with tow path bridge allowing access to a narrow canal basin running from beneath the bridge to the mill. Also clearly shown is the Amos house and shop with signs fixed to the side wall indicating both Post and Telegraph Office. Figure 39 shows top-lock from the opposite direction, clearly shown are the two telegraph lines and a busy use of the locks, with the W & S Foster Ltd boat *Trent* in the foreground. Nellie Amos shown in Figure 40, started the century

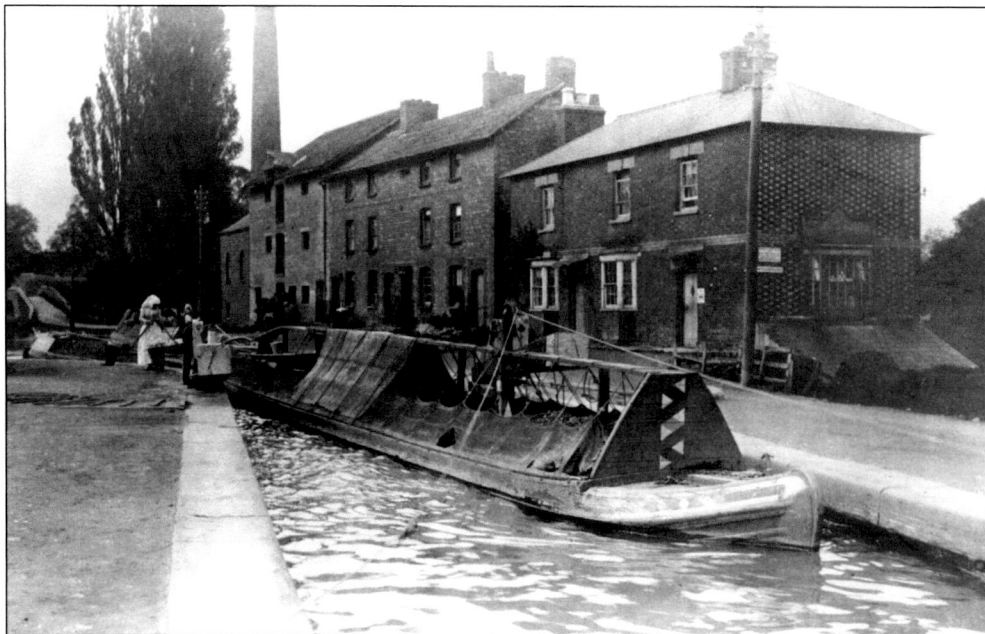

Figure 38   Stoke Bruerne top-lock (Christopher M Jones Collection)

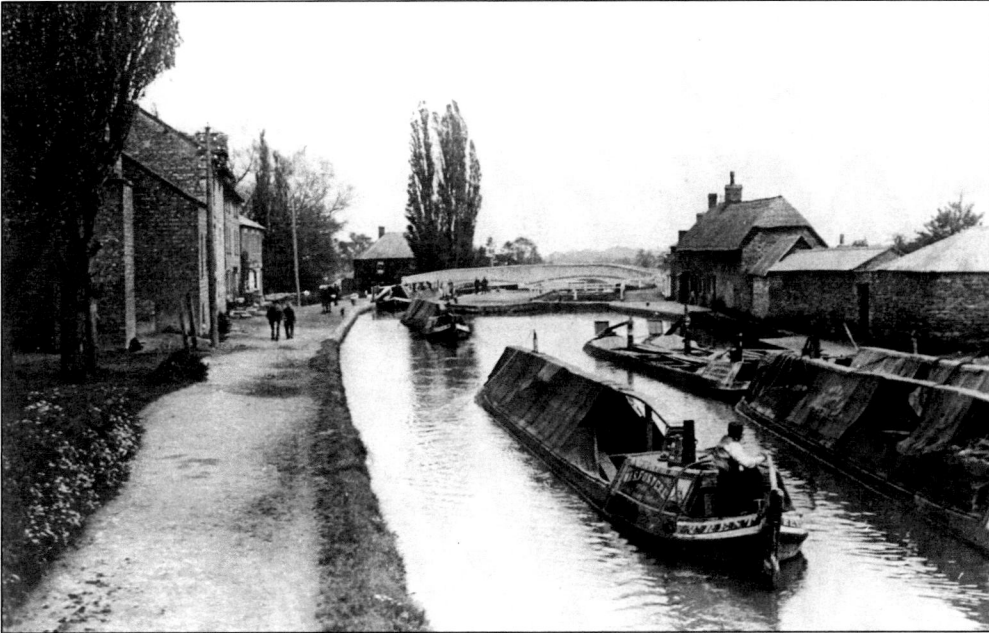

Figure 39   Stoke Bruerne top-lock showing Foster Ltd boat Trent (Waterway's Archive)

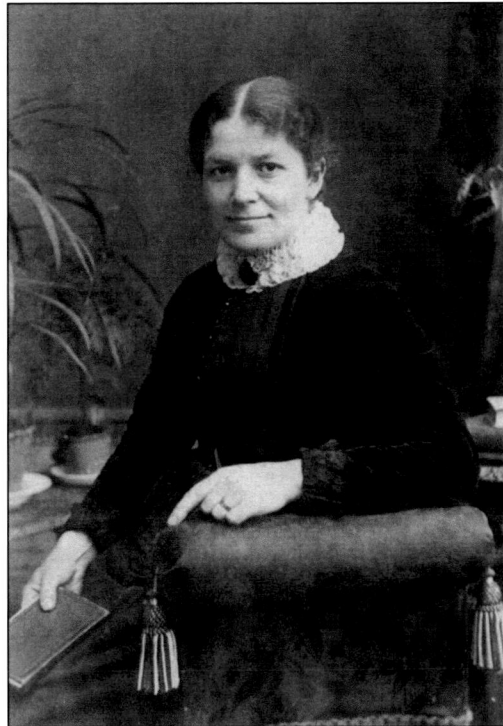

Figure 40   Sarah Ellen (Nellie) Amos
(Waterway's Archive)

with her brother-in-law Charles at a three day Good Templars Grand Lodge conference in Southampton as representatives of the Northampton Branch of the Temperance Society[200].

On census day three of the Amos daughters were with their parents, twins Mary and Ellen age 15, and Olive age 8. Mr Amos was renting the four *three storey cottages* adjacent to the disused steam mill to: Railway labourer William Welsh with his wife and two children, pensioners Joseph and Abigail Allen, farm labourer John Sturgess with his wife and son, and widower Sarah Jackson, with her daughter and grandchild. Tradesmen in the village included; a baker / confectioner, two lace makers, a carpenter, a blacksmith, four dressmakers, four grocers / shopkeepers (inclusive of the Amos shop), two butchers, an inn keeper, two shoemakers, three brick-makers (and labourers) and three masons. The village also had a number of Grand Junction Canal Company employees listed in Table 20, and Thomas Amos recorded nine boats moored in Stoke Bruerne on census night listed in Table 21, although he omitted to include the names of the boats. Nearly all the boats in the village on census night were from the West Midlands. Captain James Stokes has a total of eight on board and therefore is in contravention of the Canal Boat Registration Act, on the grounds of overcrowding, although it is possible the boats had a fore-cabin thus keeping them from prosecution for being in contravention. In the 1880's this family were working for William Foster of Tipton, but by 1900 had moved to Fellows, Morton and Clayton.

Table 20   Canal related occupations of men in Stoke Bruerne. Census 1901

Name	Occupation	Age
Thomas Woodward	Canal Boatman	39
Thomas W Taylor	Canal Boatman	18
Harry Bustin	Steam Tug Steerer	27
William Abbott	Canal Labourer GJC	41
Samuel Carter	Boatman on Canal	24
William Josiah Clark	Steam Tug Driver	41
Thomas Jones	Canal Labourer	34
Henry Allen	Lock keeper	48
George Green	Engine driver on canal	43
Frederick Warren	Canal engine tug driver	40
Richard Dyke	Lock keeper	48
James Gardner	Canal Labourer	51
George Inns	Lock keeper	35
Frances H Inns	Labourer on boat	17
George Inns	Labourer GJC	59

Table 21   Boats moored in Stoke Bruerne on census night 1901

Boat	Boat Occupants	Age	Relationship
1	George Shakels	50	Captain
	Elizabeth	40	Wife
	Rosa	20	Daughter
	Albert	12	Son
2	Frederick Kendle	26	Captain
	Annie	23	Wife
	Ellen	2	Daughter
	Edith	9 Months	Daughter
3	Edward Wenlock	46	Captain
	William Wenlock	17	Son
4	James Wilkinson	50	Captain Steam Boat
	William Tibre	45	Hand
	William Cappen	25	Engine Driver
5	James Stokes	43	Captain
	Olive	43	Wife
	Samuel	21	Son
	Salalan	16	
	James	14	
	Edward	12	
	Olive	8	
	Florey	6	
6	James Payton	44	Captain
	Katherine	48	Wife
	Eliza	14	
	John	12	
	Sarah Ann	9	
	Eadeth	5	
	Elizabeth	3	
7	John Hugh	52	Captain
	Thomas	16	
		35	Hand
8	John Coley	48	Captain
	Emma	39	Wife
	Annie	19	Daughter
	Hannah	8	Daughter
	John	6	Son
	William	3	Son
	Rebecca	2	Daughter
9	Andrew Humphries	46	Captain
	John	32	Son
	Thomas Jones	21	Servant

Thomas's brother Charles Amos lived in Roade High Street working as the village grocer and baker[201] with wife Emma, their four children were attending the Board School with Thomas and Nellie's youngest daughter Olive who re-located to Roade from a private school[202]. In 1901 Rev Masters left Roade Baptist Church in serious financial difficulty, the following year Rev. Young was appointed, Thomas Amos was Church Secretary and Treasurer[203]. Charles Amos gave up the family retail business in Roade and moved to *Grey House* Blisworth when he became an insurance agent[204], the family also transferred their Baptist membership to Blisworth Chapel. Just after Charles moved, South Northamptonshire Liberal's formed a *Blisworth and District Liberal and Radical Association*, their debut evening was held in Blisworth Lecture Hall. Mr and Mrs Amos attended the *excellent meat tea* and after dinner the Chairman gave a lively speech[205], during which *much applause and hear, hear were heard*, Mr T. Amos also gave *an earnest speech*[206]. Thomas Amos was also active in South Northamptonshire Liberal Association, being elected to serve on the executive committee in 1904[207].

Thomas and Nellie's twin daughter, 17 year old Mary Hollowell (Sister Mary's twin sister) passed away in the family home in 1902, the cause of death was recorded as cerebral thrombosis, pulmonary congestion and cardiac failure[208] the most probable cause of Mary's death being complications associated with either tuberculosis or diptheria. After Mary's death sisters Ellen and Winifred Amos were baptised at Roade[209]. Thomas Amos around this time was establishing himself as Chairman of Stoke Bruerne Parish Council[210] and Assistant Overseer of the Poor. As assistant overseer he regularly liaised with Thomas Milner the Grand Junction Canal Company engineer when he re-assessed the companies rented properties with a view to increasing the rent, an example from 1905 being when Mr Amos and Mr Milner discussed proposed rent increases for *Thomas Collins - increase to £8 from £4, and George Inns - increase to £4 from £2.12.6*[211].

In the early twentieth century Stoke Bruerne held a number of regular events in the village, including the harvest festival, various bazaars, numerous cricket matches and temperance meetings which were often held in the Wesleyan Chapel, schoolroom and the reading room. One annual event which was very popular was the *lighting fund concert* in the schoolroom, which Mr Bertie Wentworth Vernon, owner of *the big house Stoke Hall* decorated with plants and flowers[212]. The programme included performances from local musicians and those from further afield with the Amos family playing a significant part in the proceedings. Miss May Amos and Mr. Barltrop performed a novel duet *representing mechanical figures with boxes on which were printed 'Put a penny in the slot'* which caused great amusement to the audience. Mrs Nellie Amos shown in Figure 41 sang *A*

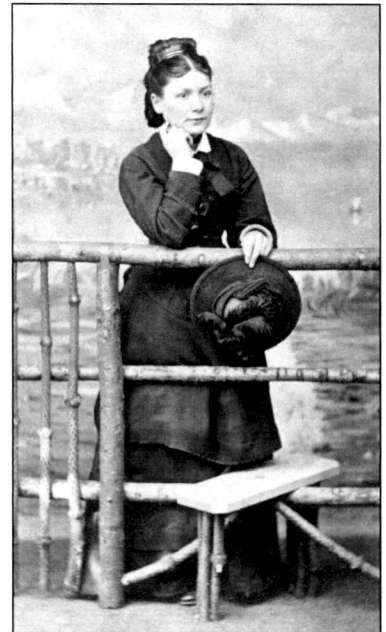

Figure 41   Nellie Amos
(Waterway's Archive)

dream of paradise with flute and violin accompaniment, and Thomas Amos gave a pianoforte solo. At the close of entertainment Mr Wentworth Vernon *heartily thanked performers for so kindly giving their services,* on returning home one of the concert goers accidentally fell in the canal, fortunately Mr Amos was able to *pull him to the side until assistance arrived*[213].

Whilst one man survived near drowning in 1904, the same year a well respected lock-keeper was not so fortunate. Fifty-three year old Richard Dyke, husband of Annie Elizabeth and father of four, died at home from fatal injuries as a result of doing his job as lock-keeper[214]. On the Friday carpenter Thomas Collins helped Mr Dyke *take the balancing pole off the lock, and put it out of the way.* the next day Dyke informed Collins *he went to move the pole and hurt himself.* Mrs Dyke called the Doctor who found *the muscles of the back enlarged and tender,* and on asking how the injury occurred Dyke told him *he was turning over some timber and the lever he was using stuck him on the shoulder* on further questioning he added *he used great force to raise the lever, and felt the muscle on the back of his shoulder go.* At the inquest Thomas Collins told the jury *the weight of the balance pole was eleven or twelve hundredweight* and the only reason he thought Dyke would have wanted to move it *was for the boat horses to get off the tow-path to the stables.* Doctor Richmond reported Dyke's condition *got gradually worse and developed diffused cellulitis,* the coroner was also informed Dyke *had a weak heart* and the *two combined probably caused death.* The jury were also informed *the muscle was partially torn off the ribs* … after which the verdict was returned, *death from natural causes, brought on by accident*[215].

The stretch of canal Richard Dyke worked is shown in two typical scenes between the locks in Stoke Bruerne. Figure 42 shows a boatman and his boy with their horse and pony towing their laden coal boat from lock 15 towards lock 16. Metal feed tins for boat horses like that shown here were common on the canals, the feed mixture was kept in bulk in a wooden box or barrel on top of the cargo. Once unloaded the pony was sometimes led aboard one of the boats into the hold down planks, then the horse was used to pull both boats back to the collieries with the pony

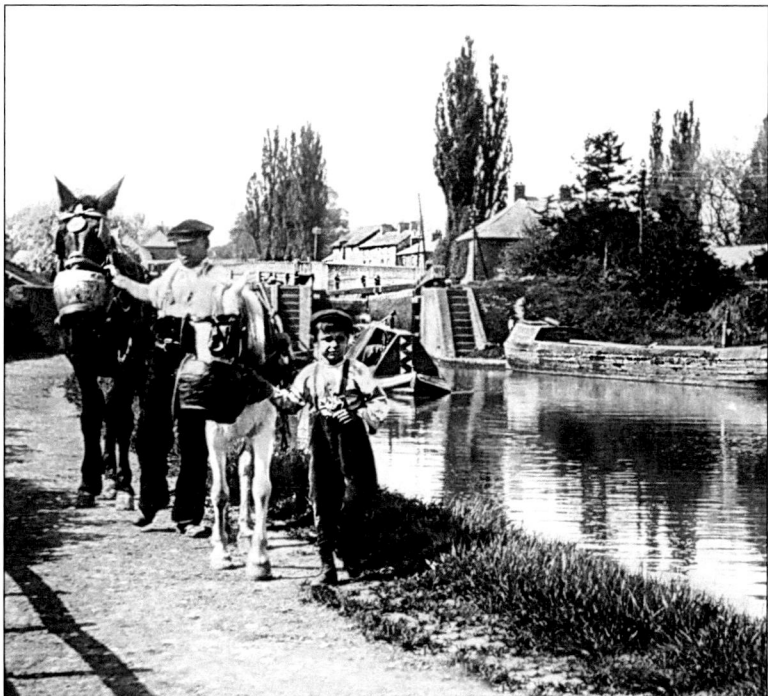

Figure 42   Father and son below lock 15 with horse and pony (Northampton Central Library)

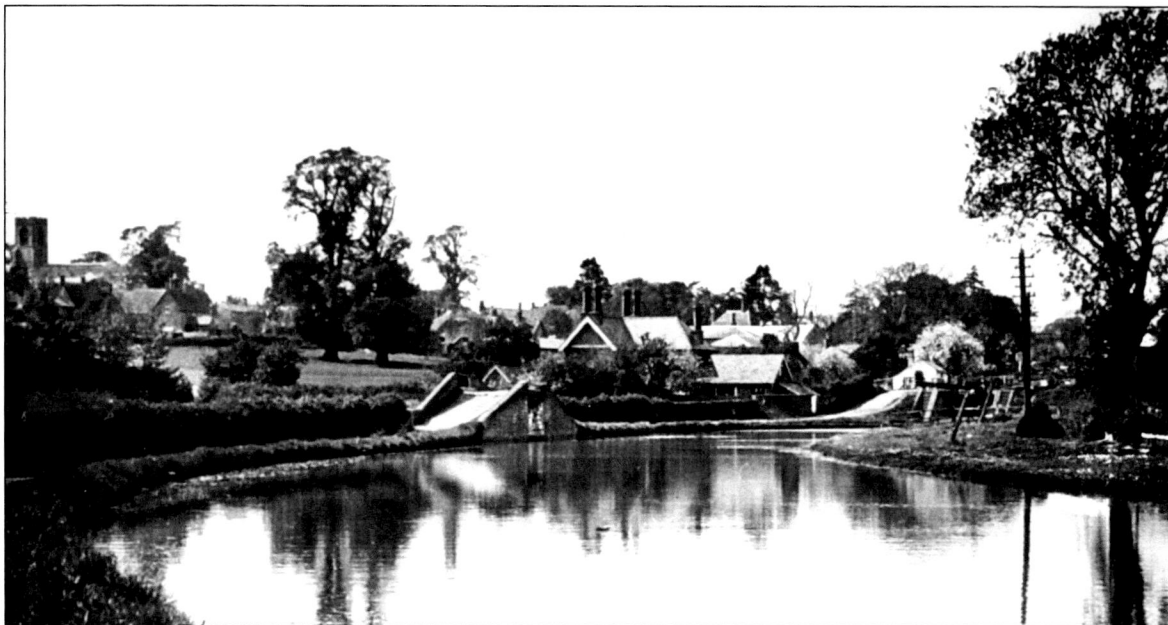

Figure 43   Towpath bridge leading to George Savage brickworks (Northampton Central Library)

as a passenger. This was done if the pony was unable to keep up with the stronger horse when running light. Figure 43 shows the tow path bridge built to enable boats to enter George Savage's brickyard basin, this is built from iron with abutments of brick. The works are out of view on the extreme left behind the hedge and trees. Lock 15 is on the right behind the telegraph pole. These two pictures were taken around the same time Mr Samuel George Savage Phipps commenced his position as Canal Boat Inspector. In 1904 Mr Phipps registered the 184th boat *Three Sisters*[216], owned by boatman and canal carrier Joseph Dunham of Tusses Bridge, who had a small fleet of craft. The boat was sold four years later to George Cutler of Bugbrooke Wharf, on which it retained the 184 registration, but was eventually re-registered at Towcester as number 245 in Cutler's name. In 1908 Mr Phipps submitted an application to the Sanitary Committee for a rise in salary, the request was granted without dispute (£10 rising to £12 guineas p.a), the following year Mr Phipps registered the 200th boat in the Towcester district.

The Amos children find their own paths …

A few miles from Stoke Bruerne in the village of Woodford Halse, post-master Mr Charles William Ward was living with his wife Emma. Charles was born to Eliza Perry in 1869 in Bath[217], after which Eliza married serving soldier Isaac Ward, Charles becoming Isaac's eldest son[218]. As Charles Ward grew up he wanted to join the army *to serve his country, but due to his small stature was denied service*[219], on his father's release from the army the Ward's moved to Leeds where Charles worked as a warehouse packer until his marriage to 27 year old Emma Parkinson[220]. After their marriage Chas and Emma Ward moved to Woodford Halse, by 1903 Chas was a tailor/outfitter and sub-postmaster in the village, and an active member of the Parish Council[221]. In his role as sub-postmaster Chas caught a 13 year old boy stealing a postal-order and three stamps, the lad pleaded guilty on his arrest. Due to the lads age he was tried under the First Offenders Act, and at the hearing Chas Ward was the main witness, the jury spared the lad imprisonment but was awarded a punishment of *nine strokes with the birch rod*[222].

When Emma was expecting the Ward's first child in 1906 they moved to School Street, Chas having secured the position of village post-master. During childbirth Emma died leaving no surviving child[223], her death cast gloom over the village of Woodford Halse …

> The deceased was well-known in the district … and was thoroughly respected, she having the good word of everyone with whom she came in contact. She was of a bright disposition, and will be greatly missed … The body of the deceased was interred at Leeds on Tuesday. The sad procession wended its way to the station at six o'clock in the morning. The coffin was carried shoulder high, the bearers being members of the Church of England Men's Society, of which Mr Ward is a prominent member. The body was followed by a goodly number of members of the society … the procession, although so early in the morning, gaining in numbers as it proceeded. At the station the coffin, which was completely covered with the most exquisite wreaths, was reverently placed in the van of the train which leaves at 6.40, en route for Leeds[224].

A few months after Emma's death, 36 year old Charles William Ward married 21 year old Ellen Hollowell Amos (Sister Mary) at Roade Baptist Church, their marriage was presided over by Ellen's uncle, Reverend James Hirst Hollowell[225], Ellen was the first of Thomas and Nellie's children to marry. Chas Ward at the time of marrying Ellen declared his occupation as *retired draper and widower*[226], after their marriage the Ward's lived at 5, Church Street, Woodford Halse[227].

In the first decade of the twentieth century some 7,466 pairs of boats and 1,570 single boats passed through Stoke Bruerne top-lock outside the front door of the Amos home, an average 170 boats each week[228], with such constant use of the canal it's no wonder restoration work was required from time to time in Stoke Bruerne, as shown in two images taken around the time of Ellen's marriage. Figure 44 shows underwater repairs being done to the base of the road bridge, including reinforcing the bank with hard-core tipped from wheel barrows. The amount of mud that needed dredging is quite substantial and would be done by hand with barrows. In 1908 lock repairs went on outside the Amos home as shown in Figure 45, workers are lifting into place a new lock gate using a crane mounted aboard this wide-beam work flat. Also visible is the tow path bridge over the entrance to the mill dock behind the tall poplar trees.

The following years saw Thomas and Nellie Amos's other children marry. After Ernest's run in with the police he moved to London and was working as a clerk where he met and married by special license Rosie Agnes Hadwell at Holy Trinity Church, Marylebone, by 1911 Ernest and Rosie were in Durham working as variety artists[229]. In 1908 Winifred Amos married Reverend

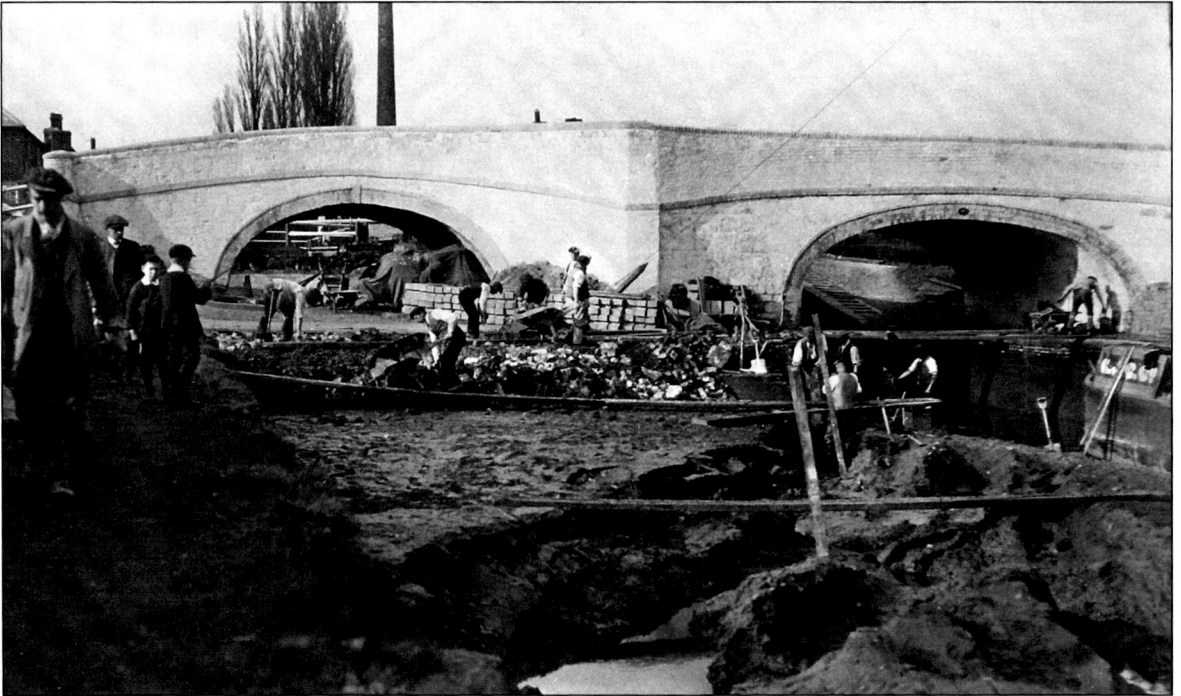

Figure 44   Canal bank repairs below lock 16 Stoke Bruerne (Northampton Central Library)

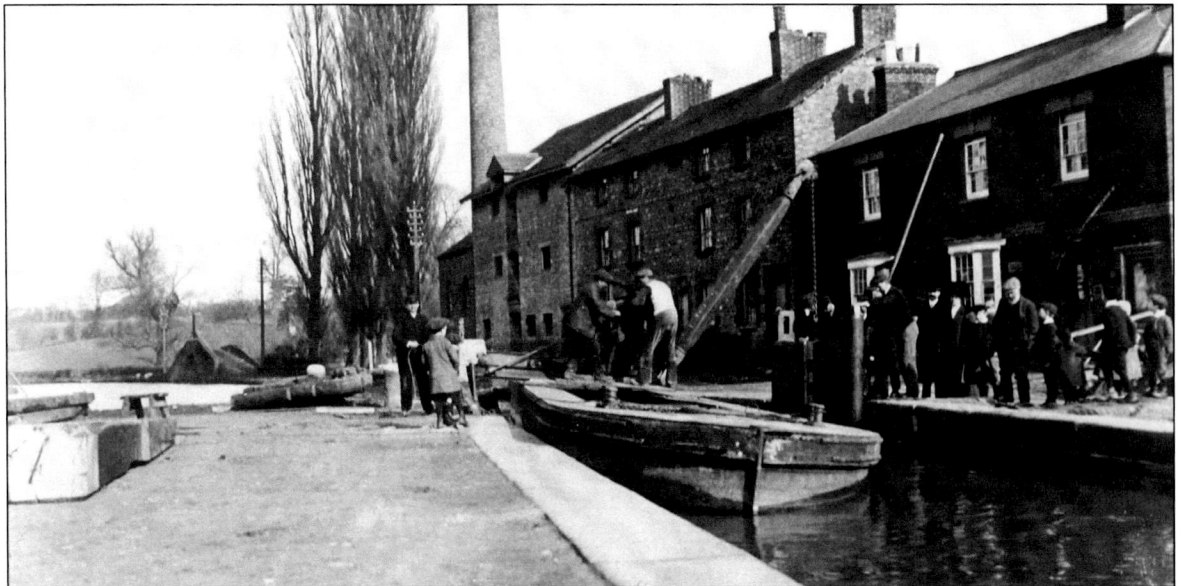

Figure 45   New lock gates at lock 16 Stoke Bruerne (Waterway's Archive)

Boyce, and no expense was spared for this special event, as indicated in the newspaper headline: *Roade. Interesting Wedding …*

> An interesting wedding took place at Roade Baptist Church … when Miss Winifred Annie Amos was married to the Rev. Arthur Ernest Boyce, Miss Amos is a daughter of Mr. and Mrs. T. Amos, of Stoke Bruerne, and previous to her marriage, she was a teacher at Vernon-terrace Council School … The Rev. A. E. Boyce is a son of Mr. and Mrs. G. Boyce. Of Cleveland-road, London … He is well-known in the southern portion of Northamptonshire, and for some time he was pastor of Silverstone Wesleyan Church. For the past few years he has been with the Rev. Gregory Mantle's Mission, a large, active organisation in Deptford, London.
>
> The Rev. James Hirst Hollowell, Rochdale, (uncle of the bride) officiated … Mr. T. Amos gave his daughter away. She made a charming figure in an Empire gown of hand-embroidered Swiss muslin, trimmed with real lace. She wore an embroidered veil, and was wreathed with orange blossom. Her shower bouquet was of white roses, stocks, and heather.
>
> There were four bridesmaids – Miss Ethel M. Amos (sister), Miss Norah S. Howe, Miss May V. Boyce (sister of the bridegroom), and Miss Olive E. Amos (sister). They wore embroidered Swiss muslin, trimmed with Valenciennes lace. Their hats were of bronze and green chip, trimmed with autumn foliage, and they had sashes to match. Their bouquets were of sweet peas and gypsophilia elegans, and they wore pearl gold-clasped necklaces, the gifts of the bridegroom …
>
> Following the ceremony a reception was held by the bride's parents in a large marquee at Stoke Bruerne. The marquee had been prettily decorated with festoons of evergreens and fancy muslins. Later in the day the happy young couple left for the Isle of Wight, where the honeymoon will be spent. The bride's going away outfit was of green Venetian cloth with hat to match. They will reside at New Cross, London, where Mr Boyce has charge of the Wesleyan Church …

The year after Winifred's marriage was busy for the Amos family, a year mixed with pleasure and sadness, commencing in the January with Nellie Amos instituting a Juvenile Temple as part of the International Order of Good Templars (IOGT)[230], followed in April by the birth of Chas and Ellen's first and only child at Brackley Maternity Home[231]. The Ward's named their baby girl Olive Mary Winifred, on registering his daughter's birth Chas was sub post-master in Moreton Pinkney. Chas Ward was also working alongside his father-in-law as a liberal sub-agent[232], positions Thomas and Chas continued well into 1910 when South Northamptonshire Liberals were working to increase the number of voters in the county as the election neared[233]. A regular speaker at liberal candidate meetings was Thomas Amos's son-in-law *the well known London Wesleyan, Rev. A. Boyce* who was once at Silverstone. In August 1909 the last of the Amos's children *flew the nest* when Ethel Margaret married drapers assistant Francis Cecil Grant at the Methodist chapel in Lewisham[234]. Olive, the youngest of the Amos children never married, for details of the marriages see Table 22.

Table 22   Marriages of the third generation Amos children

Name (AMOS)	Birth	Marriage Date	Spouse
Ellen Hollowell	1885	1906	Charles William Shepherd Perry WARD
Ernest	1882	1907	Rosie Agnes HADWELL
Winifred	1887	1908	Arthur Ernest BOYCE
Ethel Margaret	1880	1909	Francis Cecil GRANT

Whilst 1909 contained a number of joyous occasions for Thomas and Nellie these were overshadowed towards the end of the year when Nellie's distinguished brother Rev. James Hirst Hollowell died. Rev. Hollowell had for the last decade been busy campaigning on many issues in many arenas …

> … at by-elections in favour of non-sectarian education and temperance, he also took a pro-Boer position in 1900, believing the war to have been promoted by financial interest. In 1903 he took a leading part in organizing … *the passive resistance movement* … against the payment of rates and taxes, on the grounds that the Conservative government's Education Act of 1902 gave an inequitable support at state expense to church schools which taught church doctrine[235]

Rev. Hollowell *of Rochdale* published a seminal book in 1901 *What Nonconformists Stand For*[236] and in 1904 stood in a by-election for Birmingham South against the Liberal Unionist Viscount Morpeth. Although unsuccessful at the election, after the liberal landslide (1906) he became an unrelenting critic of the Liberal government's concessions to denominationalism in the education bills of 1906 and 1908. Hollowells exertion *broke down his health, and he died of cerebral apoplexy at his home* on December 24th, the funeral was held in his home town of Rochdale Mr. T Amos attended[237]. In a letter to the United Methodist Rev. Hollowell's friend and colleague wrote … *to those who knew him best he was a perfect knight in gentleness, chivalry and courage. He had a child's heart; love and loyalty were the notes of his life*[238]

Stoppages on the canal were a regular occurrence, forcing boaters to spend time in Stoke Bruerne. An example is shown in Figure 46, where a pair of Fellows, Morton and Clayton Ltd horse boats wait below Stoke Bruerne bottom lock during a stoppage at Easter 1907. The boats are *Linford* on the left, and the couple are standing in the hatches of *Portugal* which was built in 1906. *Linford* was much older being built in the spring of 1893. Stoppages were a necessary part of life on the canal when the canal companies undertook repairs to locks, bridges and other parts of the canal which required a period of temporary closure. This was usually done during bank holidays when collieries and most works were closed anyway. Several interesting features are shown in the image; the everyday working dress of the boaters, the caged bird on the cabin top, perhaps a canary or a wild songbird like a Linnet or Goldfinch. The woman to

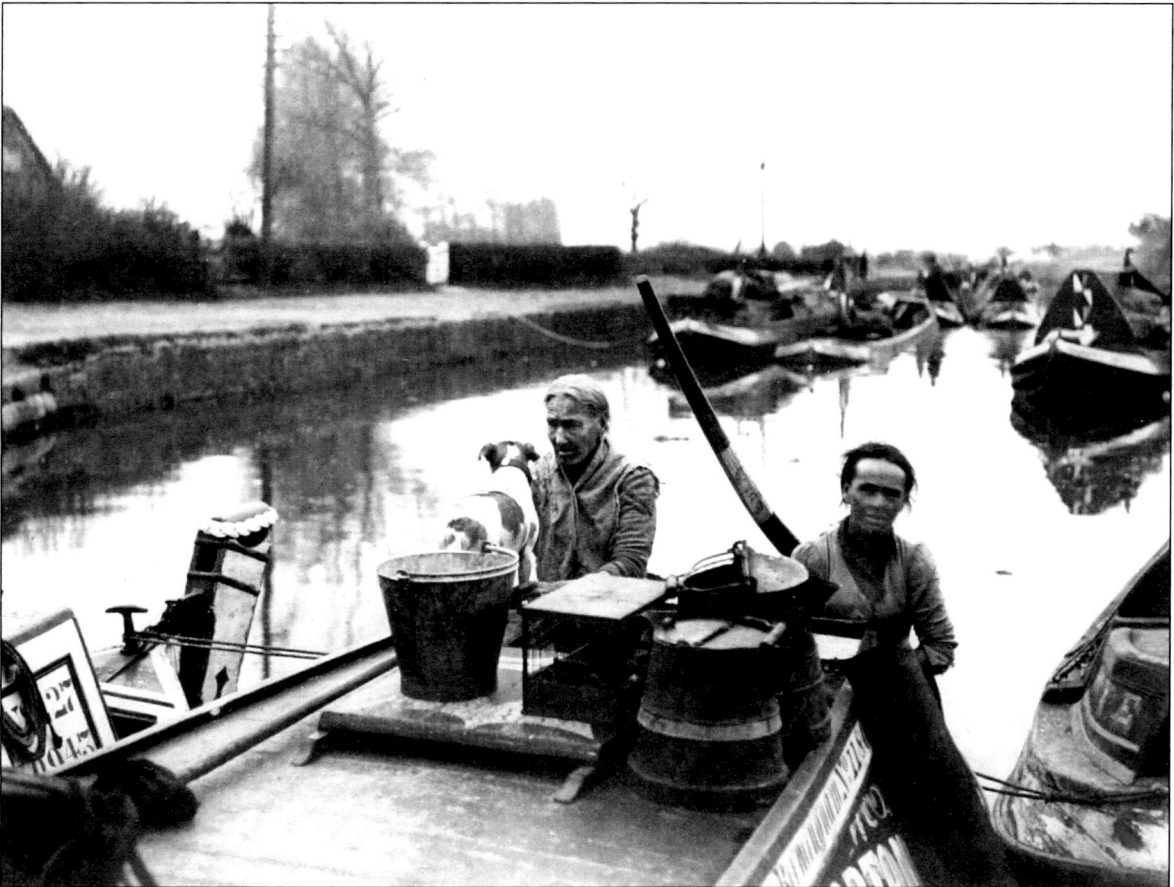

Figure 46   Caroline Yarnall and daughter Julia during a stoppage at Stoke Bruerne: (Northampton Central Library)

the left of the picture is Caroline Yarnall, one of the authors Great, Great Grandmother, next to Caroline is her daughter Julia Yarnall.   Caroline would have been 78 years old in the picture, she was a widower as her husband William died at Fazeley Street Birmingham (1891) on FMC boat *Handsworth*. Caroline took over as Captain with daughter Julia, she then had *Portugal* and *Linford* with her daughter Julia and her two grandsons Joseph and James Yarnall . Thomas Walton joined the crew as confirmed on the 1911 census, Thomas was Captain of *Portugal* and Julia Yarnall mate. Thomas Walton and Julia Yarnall married at St Gabriels Church Deritend Birmingham on July 13th 1911, Julia was 53 years old and Thomas 40. Julia's older sister Sarah married William Childs the grandson of John Childs lock keeper at Stoke Bruerne. Caroline passed away at the age of 81 in 1910, the death certificate is shown in Appendix 3.

Thomas Amos now in his mid 50's enumerated the census in 1911, at which time the Amos's had staying with them their married daughter Ethel Grant, and their two year old grand-daughter Margaret Boyce[239]. Charles, Ellen and daughter Olive (The Ward's) were sighted on the 1911 census at a boarding house in Ramsgate, at the same time Ellen's sister, brother in law and their first child were in a boarding house nearby. There are no sightings of the Ward's in the two years leading up to the war (1912 – 1914). On census day nine boats were moored in the village listed in Table 23.

Table 23   Boats moored in Stoke Bruerne on census night 1911

Boat	Occupants	Age	Occupation
The 'Kilburn'	J Brookes	?	Boatman FMC
	J Wilcock	?	Mate
The 'Earl'	Henry Smith		Master of Steam Boat
	Higgins		Engine Driver
	West		Engine Driver
	Welsh		Mate
Nantwitch (sic)	David Mills	36	Boatman
	Harriet	29	Wife
	Lizzie	12	Daughter
	Charlotte	9	Daughter
	Frank	6	Son
	Susannah	4	Daughter
	Samuel	2	Son
Polley and Heart of Oak	John Ward	39	Boatman
	Ann	49	Wife
	Agnes	14	Daughter
	Alfred	11	Son
	Ada	8	Daughter
	Mary	6	Daughter
Jersey	John Kingston		Master
	William Taylor		Mate
(not given)	George Dyes		Master Steam Boat
	William H		Engine Driver
	Guy Morris		Engine Driver
	William W		Mate
The Rose and The Mary	George Vaughan	29	Boatman
	Jemima Vaughan	29	Wife
	Nellie	9	Daughter
	George	8	Son
	Phoebe	6	Daughter
	James	2	Son
	David	4 mths	Son
'Baron'	Jo Sidwell		Master of Steam Boat
	Sam Danks		Engine Driver
	Jo Crockett		Engine Driver
	Jack Sidwell		Mate
(not given)	Edward Wenlock		Master Boatman
	James Harrison		Mate
	Jack Wenlock		Mate

Although the census return does not include much information on the boats moored, there at least two steam boats and the rest seem to be horse boats or boats being towed by the steamers. It is interesting to note there is a continuation of the families *working the boats*, as the next generation of boaters are now being noted. In St Mary's baptismal records for Christmas day 1878 Sarah Ann, daughter of James and Phoebe Vaughan was baptised. On the 1911 census is George Vaughan with his wife Jemima Vaughan (nee Stokes) with their children Nellie, George, Phoebe, James and David on *The Rose and The Mary,* son George (b.1903) carried on the family boating tradition as shown with his family in Figure 47.

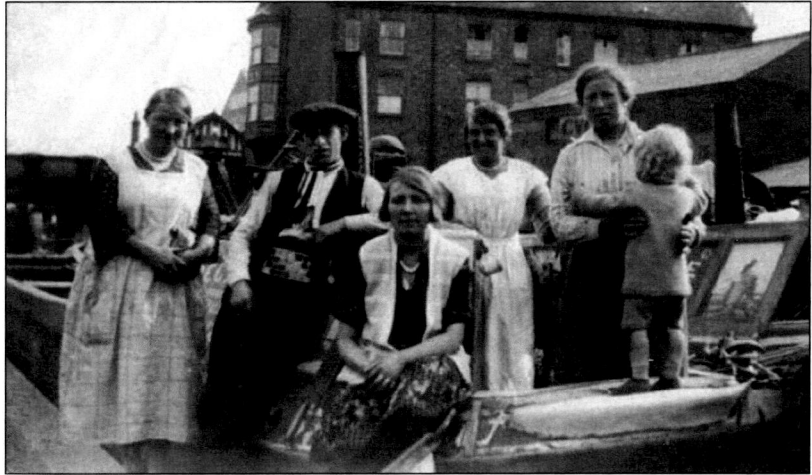

Figure 47

Young women *of the cut* wore typical dress for the era as shown by a member of the Frank's family in Figure 48, the boat girl is preparing to open the lock gate, her windlass tucked in her belt and wearing the distinctive boat woman's bonnet. In Figure 49 is Ann Stokes who was born in 1887 and shown here in a staged photograph holding a horse whip, wearing an elegantly frilled *leg-o-mutton* sleeve blouse, and a set of twisted pearls, Ann is also wearing a highly frilled white boat woman's bonnet and a spotless white apron. Ann married boatman Robert Harrison at Saint Matthew's church, Tipton in 1910[240].

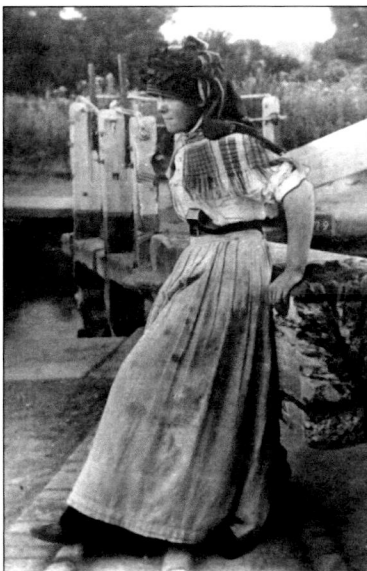

Figure 48 (left)   A boat girl from the Frank's family (George Freestone Collection)

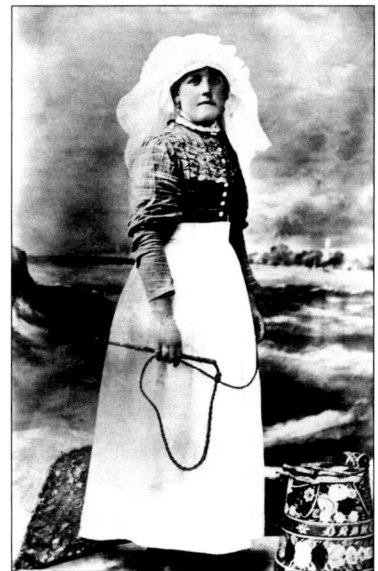

Figure 49 (right)   Boat girl Ann Stokes (Waterway's Archive)

Property ownership in Stoke Bruerne changed again in 1911 when George Savage's family drew to a close their deceased fathers Trust, when they placed three lots of freehold up for sale in the Northampton Mercury[241] (Figure 50). Thomas Amos purchased Lot 1: the steam mill and Lot 2: the dwelling house besides top lock, which the family had rented for many years. A view from Saint Mary's church (Figure 51) shows the mill chimney towering alongside the poplar trees, whilst Figure 52 shows two boats start to descend Stoke Buerne top lock, with a mule having a brief rest before continuation of their journey, immediately behind is Thomas Amos's shop, with items for sale hanging up around the entrance.

Mr and Mrs Amos continued to be involved with temperance organisations, particularly meetings of the Good Templars' Lodge in Roade where Mrs Amos regularly sang and gave recitations[242]. As Sunday School Superintendent at the Baptist Church Mr Amos organised the annual children's outing, and on a number of occasions these were canal boat trips. A particularly memorable trip took place in 1913 when the children were taken by boat through Blisworth Tunnel by one of the Grand Junction Canal Company tugs (Figure 53) to Bugbrook where they were given *a demonstration of the wireless telegraph by schoolmaster Mr Wright*[243]. The Amos's son-in-law Rev. Boyce, Wesleyan Minister for Shoreham was a regular speaker at the Baptist Chapel[244].

In Stoke Bruerne the health of canal boat inspector Mr Phipps was raised at Towcester Sanitary Committee in 1912, Thomas Amos offered to caretaker the

IMPORTANT SALE OF
FREEHOLD PROPERTIES
Comprising
A Well-built THREE-STOREY STEAM MILL,
With considerable Canal Frontage.
A Well-built DWELLING HOUSE and GARDEN
And EIGHT COTTAGES...

VALUABLE PROPERTIES:

Lot 1.- The Substantially Stone and Brick-built Three-Storey STEAM MILL, together with the Dock and Basin, situate at Stoke Bruerne, having considerable frontage to the Grand Junction Canal and containing Engine and Flour-rooms on the Ground Floor, Drying and Grinding-rooms and Lean-to on the First Floor, and Corn Store on the Top Floor, with Crane Lift from bottom; Stabling Cart, and Wagon Sheds, Yards, together with FOUR Brick-built AND Slated COTTAGES, each containing Four Rooms, Cellar, with entrance from the Mill Yard, in the occupation of Mr A Wilcox and others, at rents producing £21. The Mill is in hand.

The Machinery going with the Mill comprises a 15-h.p. Horizontal Engine, with Tubular Boiler and Shafting: Two Pairs of French Stones, Cleansing Machine, Dressing Machine, and Smutter.

The Mill, is situate in the heart of a good Agricultural Corn-growing District, is within easy reach of two Stations, and adjoins and has a large frontage to the Canal. The business to be done might be considerable, and the place could be well adapted for the manufacture of Standard Flour.

The Land Tax for 1910-11 amounted to £1 12s 3d.

Lot 2.- That Brick-built and Slated DWELLING HOUSE, situate and adjoining the above Property and containing Shop, Front-room, Living-room, Four Bedrooms, Kitchen, and Scullery, with Warehouse at the rear, and Garden: in the occupation of Mr. Amos, at an annual rental of £23

The property being well situate and close to the Mill would be a suitable house for the manger. Land Tax, £1 1s. 9d.

Lot 3.- Those FOUR Stone and Brick-built COTTAGES, situate in CHAPEL LANE, Stoke Bruerne, with Garden and Outbuildings, in the occupation of Messrs. Whitlock, Clarke, Welsh and Cox, at an annual rental of £15 12s. 0d.

Land Tax apportioned 15s. 6d.

Figure 50   Sale of property from the estate of the late George Savage (Northampton Mercury)

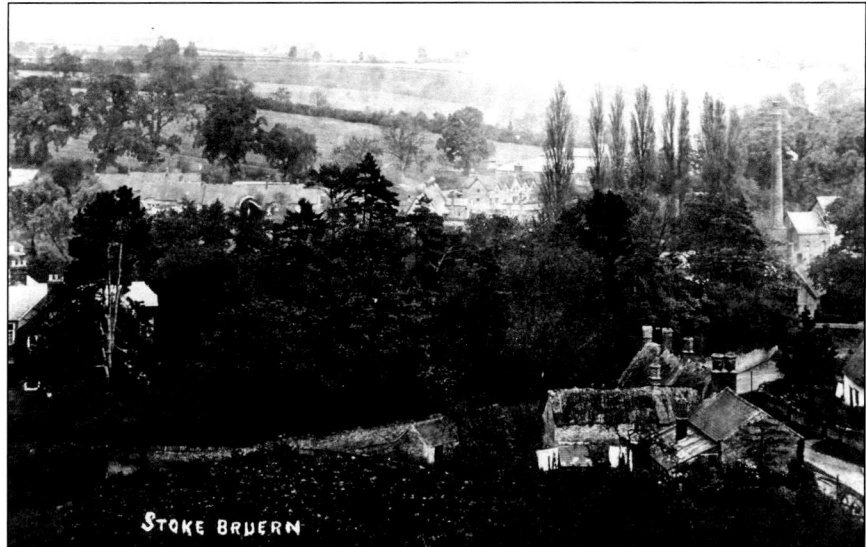

Figure 51

View of Stoke Bruerne from
Saint Mary's Church
(Waterway's Archive)

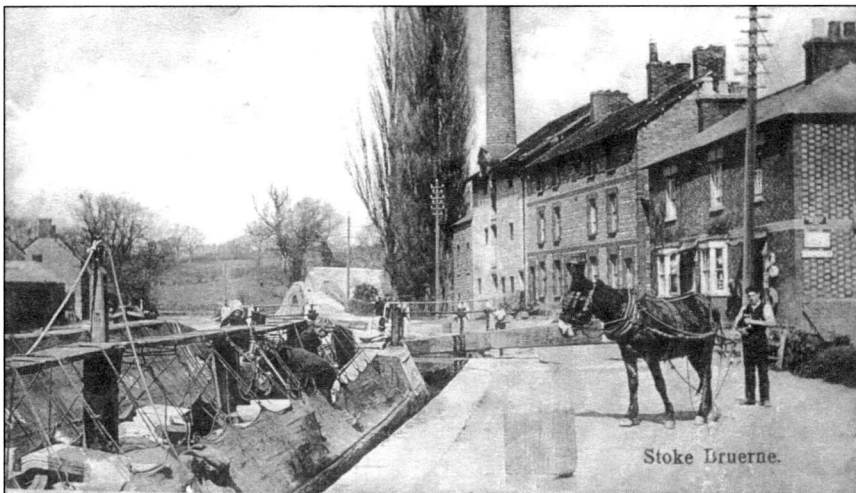

Figure 52

Lock 16 Stoke Bruerne
(Philip Garrett collection)

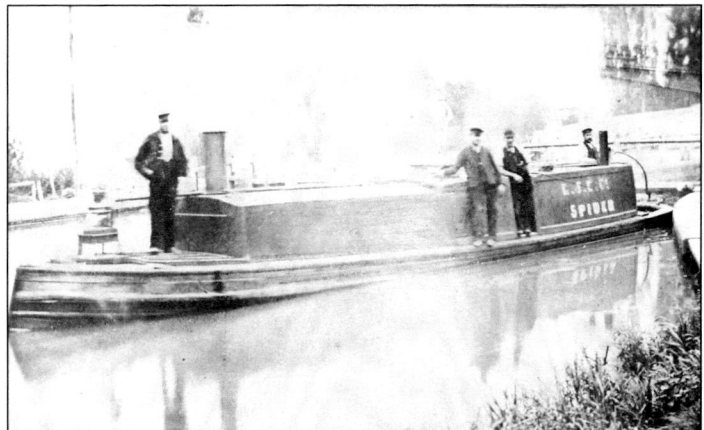

Figure 53

Tunnel tug at the north entrance to Blisworth
Tunnel (Waterway's Archive)

role, which the Sanitary committee approved[245]. Mr Phipps tended his resignation in March 1913 and passed away the following month. Mr Amos continued as caretaker until Mr Harris was appointed as Towcester Inspector of Nuisances[246], a new Local Authority position which incorporated Canal Boat Inspection. In Stoke Bruerne Annie Woodward gave up coal trading in the summer of 1913 after which she sold all but one boat[247].

Before the Great War the canal scene at Stoke Bruerne attracted a number of people who made pictorial records of the village and how the canal operated. Figure 54 shows a view of Stoke top-lock featuring an early wooden motor and butty pair exiting the lock with a tunnel lamp mounted on the motor's deckboard ready for passage through Blisworth tunnel. One point of interest is the low water level and may be the reason why the boats are waiting other than for the photographer. The boats appear to be owned by Fellows, Morton & Clayton Ltd., one of the first carriers to introduce oil-engined boats in 1912. The motor boat could be the *Lindola*, built at their Uxbridge dock, the first such craft built with a wooden hull; their other early motors being built of iron. The family nearest the camera look like Thomas Amos, his wife and possibly a member of the family standing outside of their house, shop and post office just out of view on the left.

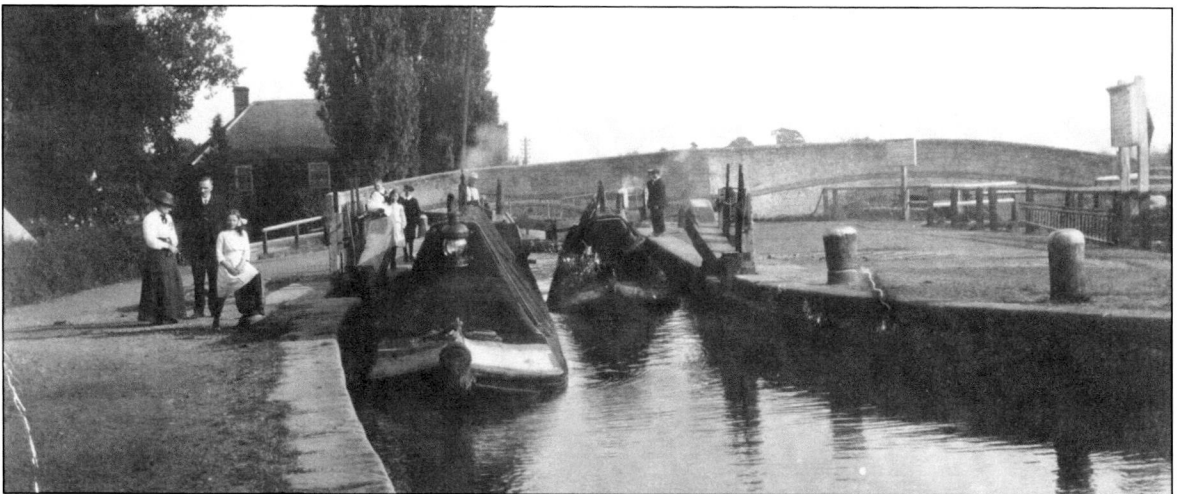

Figure 54   Early motor boat lock 16 (Phillip Garrett Collection)

Figure 55 shows two Fellows, Morton and Clayton horse drawn boats fitted with fore-cabins exiting Stoke top-lock, each one working independently by having one animal to each craft instead of one large horse pulling two boats. The former method of towing was better when these boats worked onto narrow canals north of Braunston or along the Northampton arm or Leicester canals. In Figure 56 the limitations of using horse drawn craft are exemplified in this dynamic view taken from the top of Blisworth tunnel entrance looking south east towards Stoke Bruerne about 1913. The loaded Fellows, Morton & Clayton steamer towing its butty head directly towards the tunnel entrance under their own power, whilst the horse drawn vessels in the foreground are forced to wait for the steam tug just visible in the middle distance under a cloud of steam and smoke. After all the horse boats it has just towed through the tunnel have been rejoined with their respective horses and disbursed towards Stoke, the tug has to then prepare for its next regular tow northbound through the tunnel. The boat nearest the camera is owned by Mrs. E. Riley of Foleshill near Coventry, and was usually hired out to boaters or carriers.

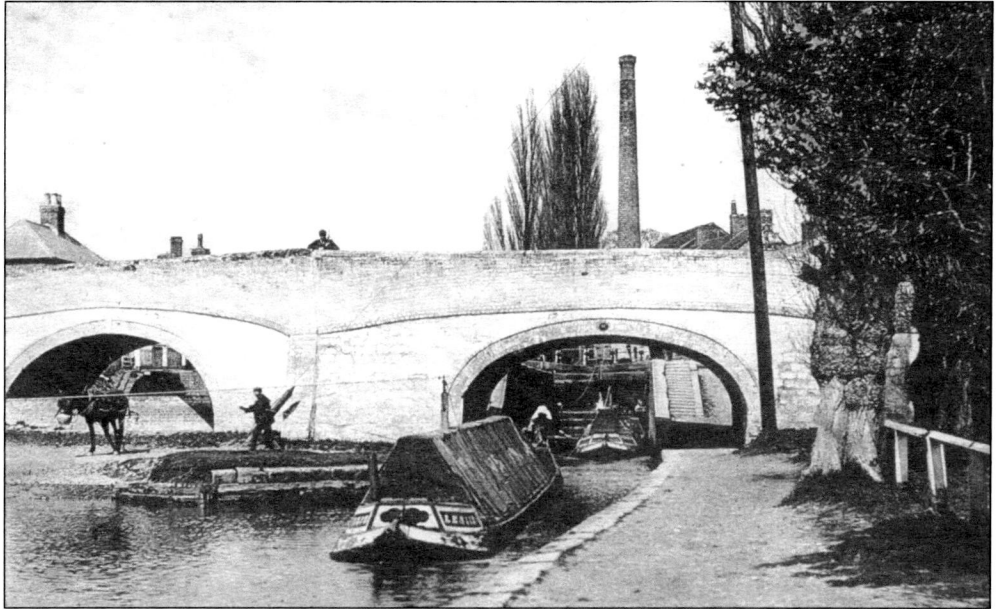

Figure 55   Two Fellows, Morton & Clayton boats exiting lock 16 (Philip Garrett Collection)

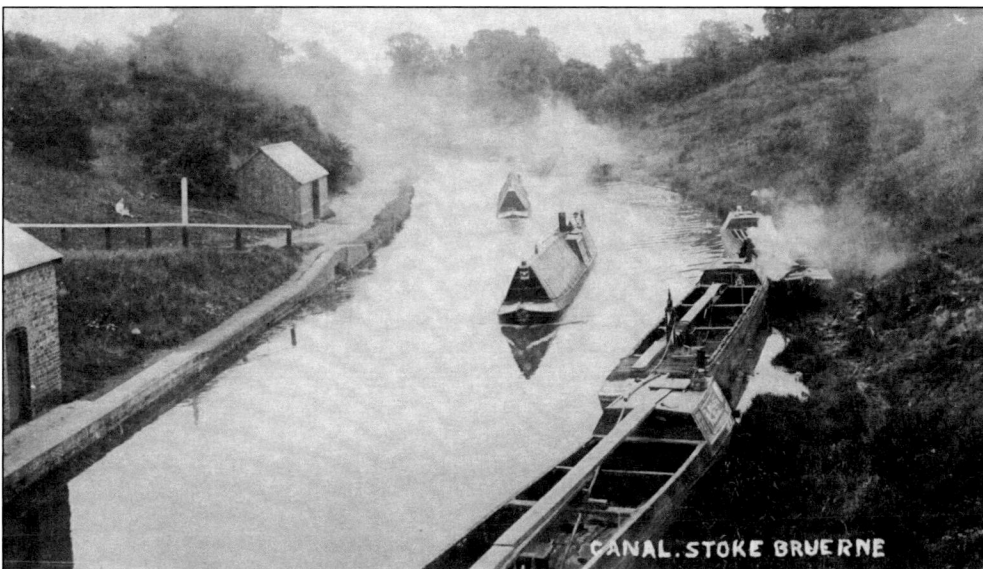

Figure 56   Horse boats awaiting tunnel tug at the southern portal of Blisworth Tunnel
(King Family Collection)

The landscape in Stoke Bruerne significantly changed before war broke out after Thomas Amos sold the disused steam mill to the Grand Junction Canal Company who demolished the mill chimney around September 1913. Figure 57 shows a close up of the preparation for the chimney being raised to the ground, with Figure 58 showing the same scene from a distance, note the chickens running round near their shed, the washing on the line at the rear of the mill and a number of outbuildings. The bridge running over the canal arm leading to the rear of the mill is seen in Figure 59 prior to it being demolished, the rubble after the chimney had been demolished is seen in Figure 60.

Just before the Great War commenced the Amos family suffered a further trauma when Nellie's 67 year older brother Richard Hollowell died, Richard was a partner in a boot and shoe manufacturing company and the first Chief Templar in Northamptonshire, this was an expected death as Richard had been seriously ill for around four years[248]. Nellie had already seen the recent deaths of her brothers Rev Hollowell and W C Hollowell.

Boater's in the first decade of the new century

At the turn of the century boaters plying long distances along the canals continued to work seven days a week, and remained at risk of health problems as a result of the changing weather and the dangers associated with boating. The Canal Boatmen's Mission was by the turn of the century well established in Brentford, having been in operation for six years in 1902[249]. The mission had a maternity room maintained by the Ladies Committee, in the year preceding the report *three little ones were born, a record for one year,* the records show a charge of 2s 6d was made for *letting a room for one week*[250].

During Owen Llewellyn's first full year of service as Chief Inspector of Canal Boats he travelled by canal between Birmingham and London *for the purpose of better understanding … the manners and circumstances of the boat people,* he also commenced an investigation into canal boat inspection books, drawing to the attention of Local Government Boards where inspection books exhibited *a record of absolutely perfect boats, with no infringements,* in his report he somewhat sarcastically commented *would that it were so*[251]. Mr Llewellyn's other concern was the *registration of fore-cabin's as dwelling*'s, which he reported to the Ministry … *as a rule, when fore-cabins (in narrowboats) are registered for occupation, children are to be found in them.* To emphasise his point Llewellyn on one occasion tried to accommodate [himself] in a fore-cabin *having 80 cubic feet of air space, for the purpose of demonstrating the possibility or otherwise of doing so, and have always succeeded only in vastly amusing the boat people,* a concern that was more than mere amusement as he went on to explain …

> Apart from their size these fore-cabins have another great defect. Many of the locks (and only those who know the canals well can form an idea of how many there are, and how frequently they occur) are of considerable depth, and when a laden boat is locked-up, her

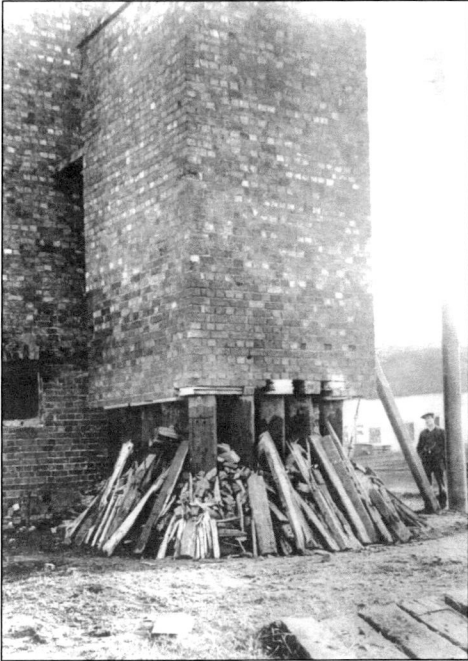

Figure 57   Mill chimney being prepared
for demolition (Northampton
Central Library)

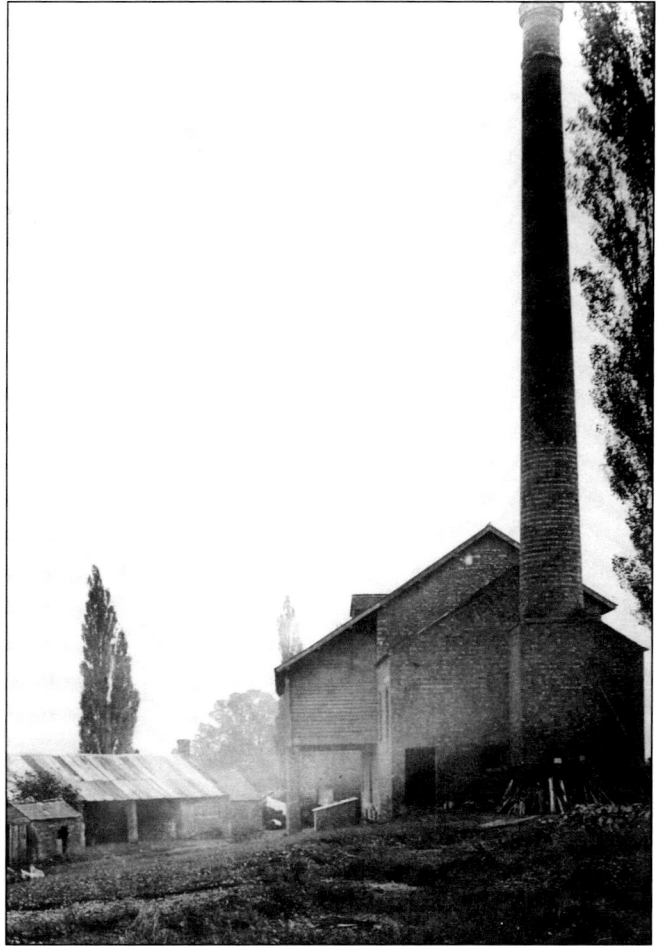

Figure 58   Mill chimney with outbuildings prior to demolition
(Northampton Central Library)

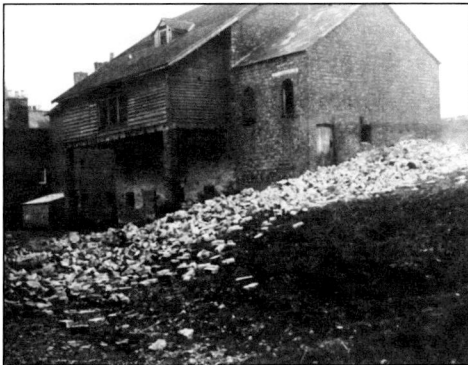

Figure 60   Rubble after mill chimney
demolished (Waterway's Archive)

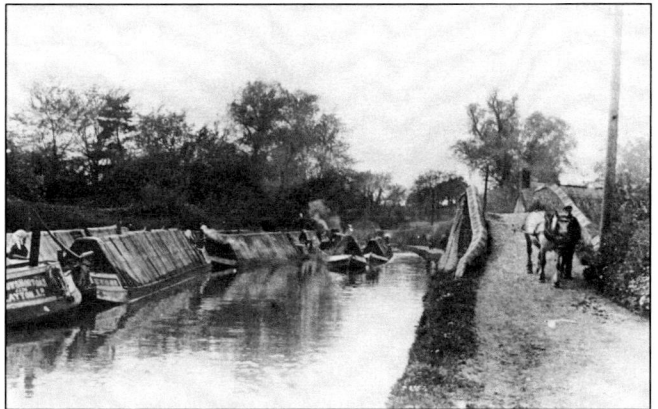

Figure 59   Ebbern bridge showing entrance to Mill Arm
(Waterway's Archive)

117

nose is amongst a rushing, squirting mass of water, boiling and heaving indiscriminately all over the forepart of the vessel, which invariably keeps the deck awash until the lock is filled, with the effect of making the woodwork perpetually damp, and unless the boat is in very excellent repair, letting a certain amount of water into the cabin, which may be occupied, and certainly cannot of the time, for mere reasons of safety, have any possible means of ventilation[252].

In response to *superficial canal boat inspection* Llewellyn send *copies of annual reports to canal boat inspectors across the country, in the hope of raising their standards of work through example*[253]. The following year he *rolled this out across the canal system*, inspection changed as a result of the appointment of *educated Inspector of Nuisances replacing traditionally appointed inspectors* which Llewellyn approved of[254]. Llewelyn also commented on his early observations regarding boaters health …

> … I think we may claim that there is apparently no more healthy occupation than boating, though I have no doubt that, if cases of infectious disease in the families of boatmen who have homes of their own as well are included, such families would be found to suffer as much as those of people ordinarily living on land. Occasionally I am informed of the presence on a boat of an adult, either blind, epileptic, imbecile, or in some manner afflicted, who is the cause of an infringement, but is retained owing to the inability of the parents to allow him on board out of their sight. Some inspectors have passed such … through, kindness, knowing there is no other refuge but the workhouse or pauper asylum. Yet, although he is able to assist to some degree … he would, in my opinion, be better off if cared for by the State, and I have not hesitated to advise inspectors to this effect.

In 1904 Llewellyn reported Education Authorities *were anxious to take much stronger measures in respect of children not attending school*[255], although he went on to discuss his own observations regarding peoples views on schooling for boat children … *there seems to be an enormous amount of ignorance, exaggeration, and misplaced sympathy now prevalent [regarding this subject]*. Two years later Llewellyn was championing the skills and abilities of boat children …

> In my view I do not exaggerate at all when I say that morally and physically the boat child is, for the most part, superior to the land child. Its open air life inures it to all weather, and its familiarity with its work from a very early age makes it reliant and strong and brings out its best qualities. The sense of responsibility from early youth which makes the British naval officer the type of a perfect public servant has a similar effect on the boat children in the performance of their work. On the boats boys and girls (whose contemporaries ashore are in their hobble-dehoyhood a source of worry and anxiety to their parents) can be found doing their duty in a quite matter-of-fact way, and taking a pride in its successful accomplishment. Undoubtedly, those ashore are more fully equipped in the matter of learning, but in application of it I do not think most of them have any advantage over the boat children[256].

The accuracy of Boat Registration statistics became an ongoing concern for Llewellyn due to his repeated observation of the *reducing number of registrations [of canal boats used as dwellings]*, which he suggested was because *a large number active on the registration list are broken up, derelict, sunk, or so entirely altered in appearance.* Llewellyn put this situation at the doors of canal boat owners, as they were under no obligation to report their disuse, with *boats seldom or never finishing their career where it had begun* …

> Canal boats are often taken for bad debts or rent; they may end by being stranded in some disused and waterless canal; old ones make admirable bonfires; some are converted into huts or fowl-houses; others are often filled with earth and used for the purpose of strengthening the banks of navigable rivers; in short, their last use is often, I fear, of more value than their first. But however obscure their fate, their names remain on the register of boats used as dwellings. For these and other reasons I retain my opinion that the number of boats now used as dwellings is not much more than half the number still on registers[257].

In 1910 over thirty unions engaged in waterside transport created the National Transport Workers Federation (NTWF), Harry Gosling was appointed President. There then followed a succession of strikes (1911-1912) which on occasions held up road, rail, canal and river carrying[258]. During the strike period the Chancellor of the Exchequer Mr Lloyd George, introduced the governments scheme for compulsory insurance against unemployment (May 1911). On launching the scheme Lloyd George outlined the extent to which the working classes already insured themselves against death, sickness and unemployment …

1. There are 42,000,000 industrial policies against death, on weekly or monthly payments. So that part of the ground is fairly well covered, and the Government scheme does not touch this class of insurance.

2. Against sickness there are more than 6,000,000 policies taken out with the friendly societies, securing sick benefits and medical aid.

3. Against unemployment only 1,400,000 workmen are insured, and only a third or a fourth of these are in the precarious trades, where the evil is most rife[259].

The new government scheme included all wage earning men, women and young persons under the income-tax paying class, that is to say, all earning less than £3 a week, with a few exceptions[260].

The War years …

Life on the cut in the south Midlands leading up to World War I apart from the strike action continued much as it had in the previous decades, although things were starting to change just enough to worry some canal company staff[261], as some trade had only been kept alive through toll reductions to stave off railway competition. The bigger issue was the slow trickle of boaters leaving the canal for better paid jobs ashore, and a lack of young boatmen coming on to the cut to replace them. Owen llewellyn went into Military Service, therefore there were no annual Canal Boat reports throughout the war years.

On August 4th 1914 Britain declared war on Germany. During the Great War boats continued to pass through Stoke Bruerne as shown in Figure 61, where two Fellows, Morton and Clayton steamer and butty pairs pass each other in the pound below Stoke top lock. The nearest craft has its towline stretching back from the steamer through a pulley block on its mast, then through three running blocks, one of which is visible tied down onto the top plank, then made fast onto an iron T shaped stud

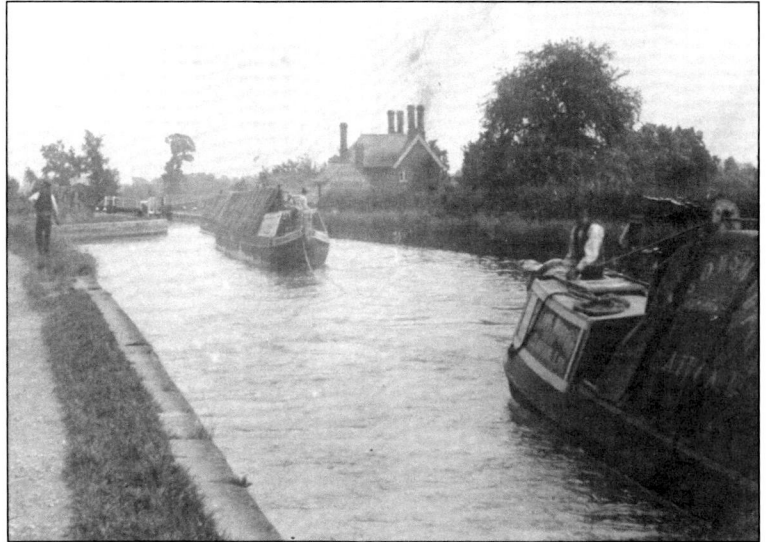

Figure 61   Short pound between locks 15 and 16 Stoke Bruerne
(Philip Garrett Collection)

bolted into the cabin roof. The use of this method of towing was said to be faster than merely tying the towline onto the fore-end of the butty, although it was dangerous if used where small children are in the cabin or on the roof. The thick coiled line or strap on the roof was used to gently stop the boat when entering a lock by coiling it quickly around a thick wooden stump set into the ground each side of the lock, to avoid the bow striking the cill or gates. The butty in the background has its strap trailing in the water to keep it wet as it got very hot with friction when used. Note the small shop advertising Grocery and Provisions next to the lock keeper's house and run by the Cakebread's, Mrs Cakebread having taken over as village post-mistress[262]. Figure 62 is an interesting action shot at Stoke Bruerne top-lock around the time of the Great

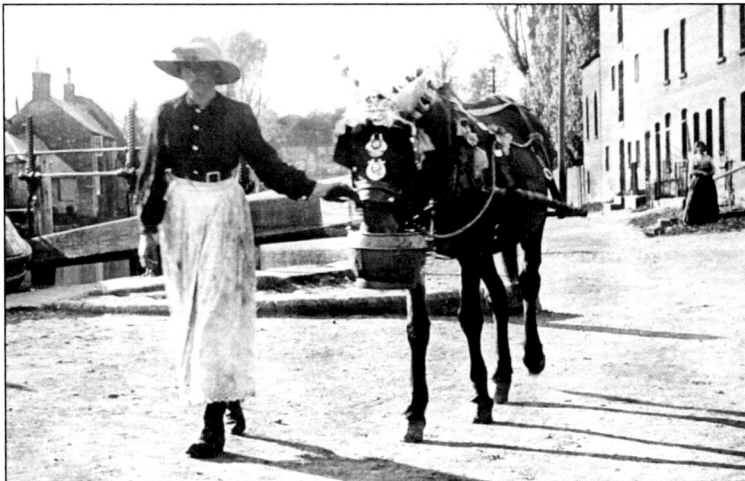

Figure 62   Boat girl leading mule in full regalia beside lock 16
(Northampton Central Library)

War, showing a woman horse driver and her well decorated mule wearing ear covers. One of the first problems to affect the canal was boatmen leaving to serve in the armed forces or for better paid jobs in factories, by January 1915 it was said boaters were becoming scarce[263]. Canal company employees were also being called-up, so much so that toll stops were closed and their work transferred to other offices.

8 Prospect Terrace
Earls Barton
June 19/1915

Dear Sir

Can you let to me, the cottage on the canal bank at Stoke Bruerne, next to the house occupied by my father-in-law Mr Thos Amos.

The circumstances under which I require a cottage just there, if possible, are rather sad ones, my wife has suffered a lot during the last three years and some three months ago this brought on slight mental derangement, she has been discharged from the institution cured, a month ago and living with her parents Mr & Mrs Amos, on the lock side.

Her visit must draw to a close and on the Drs advice I ought not to have her home to take the responsibility and worry of an establishment.

If we could have the cottage before mentioned it would solve the difficulty, as her parents would be in and out all day and every day and my wife could interest herself and manage the little place. I saw your Mr Wills this a.m. he referred me to you.

Of course sir, it is a matter of some plastering to the top room ceiling, some paper, paint, whitewash and some repairs to grate and floor tiles not a very large matter, as if the refuse in the wash house was just cleared away I should not mind anything else there.

Again, of course sir, I could not expect your company to do these things without some return and respectfully beg to offer 3/- per week instead of the 2/- they (the cottages) have been charged before.

It is a bit 'infra dig' to mention sentiment in connection with business, but the fourth generation of the Amos family is growing up beside your canal and, in addition, the circumstances in this particular case, being pathetic I trust you will let sentiment have a small place in making your decision in anticipation of your reply

I am
Sir
Yours truly
Chas W Ward

N.B. I have had to be somewhat verbose so as to thoroughly explain my need. I have one child a little girl 6 years.

Figure 63   Charles Ward letter to Mr Milner
(George Freestone Collection)

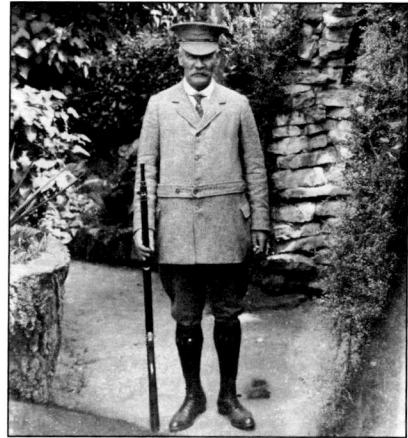

Figure 64   Mr Milner in his World War I Home Guard uniform (Waterway's Archive)

Whilst war was underway Olive Ward was living with her grandparents canalside (age 7-9) and attending with her grandfather the Sunday School at Roade Baptist Church[264]. During part of the war years Ellen Ward (Sister Mary) was also living with her parents *having been unwell the last few years.* As Ellen's stay was drawing to a close her husband Chas Ward wrote to the Grand Junction Canal Company engineer Mr Milner[265] as shown in the transcribed letter in Figure 63, requesting the renting of a company cottage next to his in-laws family home, note in the letter Chas Ward gives his address as Earls Barton. At the time of writing the letter Mr Milner was a member of Blisworth Home Guard shown in his full uniform in Figure 64. The three years Chas Ward refers to in the letter *when his wife had suffered* could be when Sister Mary underwent surgery to correct a limb deformity as reported in the *This is your Life* programme …

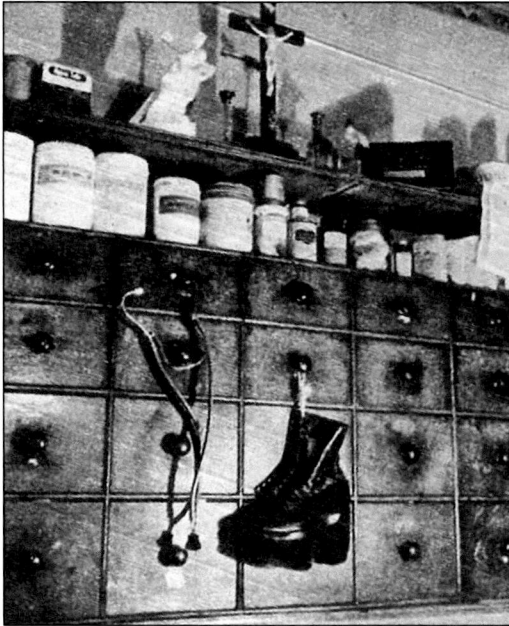

Figure 65   Surgical Boot
(Della Sadler-Moore Collection)

Tuberculosis nearly denied you that future ... after three years in plaster, and fourteen operations, it leaves you a cripple to limp in a surgical-boot. Yet there it is, hanging today in triumph in your surgery (Figure 65) – a reminder of years of patient borne suffering, and the skill of the great surgeon... who worked your cure [266].

By November 1915 war had caused many canal carriers to feel the effects of staff shortages and in the case of Thomas Clayton (Oldbury) Limited, they were given permission to display posters in toll offices advertising job vacancies for boatmen. Crewing canal boats became a 'reserved' or 'starred' occupation, and part of a national register of protected trade due to the transportation of fuel and materials being a vital part of the war effort. This did not necessarily mean all boatmen were 'starred', as the criterion for 'reserved' or 'starred' status was mainly for the transport of munitions or carrying fuel to works where munitions were manufactured, power stations and gas works[267]. The situation for boaters changed after the introduction of the Military Service Act (1916), which replaced 'reserved occupations', boaters after the act were not automatically considered protected from being called-up but had to apply for an individual exemption certificate. In the summer of 1916 some boatmen engaged in war work started to receive a War Bonus payment[268].

The difficult situation of crewing boats during the war was brought to the attention of the press when Boatman George Lemm was summoned to Tipton magistrates on account of him *not sending his 11 year old son to school regularly*[269]. Captain Lemm was working for Messrs. W & S Foster, Carriers and his son was assisting him to convey sand to munition works. The case was reported to the education committee who at the hearing stated *boy should not on any account be released from school for the purpose of industrial employment*. Mr W A Foster, the firms representative gave witness and reported *14 boats and 14 horses were idle due to a shortage of labour* at a time when *the munition works manager is clambouring for sand*, he also pointing out *it was a matter of urgent national importance that it should be delivered*. Captain Llewellyn although on military service himself returned and confirmed ... *the railways were congested, and a large number of canal boats were laid up because of inability to get men to work them. He did not think the boy could be engaged in a more useful occupation*. In his own defence young Lemm pointed out to the judge he was nearly 12 years of age. The bench imposed a fine of 10s., and concluded by expressing their opinion that *the Board of Education should so relax their regulations as to enable boys to be employed in such occupations of national importance as that in which this lad had been engaged*[270].

In 1916 the sons of Stoke Bruerne villagers who were *called up* began to return. The first Stoke man officially reported killed in action was Private John Charles Sturgess of the Royal West Kents, he was killed in action on October 29th, two others were missing and feared dead. Before joining the army in June, John worked for the Grand Junction Canal Company, he left a wife and two children[271]. The Son of Mr Batchelor of Stoke Bruerne, Private W G Batchelor of the Queen's Royal West Surrey regiment, shown in uniform in Figure 66 was wounded in France and returned to England in the November[272]. Throughout the war years injured soldiers were brought back from the front line to Northampton Infirmary and as part of their recovery were regularly entertained at Stoke Park at the invitation of Brigadier-General and Mrs H Vernon. The events consisting of musical entertainments and various games with prizes followed by refreshments before returning the soldiers to the infirmary by char-a-bancs and motor vehicles[273].

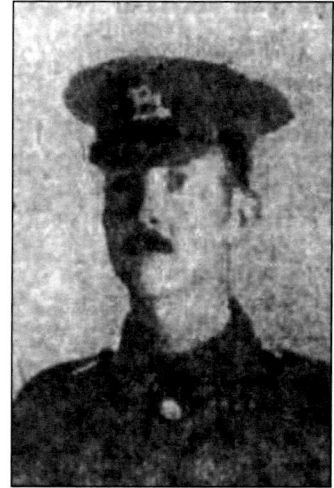

Figure 66   Private Batchelor (Northampton Mercury)

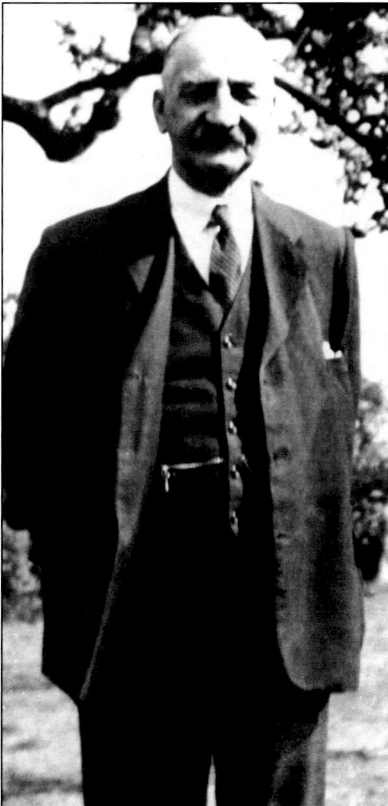

Figure 67   Thomas Amos (Waterway's Archive)

In the final year of the war Northamptonshire announced it's new county magistrates *men who have served on local authorities and are no strangers to public work*, for South Northamptonshire Thomas Amos was appointed Justice of the Peace (J.P.) shown in Figure 67. The following year at Blisworth by-election Mr Amos was returned unopposed as a member of the County Council for the Blisworth Division, in succession of the late Mr Westley, J.P., [274].

War ends, boaters unrest …

When the Great War ended (November 11th 1918), the Grand Junction Canal Company had done their bit *for the war effort* as the Roll of Honour showed many men from the company did not return[275]. It was a depressing time for the canal trade, as all except the Erewash and Warwick canals had suffered loss of traffic since 1913, government therefore continued their control of canals, preventing canal companies from raising tolls to increase income. This combined with other factors increased carrying costs, such as; the imposition of an eight hour working day for toll clerks (extra staff having to be employed to man toll offices) and wage rises due to the cost of living (including boatmen's pay). All of which led to a growth in trade union membership by working men with a more militant attitude, which brought with it a threat of strike action[276].

Post-war there was a growing concern among union leaders regarding transport workers, particularly canal boatmen. The National Transport Workers Federation (NTWF) regarded boaters as *a minority requiring special help*[277]. As a result of the union's interest in canal boat workers, on Wednesday November 12th 1919 a deputation led by Harry Gosling was received by the President of the Board of Education and representatives from both the Ministry of Transport and Ministry of Health. At the meeting Ernest Bevan gave a speech on *Canal Workers,* which he opened by asserting the need for an inquiry …

> the canal system I think it is the most medieval industry that is left in the country at the moment. I think that will be generally agreed, both from the point of view of the condition of the Canals and more particularly from the mode of life that the people have to live[278].

Bevan's speech covered a number of topics pertinent to the lives of working canal boaters, including; boat children's education, deaths associated with boat children, unhealthy cabins, poor food and clothing, no wages for the wife and children's work and legging. A transcript of the speech is provided in Appendix 5. Bevan concluded by reiterating the unions proposal for an inquiry into *the work of canal boaters,* and that this be in two parts …

> We think that there ought to be a real inquiry, in the light of what had been done in the realms of education for the children of the country, and what is being done by the Ministry of Health, or proposed to be done, from the point of view of living-conditions of the other people in the country. In other words, there should be a very distinctive inquiry into the whole position from the **social point of view**, regardless, so far as that inquiry is concerned, of whether or not it is economically sound. We feel that the **human conditions** ought to be inquired into, as has been done in the case of sweated trades, unhealthy trades, and all other trades, regardless of what the conditions of the industry might be from an economic point of view.

Having listened to Bevan the President of the Board of Trade replied *I am aware of the situation, and that government will take the matter into consideration, by taking the matter up with the newly formed Ministry of Transport*, he also acknowledged *the issue raised regarding education was important.*

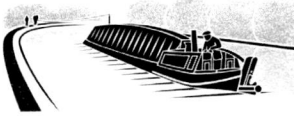

The inter-war years - father calls

Just after the Great War His Grace the Duke of Grafton placed his Wakefield Estate up for sale, twenty nine *Lots* being in the Parish of Stoke Bruerne (Lots 176 – 205). Because many Lots were currently occupied by sitting tenants the opportunity arose for the tenants to purchase these by private treaty prior to the auction. Twenty two of the twenty nine lots were sold prior to the auction, including the brickyard to the Savage Brothers, the Boat Inn with it's associated paddock, garden and smallholding to Mrs A Woodward, the rope-walk to Mr T Amos (Lot 185 rented for £2 pa, as well as a number of farms and cottages[279]. At the time of the Wakefield sale the Ward's (Charles, Ellen and daughter Olive) were living in Stoke Bruerne at *The Laurels, Chapel Lane*[280].

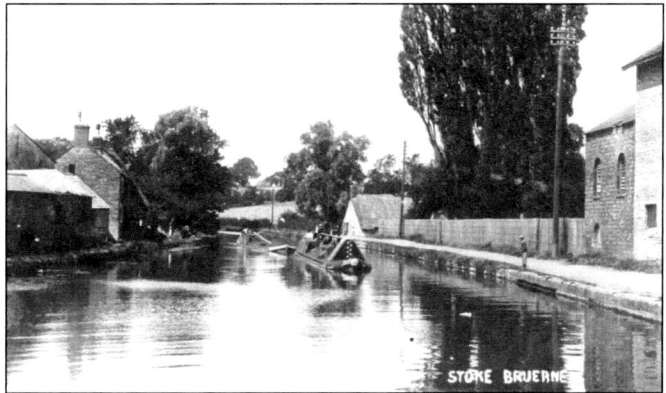

Figure 68   Two boats approaching lock 16 (Christopher M Jones Collection)

Two scenes of the Grand Union Canal the Amos's and the Ward's regularly saw from their canal side home include Figure 68, where two fully laden horse drawn boats are approaching top lock carrying small coal used in many industrial premises, probably one of the John Dickinson and Co. Ltd., paper mills in Hertfordshire. Looking closely at the picture it shows a bump on the towing path in front of the poplar trees, a reminder where the bridge once stood, which was removed and the towpath levelled around august 1913. Figure 69 shows the same pair of horse boats crossing the pound

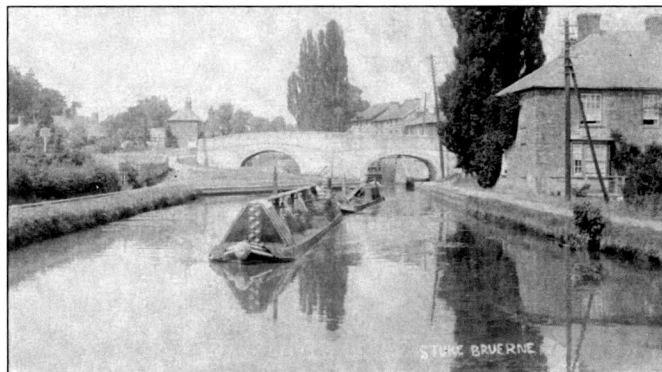

Figure 69   Coal boats exiting lock 16 (King Family Collection)

below top lock, giving a clear view of what was George Savage's house on the right against the towpath. George Savage's sons (Savage Bros.,) after purchasing the brick yard from the Duke of Grafton in 1919 the following year they placed the freehold on the market by Private Treaty for £3,000, the area comprising 29 acres, blue clay with kilns and plant[281]. The Amos shop

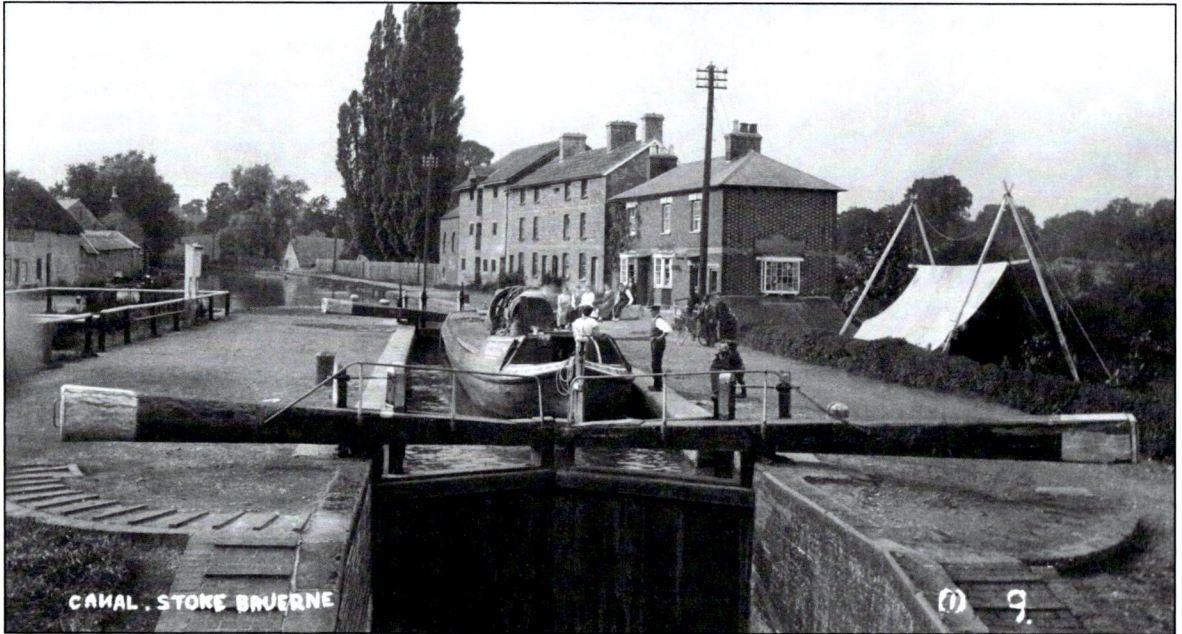

Figure 70   The Amos shop, top-lock and wide boat *Chess* (David Blagrove Collection)

continued trading in the 1920's as shown in Figure 70 where, in the lock outside the shop is the wide boat *Chess,* on this occasion running empty. The woman standing by the house immediately behind right-hand man on the balance beam is most likely Mrs Nellie Amos who ran the post-office in the near end of the house. The canvas structure on the right is most likely associated with Thomas Amos's rope business, he also

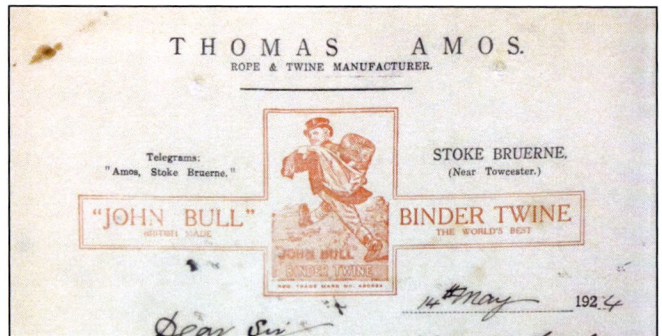

Figure 71   Thomas Amos letter headed business paper (George Freestone Collection)

made tentage and tarpaulins. The construction of sheer legs and pulleys form an A frame structure over which is a waterproofed tarpaulin it's most likely being used for drying canvas[282]. The Amos house is shown with it's *lean to* in which Mr Amos kept paraffin. The grocery and post-office were now run by Mrs Cakebread the mason's wife, although it is possible the post-office remained in the Amos shop as Mr Amos's letter head continues to indicate *Telegrams,* shown in Figure 71. The products sold in the Amos's shop, did by all accounts *keep up with the times* although not without some friendly criticism from the boaters …

> … later we bought our ready-mades and boots from Mr Aymus [Amos] shop at Stoke Bruin. He'd had the paraffin store and rope chandlery for years but in the early Grand Union days he was branchin out into ready-mades and wot-av-yer. He done the proper h'Oxford Shirtses, front gusset, warm folds, an all, and the boatee-blue stockins as well. The only trouble with his ready-made cords was, they stinked. It was summat to do with the dye. I couldn't stummick 'em in the cabin until I'd washed 'em and given 'em a good blowing along the cut. Even flappin on the line they whifted to 'igh 'eavens. Even the chaps in the Snug at the pub – and the Snug was no bed o' roses – wouldn't stummick Moy-chap in his new cords till he'd weard oorf a bit[283].

After returning from his position as Padre on the front-line in France, the Amos's son-in-law Rev Boyce, Rector of the Wesleyan Chapel, Gold-street, Northampton organised the first *Peoples Popular Service* in the Majestic Picture House. The event attracted an unprecedented number of people estimated at 1000, Rev Boyce's address was on *"Angels", where he told of many things that had been recited to him by men at the Front … and of the way in which religion caught hold of some of the men in the atmosphere in which they were[284]*. Not long after his son-in-law's concert Thomas Amos offered to retire from Roade Baptist Church, an offer the committee did not accept[285], at a subsequent meeting the pastor celebrated Mr Amos's long service …

> He had served as secretary for 41 years and in addition, filled the offices of Deacon, Treasurer and Sunday School Superintendent. The pastor felt, as others did, that some external recognition of his services was well overdue. In the name of the friends of Roade, and others interested, he had great pleasure in handing him Treasury Notes as a mark of esteem and appreciation of his labours in the Work of the Lord at Roade and also a book for Mrs T Amos.[286]

Stoke Bruerne continued to experience incidents related to the canal. At Wharf Farm Ernest Woodward on doing his evening rounds feeding the cattle, accidentally knock over an oil lamp which was close to stores of hay and straw, the fire quickly spread and ignited a petrol engine. Fortunately the fire-brigade arrived promptly and because the canal was directly behind the farm there was a plentiful supply of water quickly available. During the incident *Fireman Adams had the misfortune to lose his footings and fall into the canal, he was promptly and pluckily rescued*[287]. An incident which involved boat children during a trip through the tunnel was so significant it caused Grand Junction canal company engineer Mr Milner to convey the details to his employer[288] …

July 2nd 1923

Dear Sir,

BLISWORTH TUNNEL

I have to report that the Blisworth Tug "Hasty", on Saturday the 30th ulto, left the North end of the Tunnel at 3.30 p.m. with twelve loaded coal boats in tow going towards Stoke, they had not travelled far when a motor and butty passed them safely going North. When between the sixth and seventh (or last) shaft the Tug met a second motor, Messrs Fellows, Morton & Clayton's "Lapwing" with butty "Gambia", Steerer *Jas. Stokes*. This motor passed the tug all right, it's butty, however, got across the Tunnel and passed the Company's tug on it's wrong side, consequently the tow rope fouled the propeller and stopped it, it also put the tugs lights out. The motor and tug were signalling each other but the tunnel was so foul they could not note their respective positions. As the tugs engine could not work the motor Lapwing went stern first back to stoke with the tug and 13 boats in tow and did not reach the Southern end until 5.30.p.m. being two hours in the tunnel. During these two hours the tugs driver did not do any stoking up. While the "Lapwing" was towing this fleet of boats out, two more motors and butties, going North, passed them safely, so you will understand the atmospheric condition was not improved. No damage was done beyond the Lapwings broken tow rope.

H. Bustin was in charge of the tug and fortunately when at the North End of the Tunnel he requested the boat people to send all the children overland. *Bustin* could not state the number of children on the boats but said they looked like a regiment of soldiers on tramp; one child, however was left on a boat and this was kept going by use of damp clothes.

I have had verbal reports from *Bustin* and *Stokes* and both accounts agree that it was an accident caused through the bad atmospheric conditions at the time of meeting

You will probably hear from the boat people on the matter.

I am

Yours faithfully

T. W. M.

The most tragic event in the village occurred in 1924, when 66 year old lock-keeper William Abbott died as a result of his work for the canal company. On the Friday morning George Inns, Mr Abbott's work colleague turned up at 6am *and found the place [lock-keeper's hut] locked up.* After asking a boatman if he'd seen Mr Abbott, George called at Mr Abbott's home, as there was no reply he called for the other lock-keeper who between them opened the lock-keepers hut door *with an old key.* As there was no evidence of Mr Abbott they called the police, the events then unfolded …

> The canal was dragged, and at about 11.40 a.m the body was found outside the lock in about six feet of water … a windlass was outside the end of the lock, and the lamp which Abbott usually carried was in a hole where the concrete of the lock ended. Oil was on the surface of the water, and more came up with the body..

The coroner recorded a verdict *accidentally drowned by falling in the execution of his duty*. Mr Abbott was a native of Stoke Bruerne and *held in high respect by all who knew him*, having held the position of superintendent of the Sunday School for 24 years in the Wesleyan Chapel. The funeral service was attended by a significant number of people from the village, including Mr and Mrs T. Amos, after which Mr Abbott was buried in Stoke Bruerne. At the graveside ceremony the Wesleyan Sunday School children, led by Mrs. T. Jackson, sang the hymn, *I sing the almighty power of God*[289].

The lens focuses again on boaters

Captain Llewellyn resumed his post as Chief Inspector of the Canal Boats Acts on his return from military service in the R.A.S.C,.[290]. In his first post-war report to the newly formed Ministry of Health, Llewellyn indicated the Great War *led to deterioration in canal maintenance and a noticeable increase in the number of motor boats being registered.* He also commented on boat women and their children remaining on the canal …

> Very natural conditions act in keeping on the boats small children and young girls just over school age; parents who might otherwise leave these latter to the care of relations and strangers have very good reasons for desiring to keep them under their eye. The ordinary run of boatmen and their wives are of a very moral disposition and dislike, at any rate have no fancy for, many things that attract the ordinary shore-going classes.
>
> I am of the opinion that any compulsory separation of parents and children by making it illegal for children to live on canal boats might result in a state of affairs a great deal worse than the present, often imaginary, drawbacks. Boat people are born, not made. I have yet to come across any of them who have come on the canal from any other occupation. In the opinion of some, complete prohibition of women and children on boats would result in a discontinuation of the traffic in many places almost altogether[291].

In the aftermath of war the Ministry of Health responded to the National Transport Workers Federation request *for an inquiry into boat people* by appointing a departmental committee chaired by Neville Chamberlain, with the remit *to inquire into the practice of Living-in on Canal Boats in England and Wales and to report whether any alterations in the practice are desired.* Whilst the inquiry was underway government control of canals ceased on August 31st 1920, and the subsidy given to canal companies during the war was withdrawn[292]. Also during the inquiry Owen Llewellyn continued to express concerns regarding Local Authority Canal Boat Registration Books being *very unreliable*, he also reiterated *the canal trade* [is] *dying in most parts of the country* …

With the best intentions in the world, the inspectors are unable to account for all the boats still registered with them; for instance, during the wat many boats were withdrawn from their ordinary use and sent to Flanders and elsewhere; some have not returned, but the whereabouts of many is still a mystery.

In excuse for the uncertainty that surrounds the fate of so many boats, it must be remembered that some of them were registered over forty years ago, that their original owners are most probably dead, and that there is no necessity under the Acts to notify the sale or destruction of boats registered under them.

The canal-carrying trade is in most parts dying; for nearly a century it has held out against the railways, but with the advent of heavy road motor traction it is unable to hold its own, especially when it is required to adjust itself to legislation primarily designed for factories[293].

The *living-in* committee held twelve meetings between October 18th 1920 and March 1st 1921. At the first meeting the terms of reference were decided and a questionnaire constructed for distribution to witnesses and other's involved in canal carrying to *have their say* (transcribed in Appendix 6)*,* during the second and third meetings committee members visited *The Butts, Brentford* to see the school attended by boat children, and *Paddington Basin* where they talked to boaters. At subsequent meetings witnesses were heard (listed in Appendix 7), committee members also reviewed a comprehensive amount of correspondence, and the replies to the questionnaire.

On November 23rd 1920 at 12.30, Mr Thomas Amos J.P,. Stoke Bruerne gave evidence[294]. Mr Amos commenced by showing the committee a picture of his canal side home, after which he replied to the first question *[if the boat people] are healthy? …*

The boat people are very strong and healthy. The boys and girls too, travelling with the boats, can wind up the paddles better than the village boys and girls … they begin very young – 10 years of age, some of them [it does not do them any harm, does it?] Well, sometimes it appears to me they are too young to be struggling at it, but they seem to develop well, and they seem to get strength afterwards; I do not know whether this develops muscle. [I see you give them a good character for cleanliness?] the majority. I have noticed the boats this morning and yesterday. They clean their boats wonderfully; they are very fond of cleaning up a lot of brass work and brightening up the cabins. Of course there are exceptions; we get some very dirty ones now and again.

Mr Amos was also asked for his views on the *education of boat children*, little did the committee know of his family's connections with a leading writer on education, his brother-in-law Rev. Hirst Hollowell. Mr Amos replied …

Well, of course it is very bad, because the children have no chance of getting education. If a boy is able to write his name or do a bit, he is very proud of it. I think the children are very ambitious to learn to read and write like other children. They all seem that way if you speak to them about it. [What do the parents say about it?] Well the parents often say: "I wish I had learnt to write." I know that, because they come to me to write their letters.

Certified Nurse and Midwife Clara Jones also gave evidence[295], on this day several females joined the committee. Nurse Jones began by reported she had worked at Brentford for seven years, during which she attended around 30 confinements on [mainly] Emanuel Smith boats, Nurse Jones confirming *there were no deaths during childbirth, no cases of puerpueral fever or ophthalmia neonatorum and only one stillbirth*. Nurse Jones also enlightened the committee to the fact that prior to her being required to attend women giving birth on boats *the women were confined at the Boatmens Institute which had closed around the same time [she] came to work in the area*. A female committee member then enquired if *a boatwoman's labour more or less difficult than others?* Nurse Jones replied …

I hardly ever have a difficult case on the boats. I can recall only one case of chloroform and instruments. They are really in labour when you are sent for, and the baby is very often born before you get there. They work up till the last hour getting the boat into the dock. [The poor always work very hard to the last hour ashore and on the boats].

I have never been called to a case of an illegitimate child on the boats. Never … I find them a clean, honest, hard-working race of people, and very good to pay up. When your work is finished, there is your money for you; and very often they are confined to-day, and when you go to look for them the next day they are gone … that is the only thing I do not like about them: they are gone before you really know how they are getting on. I never heard of any wrong come to them; they just come up in another 12 or 15 months and want me again. They seem to get on alright[296].

Mrs Barton went on to asked for further information on *[boat] women working up to the last hour of labour* and about *the woman given chloroform*. Nurse Jones replied to both questions …

No, it is not right that they should [work up to the last hour before confinement] … there is no help for it; they must do that; and so must other poor mothers. [The woman with the chloroform] … I sent for Dr P___ who was not very far off, it used to be difficult, but now all doctors have agreed to come, and have signed an agreement to that effect … I only had that one case of a doctor.

It's difficult to attend a woman in a cabin … you cannot stand upright; it is very inconvenient. The chloroform case was very difficult; there was only room for two people, and when I got in there, there was not much room for anyone else, and it was a job in that case; but if I am on my own I can manage…

The boat people are very often more prepared for their confinements than some people on shore … it would be much better to be in a room [like the one that was at the Boatmen's Institute]. They are actually in a box, as it were; there is not that much depth from the ceiling of their room to the bed. When the doctor was giving the chloroform the fumes came quite over me; they could not get away.

Dame Louise Samuel asked Nurse Jones the final question regarding the *health of boat babies and the womens aftercare* ? she replied …

> [The bargee's baby] is very healthy, a very good weight indeed, I have never known a bottle-fed baby, I have very little experience of them afterwards, a few are with me the ten days. There is always another boatwoman or two there waiting to help you – the boatwomen from the other boats, they help each other wonderfully.

Neville Chamberlain concluded by thanking Nurse Jones for attending followed by the statement *your evidence is quite unique.*

The evidence received by the committee from witnesses and via written correspondence covered a vast range of issues surrounding *canal boat living-in conditions of the time*, as shown in the index to the published evidence report[297] which included many topics related to boater's health and wellbeing; accidents to boat children, cabins, cleanliness, morality, nutrition, sanitary conveniences, sobriety and the workmens compensation act, topics which demonstrate how comprehensive the committee were at *delving into all aspects of Canal Boat living-in.* The committee released their final 31 paragraph report on 11th August 1921[298]. The final paragraph of the report containing a summary of *the inquiries five recommendations*[299] listed in Figure 72. The first three relate to the *schooling of boat children*[300], the fourth *enforcement of registration,* and the fifth and final recommendation *a duty on Local Authorities to improve the availability of sanitary conveniences for boaters.*

---

1. Children of school age, that is, at present, between the ages of 5 and 14, should in future be prohibited from living-in on canal boats during the term times of the schools which they are attending.

2. A period of grace of twelve months from the date of the passing of the Act or the making of any Regulation to enforce this prohibition should be allowed before it comes into operation.

3. The head teacher of any school attended by a child of parents living-in on a canal boat should be required to deliver to either parent on application a certificate giving the dates of the commencement and termination of each holiday period, and the prohibition should not apply to any child during such holiday periods.

4. The owner of every boat used as a dwelling should be required to take out an annual licence in the prescribed form, procurable at any time during the first two months in each year at certain toll-offices to be agreed upon between the Ministry of Health and the Canal Companies concerned, on payment of a fee of 1s. per boat to the canal company.

5. It should be the duty of local authorities to provide such sanitary conveniences as may be necessary in the neighbourhood of important stopping places on canals, and their attention should be drawn to the matter.

Figure 72   Recommendations from the committee on living-in on canal boats 1921

After the report was published Owen Llewellyn commented on the recommendations in his annual report…

> The conclusions of the recent Departmental Committee on living-in on canal boats have … caused boat-owners to look carefully at the proposals for further use of canals, although at present no legislation has been set on foot to comply with the recommendations. At the same time I am under the impression that more boat people now realise the value of education for their children, and, were it not for the difficulties and expense of securing houses on shore, would take them off the boats when possible. In the present condition of affairs, however, there is a greater tendency now than there has been for some time past to utilize narrow boats as the only home[301]

The same year as the *living-in* report was released, boatmen's pay peaked even after their expenses such as horse feed started to fall, leading canal companies to collaborate with carriers and traders who collectively, and gradually, forced boatmen's pay rates down to a more competitive level, all of which was occurring at a time when the National Union of Transport and General Workers (NUTGW) became officially functioning (January 1st 1922), with Harry Gosling as president (also Secretary to the Waterways Trade Group), and Ernest Bevin Secretary to the union (also its Docks Trade Group)[302]. Nine months after the union became fully operational (August 13th 1923) the union called out on strike those of its members employed by Fellows, Morton and Clayton (FMC), one of the country's largest canal carrying companies[303]. As a result of the dispute the movement of long-distance commercial traffic on canals linking London, the Midlands and north-west England came to a virtual standstill.

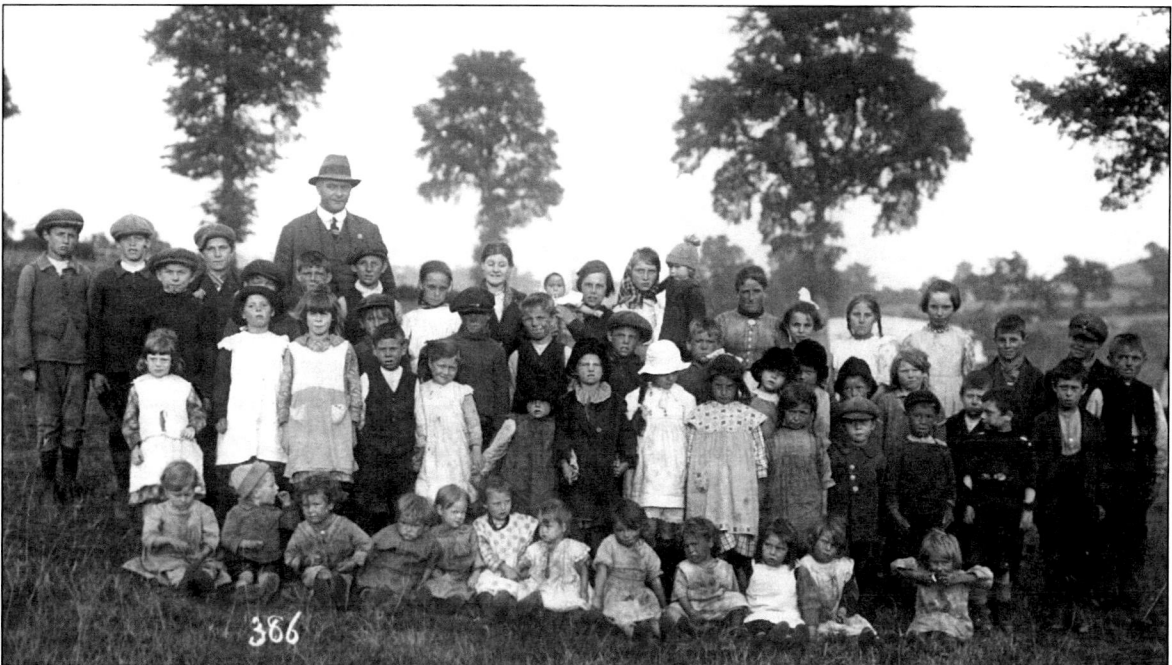

Figure 73   Boat children attending school during the Braunston strike 1923 (Lorna York collection)

On the Grand Junction Canal, and at the canal-side settlement of Braunston, the strike lasted fourteen weeks, during which 66 boats lay idle and 110 men waited there while their wages and living conditions were in dispute. Altogether 375 men, women and children came to a stop at Braunston as a result of the strike, it was reported *the striker's behaviour being impeccable throughout the dispute … they have behaved in the most orderly way, forming a little colony of their own, interfering with no one*[304].   Due to a significant number of children being caught up in the strike, the Union set up a special class for boat children in the village school. The children attending the special class are shown with Mr Sam Brookes in Figure 73. Mr Brookes was the union representative responsible for setting up the school and for employing the additional teacher, the names of the children shown in the picture are given in Table 24[305].

Table 24   **Names of the boat children attending Braunston School during the 1923 strike**

Surname	Childs First Name	Date of Birth	Fathers Name	Boat Names
Ball	Albert	24th May 1910	Jacob	Buckingham / Laurel
	Jacob	1913		
	Sarah	1915		
	Priscilla	1919		
Bland	Jack	24th February 1911	William	Digby / Poplar
	Eva	31st March 1914		
	Harry	23rd December 1917		
Clutterbuck	William	1915	William	Rose Agnes
	Dorothy	1918		
Davis	Alfred	14th January 1912	William	Mars / Jupiter
	John	1913		
	George	1914		
	Frank	1917		
Edwards	Henry Bert	12th February 1910	William	Kilsby / Japan
	Lucy May	3rd July 1911		
Estep	Violet	13th July 1910	Walter	Prosperous / Violet
Higgins	Eliza	25th September 1911	Thomas	Penguin / Nanchurch
Hough	Florence May	24th May 1906	John	Frank / Lyn
	Albert	30th September 1910		
	Thomas	4th August 1912		
	Lily	14th March 1919		
Knibbs	James	5th April 1919	Arthur	

Mees	John	1913	Jack	Egypt / Plover
	George	12th July 1915		
	Sam	16th February 1917		
Mitchell	Sarah	28th September 1911	Thomas	Norway
Powell	Rene	11th June 1909	Edward	Grange / Urmston
	Ivy Cordelia	21st May 1911		
	Harriet	16th May 1916		
	Betsey	15th June 1919		
Ray	Louisa	21st December 1910	William	India / Greet
	Rosie	7th June 1914		
	Alfred	13th August 1916		
	Frank	4th September 1916		
Richards	Mary	28th September 1918	James	
Roberts	Sarah	22nd August 1910	William	Robin / Denmark
	Charles	12th August 1911		
	Edward	1914		
	Eliza	1915		
	Olive	1917		
Russon	Ernest	17th July 1913	Albert	Columbia / Lion
	Albert John	18th March 1912		
Shaw	Martha	1915		Flint
Webb	Mary Ann	12th September 1911	Thomas	Lemon

For one young boat lad, 12 year old Edward Walker the strike made no difference to his working life because the Walker family were independent boaters from Bugbrook with a home in the village, during the strike the family were working under a sub-contract to Fellows, Morton and Clayton. Young Edward Walker drowned at Braunston during the strike, Edward's father identified the body and at the inquest gave an account of the events surrounding his son's death …

… about 7.30 on Thursday morning he was driving a motor boat and towing a butty boat. His eldest daughter was in charge of the second boat. When last seen he was having his breakfast. Having called him and received no reply his daughter set out to look for the deceased but could not find him.

[Father] obtained assistance from other barges and searched for three-quarters of an hour, but with no result. The body was later recovered by means of a drag. Deceased was liable to fits, but had not had one for six years. He could not swim. Elizabeth walker, the little boy's sister, corroborated.

The coroner returned a verdict *Accidentally Drowned*. The following Monday a moving funeral took place in the village with *the men, women and children forming a mournful procession, at the head of which was the little coffin of Edward Walker … walking slowly from Castle Inn, where the body had remained, to the church.* A reporter captured the devastating mood cast over the boaters at this sad time …

> It was purely a barge people's affair, and it was surely the oddest assembly that ever occupied the church-swarthy faced women, many of whom had acquired black fur coats for the occasion, and rugged men. They were reverent and attentive while the rector … recited the words of the burial office.
>
> At the side of the coffin were placed a score or so of wreaths and posies, mostly made up of simple flowers by the givers. When the last words had been said the rector walked aside to where the barge men were standing in double file and addressed a few kindly words … the men were obviously touched by the rector's sympathetic words, and some exclaimed "Hear, hear"[306].

Captain Joseph Green age 65 from the boat *Flint* also passed away at Braunston during the strike. Joseph was born in Staffordshire and married Annie Grant in June 1884 at St James, Lower Gornal, after which they had eight children[307]. Joseph's funeral cortage passing across the lane in Braunston is shown in Figure 74 and in Figure 75 the funeral cortège is seen outside Braunston Church. On a happier note a Boatmen's concert was organised during the strike by *Rev Davis, Mr Dixon and friends from Rugby*. The concert was held in Braunston Memorial Hall, attended by 120 boat children who

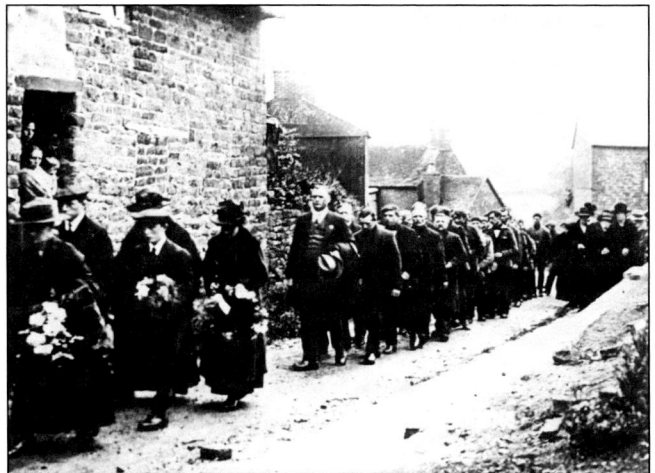

Figure 74   Funeral cortège for Captain Joseph Green during Braunston strike 1923 (Waterway's archive)

sat on low seats at the front of the hall, with the adult boater's behind them, the remaining space was filled by parishioners. In total the reporter estimated the hall was filled *with upwards of 450 people,* the programme being *long and most entertaining,* afterwards the women and children were given sweets and the men smokes[308].

According to several articles about the strike (mainly Ken Sherwood) it was concluded by arbitration. The strike also effected Brentford whereby Fellows, Morton and Clayton (FMC) issued a writ against a union official for trespassing on one of their boats to delay unloading. The judge suggested an adjournment so both FMC and the Union could come to some agreement, which is what happened. The union agreed to a return to work by boatmen under FMC's old terms if FMC agreed to abide by an arbitrators decision which they hitherto refused to do.

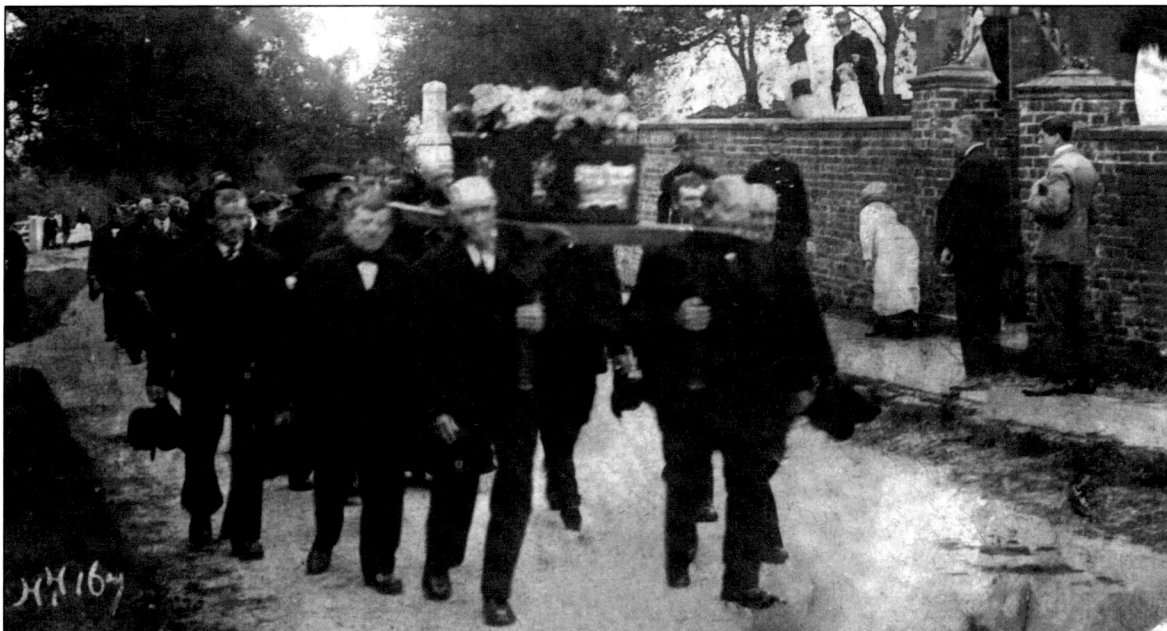

Figure 75   Funeral cortège for Captain Joseph Green during Braunston strike 1923 (Lorna York collection)

FMC wanted a 6.5% cut in boatmen's pay which the arbitrator said was to much, but agreed a 5% cut was more reasonable on those rates of pay that were in effect in January 1923, made in two instalments of 2.5%, one immediately in November after which the boats started to move, and the second on 19th December 1923. No further strike action was taken by the boatmen as this was the arbitrators decision[309].

Some evidence survives to suggests boatmen working for carrier companies in the 1920's were insured regarding accidents and injuries. For example the company records of Samuel Barlow (Tamworth) Ltd.,[310] indicate the company had a policy regarding compensation, although payment for the policy led to some problems for the company …

> … it was decided in view of the high premium for workmens insurance to allow policy to lapse as from October 4th. Some amount later to be decided upon shall be placed into a contingency fund to meet any claims made after risk is undertaken by the company.

In July of the following year Samuel Barlow (Tamworth) Ltd., received a compensation claim from Boatman F. Baxter [311] *for incapacity arising from back strain*, this was dealt with by Mr Brown and Mr Harries, after which the claim was agreed *not to exceed £80*. In the September *the manager reported a satisfactory agreement of compensation for Fred Baxter for redemption sum of £75 having been agreed by the court*[312]. In 1924 the committee at Samuel Barlow (Tamworth) Ltd discussed the position of captains wives and the Unemployment Insurance Acts. The secretary being instructed in May 1924 to obtain quotes from insurance companies under the Workmen's Compensation Acts 1908-1923, details of the policy with Midlands Employer's Mutual Assurance Ltd from June 26th 1924 covered all staff except 'clerical'[313]

Boaters health and well-being remained on the Ministry of Health agenda after the Committee on Living-In reported their conclusions, mainly as a result of it being noted the existing regulations covering canal boats had not been updated since coming into operation on March 20th 1878. Regarding *Habitable Cabins*[314] the regulations were reviewed as to *whose responsibilities related to certain aspects of periodic registration.* With the canal boat regulations committee concluding *the habitable condition of a canal boat (except as regards the periodic painting of the interior of the cabins) is placed entirely on the master of the boat,* although they acknowledged …

> Circumstances may arise in which it is desirable that proceedings should be taken against the OWNER of a boat in respect of defects in habitable conditions, particularly structural defects. Regulation 3, has therefore, been amended so as to place upon the OWNER of a canal boat the responsibility of maintaining the boat in the condition required at the time of its initial registration.

The Act was subsequently amended to include a new paragraph after Regulation 3 placing the responsibility for *Habitable Cabins* firmly under the remit of the boat owner …

> The owner of a canal boat shall maintain it in the condition required for the purpose of registration under this Regulation and if such owner be convicted of default in so doing the Court of Summary Jurisdiction may (in lieu of or in addition to imposing a penalty) order the suspension or cancellation of the registration (Regulation 4 of the 1878 Act hereby repealed)[315]

Less than a year later Owen Llewellyn reported the Amendment Regulations were *already having a good effect on the state of the cabins,* as well as being of *great value to the inspectors in carrying out their duties.* Concluding he had observed boat-owners *now realize that it is their business to keep the cabins of their boats in proper condition, and repairs ordered by inspectors appear to be carried out much more promptly than in the past*[316]. Two years later Llewellyn again reported continued improvements in *the habitable state of boats* and *the inspection of these by Local Authorities.* Llewellyn also reported disease on canal boats to be *a very rare occurrence* and prosecutions almost more uncommon …

> The Canal Boats Order of 1925 has had a most beneficial effect on the condition of the boats, in that it is now realised by their owners that they themselves are responsible for their repair and general "habitableness", instead of, as formerly, this being the duty of any boatman who might at the time occupy the position of master[317]

Nurse Ward the Earls Barton year's

Ellen, Charles and Olive Ward returned to Earls Barton c1925, a rural village 14 miles from Stoke Bruerne, it's main industries being farming and boot and shoe manufacturing. Ellen Ward (Sister Mary) worked for Doctor Joseph William Baird as Doctor's Assistant (Nurse Ward). Doctor Baird a Physician Surgeon and member of Edinburgh Obstetrical Society[318] moved to Earls Barton in 1904 when he purchased an established General Practice on the retirement of

Dr Lawrence, after which he married Margaret Palmer[319]. Initially the Baird's lived in rented accommodation, where their daughters *Mary Josephine (b.1907) and Margaret Palmer (b.1908)* were born. Due to the Baird's expanding family and their thriving General Practice they had a home built in North Street (c.1910), after moving in their third child *John Palmer (b.1913)* was born.

Dr Baird was appointed Chief Inspector under the factory and Workshop Act[320], which required him to inspect the local boot and shoe workshops, provide care for workers injured or ailing as a result of their employment, and report to the County Medical Officer on factory and Workshop matters. It is possible the Baird's knew the Ward's before Ellen commenced her employment at the surgery because Charles Ward (Sister Mary's husband) was a resident in Earls Barton in 1915, giving his address as 9, Prospect Terrace, in the letter he wrote to Thomas Milner (Figure 63). In 1918 Dr Baird was lecturer for St Johns Ambulance Home Nursing course[321], the same year he extended the family home to include a dispensary, surgery and waiting room, he also added an entrance to the surgery from the main street. Charles and Ellen Ward were residing in Northampton Road, Earls Barton in 1918[322] by 1925 the Ward's were at King Street[323], Ellen was employed by Dr Baird as Doctor's Assistant / Nurse, a position usually undertaken by the Doctor's wife[324]. As Mrs Baird was raising three children and busy managing an increasing number of positions in the village and beyond this is the most likely reason why she was unable to assist her husband in his rural General Practice.

Dr Baird's General Practice during the 1920's-1930's would have been run in a fairly regular manner; *general appointment* sessions two or three times a week, a session for *minor surgical procedures*, dedicated time when Dr Baird *did his rounds* and at least one *ante / post-natal* clinic a week. Dr Baird would also be fulfilling his Factory Inspector duties and not to forget he would be *on-call* in the event of a local emergency. From Nurse Ward's surviving *Surgery Dressing Book[325]* her role in the General Practice included …

- Managing Dr Baird's appointments,
- Dispensing medications prescribed by Dr Baird,
- Managing the surgery stock: Dressings, medicines, lotions and instruments,
- Chaperoning patients when being attending by Dr Baird,
- Assisting Dr Baird when he was performing surgical procedures,
- Cleaning, sterilizing and safely storing surgical instruments,
- Recording patients clinical observations (particularly temperature and pulse) and
- Wound Care.

By far the most common aspect of Nurse Ward's work was the management of wounds, as indicated in the meticulously maintained *Surgery Dressing Book[326]*. Nurse Ward held daily *dressing clinics* at the surgery, she also managed patients who attended the surgery on an impromptu basis, usually as a result of an injury or minor ailment. Patients presented to the General Practice with a vast range of conditions related to almost every aspect of the body, the range of conditions Nurse Ward provided wound care was also vast, as such a more detailed account is provided in Appendix 8. Taking one week from the *Surgery Dressing Book* shown in Table 25, exemplifies how busy Nurse Ward was in relation to managing wounds and injuries. In the course of this one week she treated 24 different patients, some she saw only once, whilst others were treated daily or every other day, she provided care on a Saturday and a Sunday, and on many occasions cared for patients in their own home.

Table 25   A week in the life of Nurse Ward's wound management May 193)

Patient Number	Presenting Condition	Wound Care
Monday 6th May		
1	Eczema of Arms	Wet Dressing. Bandaged
2	Cyst of Scalp: Septic (Incised 3rd May … Day 3)	Wet Dressing. Bandaged
3	Cyst of Neck	Observe. Medicine
4	Septic Finger	Wet Dressing. Bandaged
5	Septic Finger (continued from previous book)	Dry Dressing. Bandaged
6	Septic Fingers (Incised 5 days ago)	Wet Dressing. Bandaged
7	Ulceration of both legs	Wet Dressing. Bandaged
8	Cyst of Nose	Dry Dressing.
9	Accident: Strain of foot	Bandage.
10	Cysts of Scalp	Dry Dressing.
11	Cyst of finger: Enlarged Glands	Wet Dressing.
Tuesday 7th May		
1	Eczema of Arms	Wet Dressing. Bandaged
2	Cyst of Scalp: Septic (Incised 3rd May … Day 4)	Wet Dressing. Bandaged
12	Glands of Arm and wart of Finger	Observe.
4	Septic Finger	Wet Dressing. Bandaged
13	Injury to Knee	Observe
14	Septic wound of Ankle (old accident)	Dressing. Bandage. Medicine.
15	Eczema of Hands	Wet Dressing. Bandaged
16	Eczema of both hands and five fingers	Dressing. Bandage. Medicine.
5	Septic Finger	Dry Dressing. Bandaged
17	Ulceration of Leg	Wet Dressing. Bandaged
18	Conjunctivitis	Neoprotosil
19	Accident wound of arm	Dry Dressing. Bandaged

6	Septic Fingers (Incised 6 days ago)	Wet Dressing. Bandaged
7	Ulceration of both legs	Wet Dressing. Bandaged

Wednesday 8th May

5	Septic Finger	Dry Dressing. Bandaged
20	Glands Enlarged	Dressing
7	Ulceration of both legs. Rheumatism	Wet Dressing. Bandaged
8	Cyst of Nose	Dry Dressing.
11	Cyst of finger: Enlarged Glands	Wet Dressing.

Thursday 9th May

1	Eczema of Arms: Septic	Wet Dressing. Bandaged. Medicine
2	Cyst of Scalp: Septic (Incised 3rd May … Day 6)	Wet Dressing. Bandaged
21	Fracture of Radius (6 days ago)	Electric and Massage
3	Cyst of Neck: Removed today	Dressing. Medicine
12	Glands of Arm and wart of Finger	Observe.
4	Septic Finger	Wet Dressing. Bandaged
13	Injury to Knee	Observe
14	Septic wound of Ankle (old accident)	Dressing. Bandage. Medicine.
15	Eczema of Hands	Wet Dressing. Bandaged
16	Eczema of both hands and five fingers	Dressing. Bandage. Medicine.
5	Septic Finger	Wet Dressing. Bandaged
17	Ulceration of Leg	Wet Dressing. Bandaged
18	Conjunctivitis	Neoprotosil
6	Septic Fingers (Incised 8 days ago)	Wet Dressing. Bandaged
7	Ulceration of both legs. Rheumatism	Wet Dressing. Bandaged

Friday 10th May

1	Eczema of Arms: Septic	Wet Dressing. Bandaged. Medicine
2	Cyst of Scalp: Septic (Incised 3rd May … Day 7)	Wet Dressing. Bandaged
22	Fracture of Arm (3rd May)	Electric and Massage
3	Cyst of Neck: Removed yesterday	Dressing. Medicine
4	Septic Finger	Wet Dressing. Bandaged
13	Injury to Knee	Observe
16	Eczema of both hands and five fingers	Dressing. Bandage. Medicine.

5	Septic Finger	Wet Dressing. Bandaged
17	Ulceration of Leg	Wet Dressing. Bandaged
20	Glands Enlarged	Dressing
18	Conjunctivitis	Neoprotosil
6	Septic Fingers (Incised 9 days ago)	Wet Dressing. Bandaged
23	Baby: Eczema of scalp, face, hands and feet	
7	Ulceration of both legs. Rheumatism	Wet Dressing. Bandaged
8	Cyst of Nose	Dry Dressing.
9	Accident: Strain of foot	Bandage.
10	Cysts of Scalp	Dry Dressing.
11	Cyst of finger: Enlarged Glands	Wet Dressing.
Saturday 11th May		
1	Eczema of Arms: Septic	Wet Dressing. Bandaged. Medicine
2	Cyst of Scalp: Septic (Incised 3rd May … Day 8)	Wet Dressing. Bandaged
3	Cyst of Neck: Removal 2 days ago	Dressing. Medicine
14	Septic wound of Ankle (old accident)	Dressing. Bandage. Medicine.
15	Eczema of Hands	Wet Dressing. Bandaged
5	Septic Finger	Wet Dressing. Bandaged
18	Conjunctivitis	Neoprotosil
19	Accident wound of arm	Dry Dressing. Bandaged
23	Baby: Eczema of scalp, face, hands and feet	
7	Ulceration of both legs. Rheumatism	Wet Dressing. Bandaged
24	Accident wound to arm. Septic	Dry Dressing. Bandaged.
Sunday 12th May		
1	Eczema of Arms: Septic	Wet Dressing. Bandaged. Medicine
2	Cyst of Scalp: Septic (Incised 3rd May … Day 9)	Wet Dressing. Bandaged
3	Cyst of Neck: Removal 3 days ago	Dressing. Medicine
12	Glands of Arm and wart of Finger	Observe. Discharged
4	Septic Finger	Wet Dressing. Bandaged
13	Injury to Knee	Observe
16	Eczema of both hands and five fingers	Dressing. Bandage. Medicine.

5	Septic Finger	Wet Dressing. Bandaged
20	Glands Enlarged	Dressing
18	Conjunctivitis	Neoprotosil
6	Septic Fingers (Incised 10 days ago)	Wet Dressing. Bandaged
10	Cysts of Scalp	Dry Dressing.
11	Cyst of finger: Enlarged Glands	Wet Dressing.
24	Accident wound to arm. Septic	Dry Dressing. Bandaged.

Upper limb ailments were very common, including crushed, lacerated, septic, severed and on some occasions septic fingers and thumbs. Many patients with upper limb problems presented to the surgery with a swollen neck and/or axilliary glands as a result of sepsis, most likely due to their delaying seeking medical attention. Given the nature of the hand wounds Nurse Ward treated in the Earls Barton General Practice the most likely cause was the patients employment in the village boot and shoe factory, where hand work was prevalent . Patients with head and neck complaints were also regularly seen including abscess's, carbuncle's and cysts. Skin conditions were common, including eczema, blistering and dermatitis, with the most probable causes of skin irritations being from the boot and shoe manufacturing processes which used a considerable number of chemical products; abrasives, adhesives, oils, acids and glues to name a few[327]. Eye conditions were a regular problem requiring Nurse Ward on some occasions to remove a foreign body, cleanse eyes due to conjunctivitis or give first aid as a result of an eye injury. Nurse Ward also managed members of the village community with long-standing medical problems, particularly women with problems related to their lower limbs; ulcerated leg(s) (one or both), swollen (bulbous) legs and inflamed legs (phlebitis). For most of the women re-dressing their wounds was done daily, when the ulcer / wound showed signs of improvement the frequency of the dressing changes was reduced to every other day or every third day. For one lady with a severe leg ulcer Nurse Ward dressed the wound on 54 occasions[328].

Nurse Ward also cared for women before and after confinement, in conjunction with the visiting Midwife[329], these women required ongoing care due to *breast problems* of quite a severe nature, as one case study reveals. On Tuesday May 31st 1932 Nurse Ward saw a lady for the first time, the woman was examined and the right breast was found to be *hard with reduced milk,* the woman had a raised *temperature of 102.9, a wet dressing [was] applied.* The following day the woman's temperature was slightly higher at *103* Nurse Ward noting the breast *looks like [an] abscess.* The following day Nurse Ward visited the woman three times, on the fifth day Dr Baird incised the abscess and inserted a *plug and drain.* After the surgical procedure Nurse Ward cared for the wound daily, the woman's temperature began to return to normal and the records show the wound to be *greatly improved,* although three weeks after the initial visit, the wound continued *pouring much pus.* Daily dressings continued for a further 12 days when *milk again in both breasts … improving,* Nurse Ward making the comment *still very stubborn,* as to whether she was referring to the wound or the patient will never be know, daily wound care continued till Saturday July 23rd[330].

Nurse Ward also managed Dr Baird's surgery finances, including collecting payments from patients, and *dues* from members of the *Northampton District Friendly Society (NDFS)* which she passed on monthly to the societies local representative. Ellen Ward was also socially active in the village, hosting teas[331] and other events[332], whilst her husband Chas was a member of the committee at the *United Working-men's club and institute*[333] and honorary secretary of *Earls Barton Hospital Committee*[334].

During Ellen's employment in the surgery, Mrs Baird became increasingly active in local, county and national organisations, Marjorie being elected Chairman of the Earls Barton Women's Institute in 1927[335] and President in the early 1930's[336], as well as a prominent Northamptonshire Spiritualist, she performed the opening ceremony at the new Moor Street Spiritualist Church in Rushden[337]. Mrs Baird regularly lectured at Divisional Liberal Party events, on such topics as *proportional representation*[338] and *slavery in our times*[339]. In 1928 the Baird's suffered a tragic loss when their 15 year old son was killed in a motorcycle accident[340], John at the time of his death was the same age as the Ward's daughter Olive. Olive Ward and the Baird daughter's spent their teenage year's together, regularly organising fund raising dance's[341] and concerts[342] in Earls Barton. At one annual event in aid of the *Help for Hospitals* scheme the three girls entered the fancy dress competition[343], Olive won second prize as a Sea Nymph, Molly Baird third prize, as a Manchu Princess, and the consolation prize went to Peggy Baird as a Snow Queen.

Olive married Eric Arthur Drage[344], a local lad who worked alongside his family in the boot and shoe industry. After their marriage Eric and Olive moved to London, but returned briefly to Earls Barton so she could perform her duties as Matron of Honour at the Baird's youngest daughter's marriage[345]. Chas and Ellen in the last two years of their time in Earls Barton moved to West Street, possibly in the house built in the garden of the Baird's home and surgery. The Ward's left Earls Barton in January 1935[346].

Ageing in Stoke Bruerne - father calls

In May 1928 whilst the Ward's were in Earls Barton, Emma Amos, the sister-in-law of Thomas Amos passed away suddenly during a visit to her daughter in Birmingham, Mrs. C Amos *had been an untiring worker for the Baptist Church at Blisworth*[347]. Thomas Amos attended the funeral, his wife Nellie was unable to attend with him *due to failing health*, she was at the time being cared for by her married daughter Ethel Margaret. Nellie Amos (Sister Mary's mother) passed away in her canal side home just two months after Emma died, Nellie was 72[348]. The funeral was held at Roade Baptist Church, attended by family mourners from all parts of England as well as representatives from organisations Mrs Amos had taken a leading part in, *Stoke Bruerne and Shutlanger Chapels, The Mothers Meeting Stoke Bruerne, Roade Baptist Chapel, Band of Hope Union and the Good Templar Order.* A particularly moving part of the service was the hymn sung by Mrs Coates, *I heard the voice of Jesus say* reminding *those present of the voice now stilled, that has so often given pleasure in song at meetings of causes with which she was associated*[349].

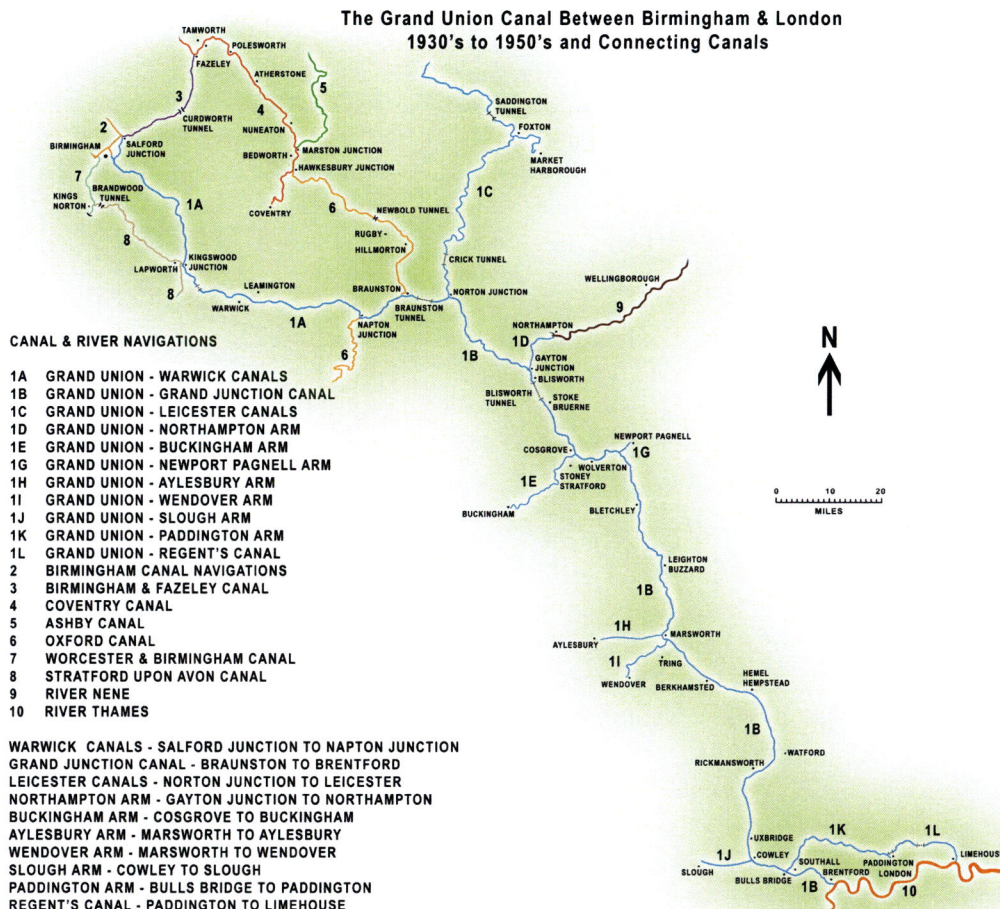

Figure 76   Map of the Grand Union Canal (Christopher M Jones)

At the time of Emma and Nellie's deaths the Grand Junction Canal was changing, mainly as a result of an Act receiving royal assent in August 1928 for the amalgamation of a number of canal companies. From midnight December 31st the Grand Junction Canal Company came to a conclusion, the Regents Canal Company was absorbed into the Grand Union Canal Company and at the strike of midnight (January 1st 1929) the Grand Union Canal came into being, the longest canal in the country and a unified inland waterway from London to Birmingham, formed from an amalgamation of a number of canals: Birmingham and Warwick Junction, Warwick and Birmingham, Warwick and Napton, Grand Junction Canal (minus Paddington Estates Property) and a 5 ½ mile stretch of the Oxford Canal from Napton to Braunston shown in Figure 76. The same month the Grand Union Canal came into being Thomas Amos retired from his position as County Councillor owing to ill-health and increasing age[350].

After amalgamation of the canals Owen Llewellyn reported he had undertaken a *special investigation into the treatment of children on canal boats* because *an impression seems to prevail in some quarters that parents are indifferent to the well-being of their children, and put them to tasks beyond their strength.* Llewellyn in his report defended the position of boat families in relation to their offsprings …

> My own experience is that canal boat people are solicitous for their children's welfare and look after them properly, and that there has been a great improvement in conditions generally in recent years. Exceptional cases no doubt occur, as in other classes of the community, but they are rare.

> These are my own views, based on a long and intimate experience. In view of statements which have been made I have made special inquiries of other persons on whom I can rely, who are familiar with canal boat people and their lives, and in every case their views were in full agreement with those which I have just expressed.

> My attention has been directed to the fact that many persons still are anxious that children should not be allowed to dwell in canal boats. I do not agree that the time is yet opportune for this step in spite of the fact that undoubtedly the education of the children to some extent suffers. My principal reasons are that the housing problem is not easier for this class of folk, that family life would be broken up (the wives would have to go with the children), and that the pay of the boatmen would not cover the extra expenses to be incurred- including the cost of a mate to take the place of a wife. (Family canal-boat life can be a very economical one.) Motors on boats are in themselves a form of education to a most important profession; both parents and children are anxious to take advantage of the opportunities afforded the children to attend such schools as exist; teachers seem keen to get hold of them, and finally, the decent, kindly, and healthy status of the boat-people as a whole is proof that there can be little wrong with this mode of living and that their chief desire is to be left alone[351]

Regardless of Mr Llewellyn's observations Harry Gosling continued his mission to change the *conditions of the canal boaters.* In March 1929 Gosling presented to parliament a Canal Boat Bill, aimed at amending the Canal Boats Acts of 1877 and 1884. The Bill went to a second reading in 1930 and on the day the Bill was read boaters in their *Sunday Best* protested outside parliament as shown in Figure 77 and

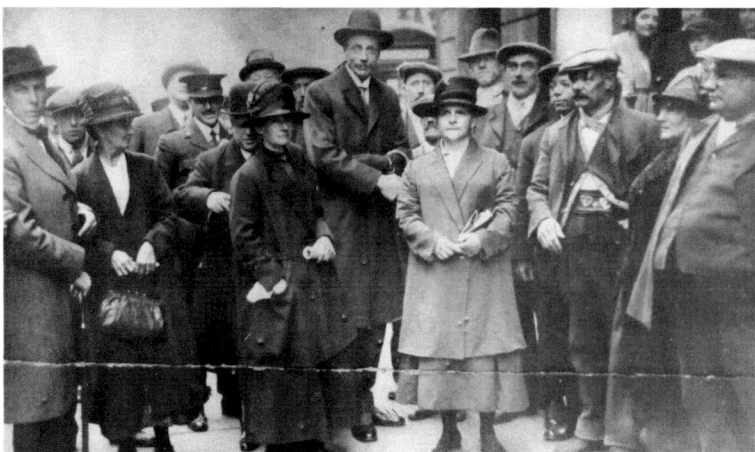

Figure 77   Boaters protest outside the House of Commons 1930 (Waterway's archive)

Figure 78. In the latter picture the caption reads …

BARGEES PROTEST. – Earl Winterton greeting yesterday at the House of Commons a deputation which came to protest against the Canal Boats Bill. The Bill states that children under 15 may not live on the boats.

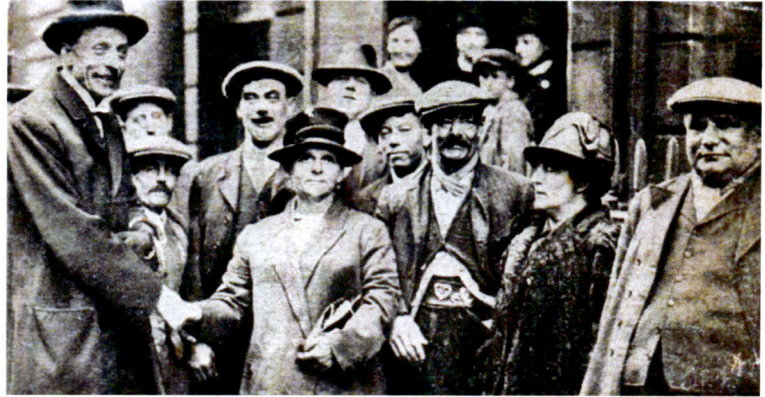

Figure 78   Boaters protest outside the House of Commons 1930 (Della Sadler-Moore collection)

In 1931 Owen Llewellyn retired from his position as the second Chief Inspector of Canal Boats. In what was his thirty second and final report Mr Llewellyn wrote *he trusted he be allowed to make it's substance more recapitulatory and discursive than usual,* from which the following is recounted …

… during my inspectorship, circumstances and surroundings connected with canal boats and water transport have altered probably to a greater extent than ever before since the invention of locks.

When motor engines first came in, it was imagined that boats fitted with them would necessarily be worked only by men to the exclusion of women and children. This idea, however, was soon found to be incorrect, with the result that most of the young folk on the boats have become quite skilled engineers as well as navigators. Incidentally, mechanically propelled boats have proved themselves less dangerous than the old horse-drawn type, as there is not the same necessity for crew to be for ever jumping on and off the boats, a fruitful cause of accidents between locks.

During the period of my inspectorate many hundreds of miles of canals have become derelict or have fallen into disuse. Owing to the impossibility of knowing where once-registered boats may have gone and what may have happened to them, it has always been impossible to state with any certainty how many boats still exist and are at work. Many old boats are used to strengthen the banks … some have been turned into houseboats; they make excellent bonfires, and after big floods are often found in fields many miles away from the places at which they were left …

From his *long services with* the boat people, Owen Llewellyn concluded by summing up how he felt about boaters on his retiring …

And I am even more sad to leave the boat-people, folk from whom in all my time I can honestly say I have never had one cross word, let alone the type of language that ignorant humorists think it witty to attribute to them. "Bargees" are decent folk in the best sense of the word, and the fact that they take very little interest in what other folk do and say, and are content to get on with their work, is a clear proof of it. The debates and the correspondence aroused on the occasion of the late Canal Boats Bill showed that no class of worker stood in less need of supervision and their morals and morality were held up to public approval[352]

After Llewellyn retired the Minister for Health divided the country's waterways into districts, and distributed Llewellyn's duties to a number of General Inspectors of the Ministry as listed in Table 26[353], each appointees being issued a *warrant of appointment as a canal boat inspector.*

Table 26   Appointees following the retirement of Owen Llewellyn

Names: General Inspectors	District: Responsibilities
Sir A. B. Lowry, C.B. (Chief Inspector)	
Mr. A. P. Hughes Gibb, O.B.E.	Beds., Berks., Northants., Oxon.
Mr. C. F. Roundell, C.B.E.	London, Middlesex, Herts.
Mr. G. R. Snowden	Kent, Hampshire, Sussex, Surrey.
Mr. W. D. Bushell	Cambs., Essex, Hunts., Norfolk, Suffolk.
Mr. R. H. A. G. Duff	Cornwall, Devon, Dorset, Somerset.
Mr. H. K. Nisbett, O.B.E.	Glos., Warwickshire, Wilts, Worcs.
Mr. W. P. Elias	Cheshire, Herefordshire, Salop, Staffs.
Mr. W. J. T. Turton	Derbyshire, Leicestershire, Lincs., Notts., Rutland.
Mr. C. J. Maslin, O.B.E.	Cumberland, Lancs., Westmorland.
Mr. A. G. Hayward, M.C.	Yorks (E. and W. Ridings).
Mr. N. B. Batterbury	Durham, Northumberland, Yorks (N. Riding).
Mr. J. Evans	Wales and Monmouthshire.

At the time of appointing the new inspectors the Grand Union Canal passed through sixty one District Councils shown in Figure 79.

Thomas Amos was now in his late 70's and having resided all his life in Stoke Bruerne Thomas and Henry Valentine were appointed Trustees of the United Parish Councils for Stoke Bruerne and Shutlanger[354]. In recent years at Roade Baptist Church Mr Amos had been assisted in his role as Church Secretary by his daughter, on nearing his 80th birthday he resigned from his position, although his daughter continued in the role for a short while. Mr Amos was appointed Life Deacon to the church in 1934, the congregation presented him with a Westminster chime clock in recognition of 52 year service as secretary and treasurer[355]. As Thomas's health began to fail a chance remark to his daughter Ellen, changed the course of [her] life … *it would be great work for you to look after the canal-boat people[356].* Chas and Ellen Ward returned to Stoke Bruerne, after which Ellen took over the care of her father from her sister, whilst Chas ran the Amos family business. As one boat woman recalled Mary's return to Stoke Bruerne was very welcomed …

> Mary had come home to nurse her father, Mr Aymus, now he was goin blind … her dad wasn't a lot of trouble, her husband was copin well with her Dad's shop, and her daughter

District Councils Through Which The Main Line Of The Grand Union Canal Passed 1930's to 1950's

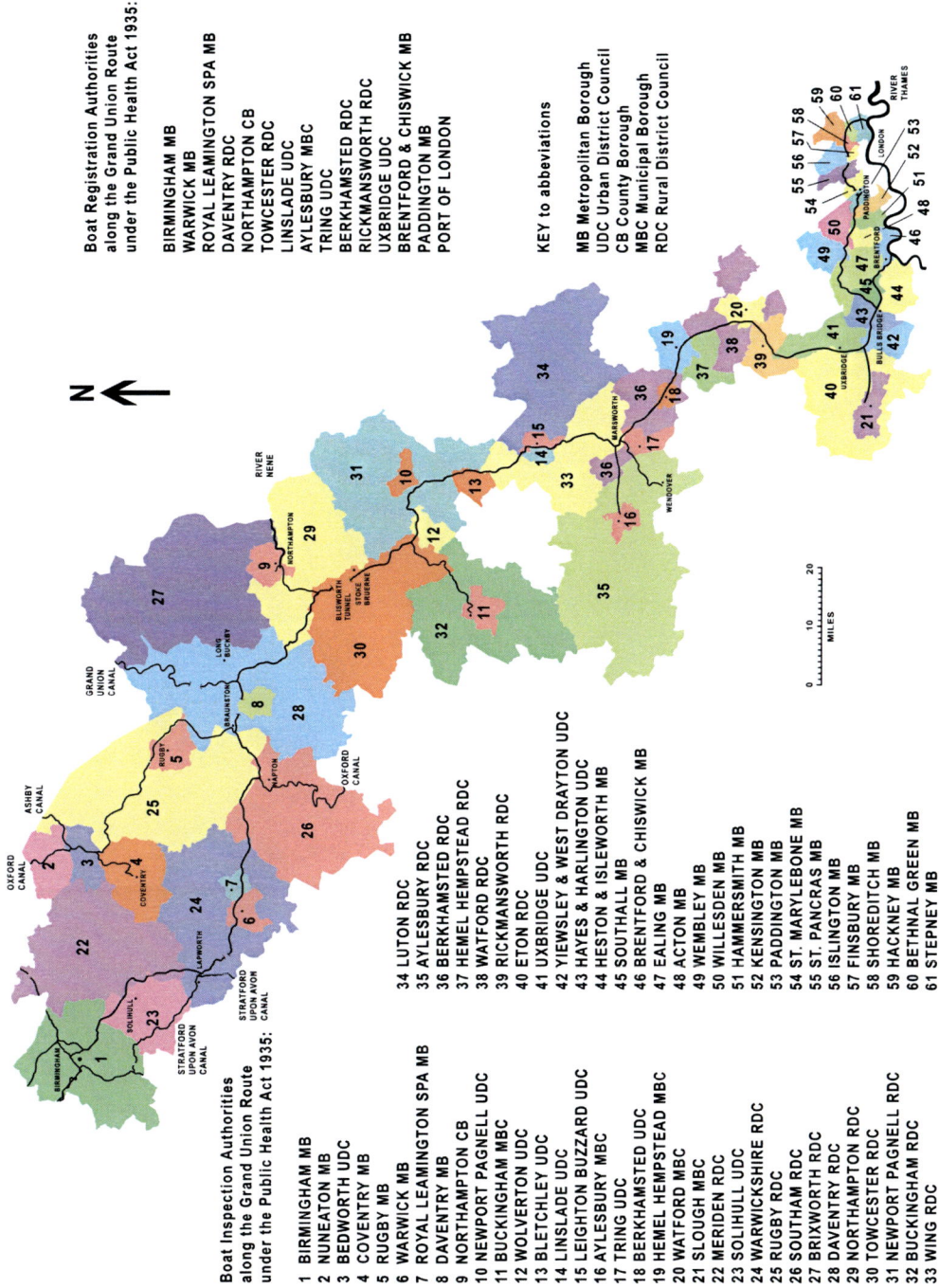

Boat Registration Authorities along the Grand Union Route under the Public Health Act 1935:

BIRMINGHAM MB
WARWICK MB
ROYAL LEAMINGTON SPA MB
DAVENTRY RDC
NORTHAMPTON CB
TOWCESTER RDC
LINSLADE UDC
AYLESBURY MBC
TRING UDC
BERKHAMSTED RDC
RICKMANSWORTH RDC
UXBRIDGE UDC
BRENTFORD & CHISWICK MB
PADDINGTON MB
PORT OF LONDON

KEY to abbreviations

MB Metropolitan Borough
UDC Urban District Council
CB County Borough
MBC Municipal Borough
RDC Rural District Council

Boat Inspection Authorities along the Grand Union Route under the Public Health Act 1935:

1 BIRMINGHAM MB
2 NUNEATON MB
3 BEDWORTH UDC
4 COVENTRY MB
5 RUGBY MB
6 WARWICK MB
7 ROYAL LEAMINGTON SPA MB
8 DAVENTRY MB
9 NORTHAMPTON CB
10 NEWPORT PAGNELL UDC
11 BUCKINGHAM MBC
12 WOLVERTON UDC
13 BLETCHLEY UDC
14 LINSLADE UDC
15 LEIGHTON BUZZARD UDC
16 AYLESBURY MBC
17 TRING UDC
18 BERKHAMSTED UDC
19 HEMEL HEMPSTEAD MBC
20 WATFORD MBC
21 SLOUGH MBC
22 MERIDEN RDC
23 SOLIHULL UDC
24 WARWICKSHIRE RDC
25 RUGBY RDC
26 SOUTHAM RDC
27 BRIXWORTH RDC
28 DAVENTRY RDC
29 NORTHAMPTON RDC
30 TOWCESTER RDC
31 NEWPORT PAGNELL RDC
32 BUCKINGHAM RDC
33 WING RDC
34 LUTON RDC
35 AYLESBURY RDC
36 BERKHAMSTED RDC
37 HEMEL HEMPSTEAD RDC
38 WATFORD RDC
39 RICKMANSWORTH RDC
40 ETON RDC
41 UXBRIDGE UDC
42 YIEWSLEY & WEST DRAYTON UDC
43 HAYES & HARLINGTON UDC
44 HESTON & ISLEWORTH MB
45 SOUTHALL MB
46 BRENTFORD & CHISWICK MB
47 EALING MB
48 ACTON MB
49 WEMBLEY MB
50 WILLESDEN MB
51 HAMMERSMITH MB
52 KENSINGTON MB
53 PADDINGTON MB
54 ST. MARYLEBONE MB
55 ST. PANCRAS MB
56 ISLINGTON MB
57 FINSBURY MB
58 SHOREDITCH MB
59 HACKNEY MB
60 BETHNAL GREEN MB
61 STEPNEY MB

Figure 79   District councils through which the main line of the Grand Union Canal passed 1930's-1950's (Christopher M Jones)

> was growed oop. Mary, bein used to havin her 'ands full of nursing, wanted more to do.
>
> The boat people are always turnin to you for help', her Dad sez. "You said yourself that the shop was full of wounded this morning. Why don't you turn the shop into a surgery and be a proper nurse to the boat people?" And that's just what Mary did[357].

Figure 80 shows one of the last pictures of Ellen with her father on the Buckingham Arm of the Grand Union Canal. Evidence survives in the form of a shop receipt to confirm Chas Ward was running the Amos shop in the mid 1930's, the receipt shows Chas's signature on a sale worth £121 16s 9d shown in Figure 81[358].

The receipt was analysed by Ken Sherwood, his account of this is reproduced in Figure 82 which gives an insight into the products Chas had on sale[359].

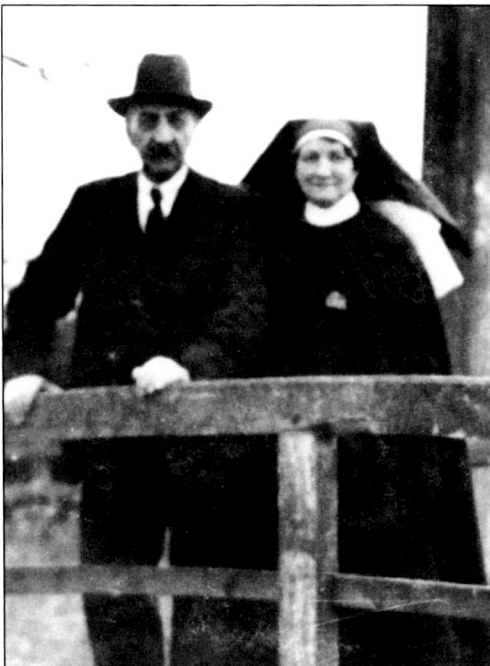

Figure 80 Thomas Amos with daughter Ellen Ward (Waterway's Archive)

~~RECEIPT AND PAYMENT BOOK~~ Page 4

~~the day of 19~~

Binder ~~PAYMENTS~~ Twine

ITEMS		£	s.	d.
		17	11	11
1¾ c Binder Twine	c 36/-	3	3	-
2½ c Hay Cord	c 34/-	4	5	-
5 Rolls Coir Yarn	c 1/6	-	7	6
4 Cotton Towing Ropes	c 20/-	4	-	-
6 Coir Scrubbers	c 18/-	5	-	-
2 Manila Towing Ropes	c 18/6	1	17	-
2 Up Hill Straps	c 6/6	-	13	-
2 x 4 gall Water Cans	c 8/6	-	17	-
3 x 3 gall do	c 7/6	1	2	6
		£38	16	11
	25% dis =	9	14	3
		£29	2	8
Net Price - cost				
82 do 2½ in Best Manila	c 32/-	1	3	3
26 ps 1½ " do	c 32/-		7	6
16 5ft 3½" Manila Rope	- 28/6	1	10	-
General List		£32	3	5
Grocery & Drapery Brought Over from other list		89	13	4
		£121	16	9

Signed Chas W. Ward
Sept 30th 1935

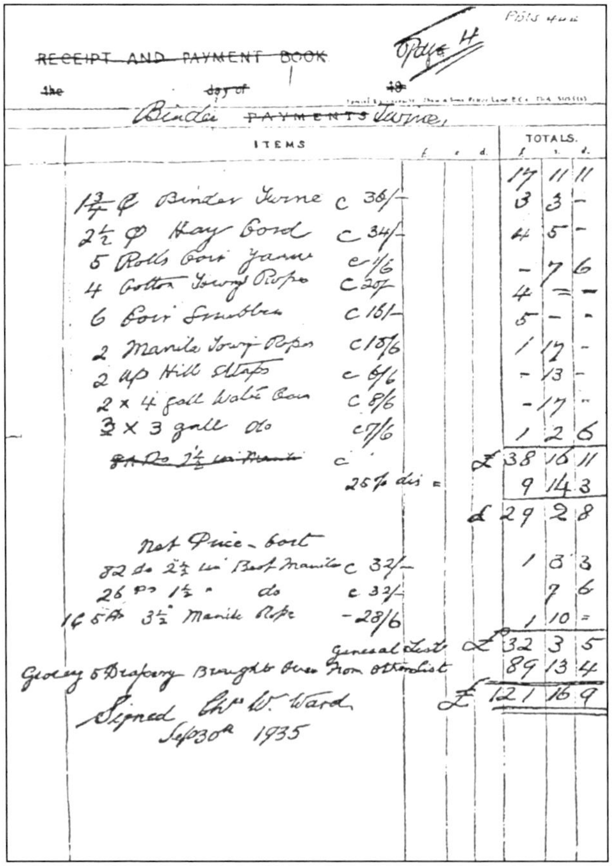

Figure 81 Chas Ward shop receipt (Ken Sherwood collection)

> **A note on the shop stock book**
> The entries in the shop stock book contain references to specific kinds of rope which had particular functions for the working boatmen.
> Straps were short lengths of rope, usually about 9 yds (8.23m) long. A 'short' strap was used to help a pair of boats negotiate locks, one end of the rope being attached to the T-head pin, or stud on the butty boat's deck and the other end looped and fastened to a hook at the stern end of the motor boat. As the motor entered the lock the loop was detached allowing the butty to swim in alongside. As it passed the motor the strap would be placed in the fore-end of the butty and then carefully reattached to the motor as it left the lock.
> Downhill and uphill straps were used, as these names suggest, when locking, and their main function was to stop and hold the boat in the lock. The looped end of the appropriate strap would be fastened to the stud on the boat and the other end wrapped around a stump or bollard 'on shore'.
> Snubbers were 70 ft (21.35m) long ropes, usually made of coconut fibre, and were used for towing the butty in long pounds. The reason for their great length was that the butty boat was kept clear of the wash from the propeller of the motor boat whilst the motor was well clear of the tow.
> Towing ropes were sometimes used as an alternative to short straps when locking. A long length of rope was carried from the motor boat through a series of running blocks along the length of the butty boat to the steering position at the stern end. As the motor boat left the lock the steerer on the butty would pay out the rope, gradually taking the strain with a turn on the T-stud until sufficient distance between the motor and the butty was achieved when a few more turns on the stud would secure the rope.

Figure 82   An interpretation of ropes and boaters (Ken Sherwood)

By the 1930's the motor boat was becoming more common on the Grand Union Canal. The dangers associated with this new form of canal boat propulsion stimulated the Ministry of Health in December 1934 to set up a committee on Canal Boat Regulations in response to *concerns regarding the effects on boaters health of the rising number of mechanically propelled crafts bringing about conditions not contemplated when the existing regulations were framed*[360]. This danger, together with other considerations led the committee to compare the design of the horse boat shown in Figure 83, with that of a motor boat shown in Figure 84[361]. The illustrations produced by the ministry show the side-elevation and plan view of a typical "Old Type Horse Drawn Narrow Barge" (sic), and a "New Type Mechanically Propelled Narrow Barge" (sic) dated June 1935. These two images clearly show the difference in shape between the horse or butty boat and the motor boat, with the propeller shaft from the engine to the propeller passing beneath the cabin floor of the living cabin, hence the cabin has been raised and the cabin sides made taller when compared with the butty. Some early examples of motor boats had the engine room aft of the living cabin, giving the latter more headroom inside, however this arrangement never caught on and most motor boats were arranged as shown[362].

The committee held eight meetings, during which they invited a number of expert witnesses, one of the experts was Mr Lesley Morton, manager of the Grand Union Canal Company fleet. The committee considered four main issues: 1) the *relative position of engine room and cabin, 2) the ventilation of engine-room, 3) the ventilation of cabin and, 4) the amount of cubic air space in cabin.* Regarding the diesel or semi-diesel type engine on canal boats the committee agreed …

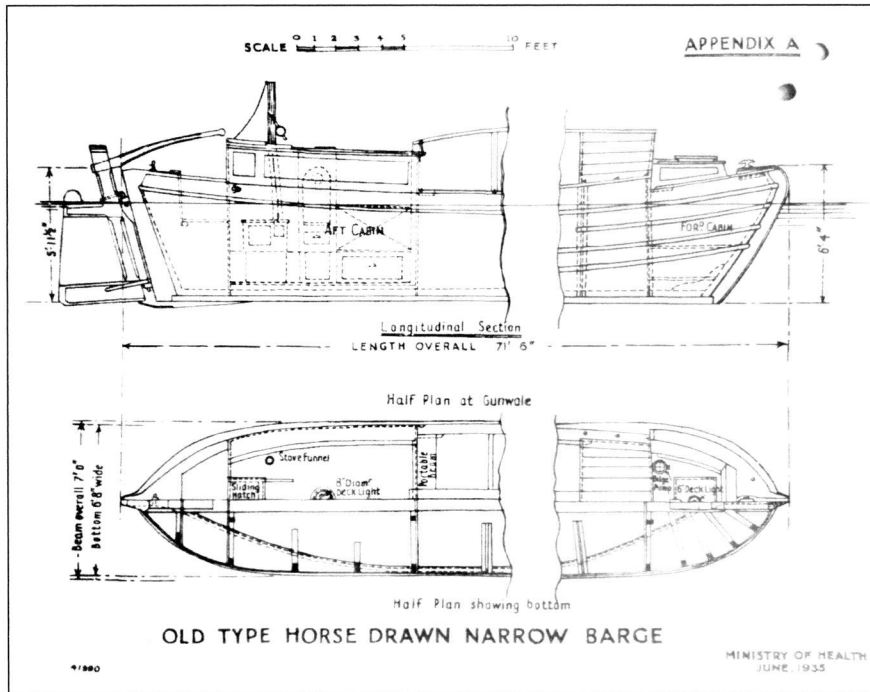

Figure 83   Horse Boat 1935 (Christopher M Jones Collection)

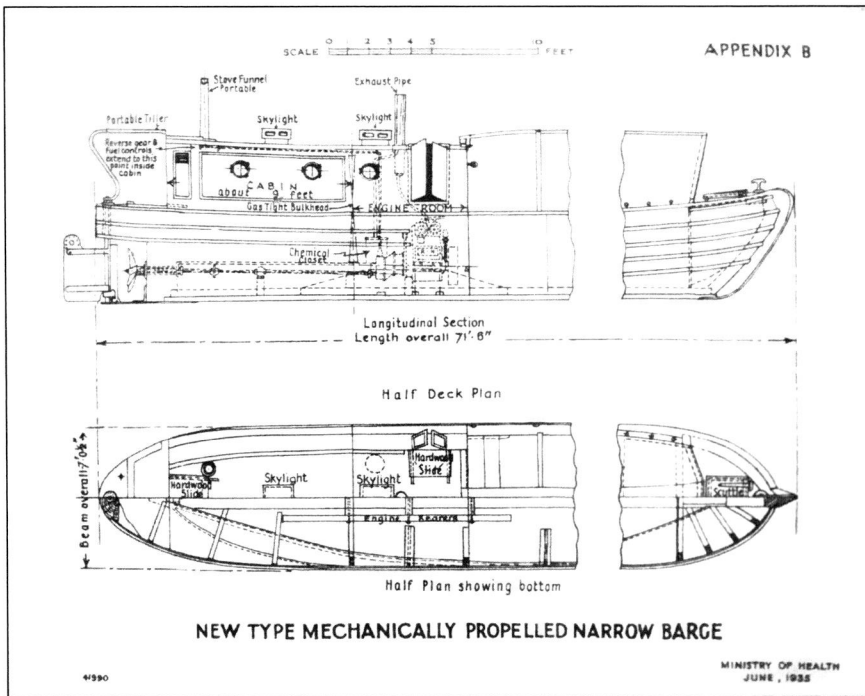

Figure 84   Motor Boat 1935 (Christopher M Jones Collection)

In our view the available evidence shows that there is danger to the health of the crews and families from the fumes from the engines if proper means are not taken to exclude such fumes from the living quarters ...

After the final meeting in June 1935, the committee issued an *Interim Report* due to the *seriousness of the identified problems to boaters health,* transcribed in Appendix 9. The report contained 28 points related to the original four issues (1-4 above), but, during the inquiries the committee added a further seven issues; *5) Lighting; 6) Fire extinguishers 7) Design of the main cabin 8) Use of the fore-cabin for sleeping arrangements; 9) Latrine accommodation; 10) Water supply; and 11) Oil wastes and bilge water.* In the final two points of the interim report the committee concluded ...

27. We do not suggest that the conclusions which we have reached should, for the present, form the subject of amending Regulations, particularly as we are impressed by the developments now taking place in the design of new boats. We are happy to record that many of the suggestions which we have made are being incorporated in many new boats now under construction.

28. We suggest, however, that the recommendations outlined in paragraphs [...] of this Interim report should be embodied in a memorandum to be sent to owners, designers, builders, canal companies, etc.

> We have the honour to be Sir,
>
> Your obedient Servants,
>
> Ministry of Health, Whitehall, S.W.1,
>
> 21st June 1935.

The memorandum referred to in Point 28 was issued as a CIRCULAR by the Ministry of Health in August 1935[363].

Sister Mary's surgery becomes established ...

There are no records to verify when Sister Mary was appointed *Consultant Nurse to Long Distance Boat families* by the Grand Junction Canal Carrying Company, as shown on her calling card in Figure 85. It is possible the investigation into canal boat regulations and the subsequent issuing of the Ministry of Health Circular / Recommendations to Canal Companies led Mr Lesley Morton, fleet manager for the Grand Union Canal Carrying Company to employ Nurse Ward on a contractual basis, as this was a period when Industrial Health was becoming increasingly recognised as everybody's business[364]. The first entry regarding a boaters' care

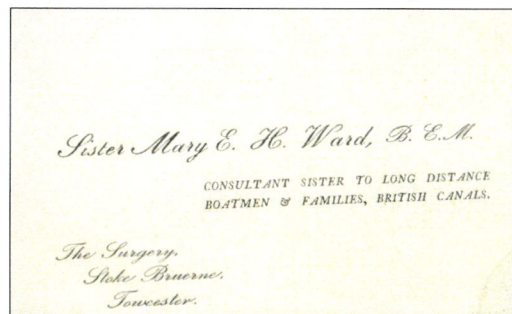

Figure 85   Sister Mary's calling card
(Waterway's Archive)

by Sister Mary in Stoke Bruerne is recorded in the *surgery dressing book* she brought with her from Earls Barton, dated April 10th 1936. The patient was a boat woman who presented with an *ulcerated leg,* Sister Mary cleaned and dressed the wound that day, and on a number of other occasions when the boat tied up in Stoke Bruerne. This arrangement continued for the next three months, by which time a note in Sister Mary's case book indicates the wound required only a *dry dressing.*

After Ellen and Chas returned to Stoke Bruerne Thomas Amos began to withdraw from public duties in 1936, resigning his position as trustee to two of the Stoke Bruerne charities for the poor; The Thomas Kingston Charity and the Bozenhoe Charity[365]. That same year Thomas saw the Grand Union Canal Carrying Company tunnel tug service withdrawn as a result of the rapid expansion of motor propulsion replacing horse boats, after which the remaining horse drawn boats would pass through Blisworth Tunnel either by *begging a tow* from a motor boat or by the time honoured tradition *legging*. A typical scene in Stoke Bruerne where boats are tied up outside the mill is shown in Figure 86. The 1930's and 40's saw many new narrow boats passing Stoke Bruerne after creation of the Grand Union Canal Carrying Company, as can be seen here with two pairs of their boats moored against the former mill. But as this might be seen as a new beginning it was at a time of increasing neglect of the canal as is evident here above and below the water level. The tow path is unkempt and reeds grow on the opposite bank whilst the boats cannot be tied-up directly against the tow path due to lack of maintenance.

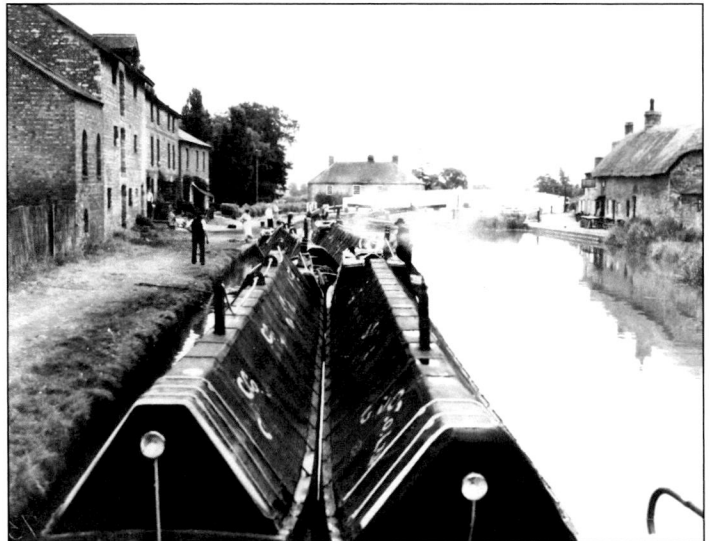

Figure 86   Boats moored beside mill building Stoke Bruerne (Waterway's archive)

As the surgery became established entries in the case book show Sister Mary consulted with, and physically examined boater's in her boatmans surgery (in the Amos family home), or in the boater's home (the narrow-boat back cabin). Sister Mary's nursing assessments included: Taking a medical history from the boater; *where necessary* measuring a boaters temperature and pulse; asked about the boater's bowel activity; assessing the condition of the skin (including wounds), enquired about the boater's general and emotional well-being, and in some cases testing a boater's urine. The frequency of boater's visits to Sister Mary depended on their presenting complaint / condition and her nursing assessment. Some attended on only one occasion, whilst others were visited in their home (the back cabin) up to four times a day after she *laid them up* due to an acute illness or injury. This would allow Sister Mary to monitor a boaters condition closely, give treatment on a regular basis, and for her to re-assess if the situation was improving or deteriorating.

Dispensing was part of Sister Mary's role, each time a medicine or treatment was given to a boater the name(s) and quantities dispensed (or dressing materials used) were noted in the case book using the abbreviations of traditional apothecaries weights and measures. Sister Mary's dispensing role was diverse, including; Mixtures, tablets, throat spray and wound products. From her *Surgery Account Ordering Inventory* the surgery was stocked with a comprehensive range of products; Gamgee Tissue, White Lint, Cotton Wool (best and swabs), Bandages (different sizes), Elastoplast (different sizes), Dressing strips, Jaconet, Boric lint, Iodine gauze, Sterile gauze, Triangular bandage, Absorbent wool, Zinc oxide strapping (different sizes), Sofra Tulle, Kaolin poultice, Thermometers, Rubber catheters, Dr's forceps, Feeding cup, Labels, Rubber gloves, Johnsons (Soap , Powder, Cream), Dettol and Dressing scissors.

In the first eight months of opening the surgery Sister Mary treated an every increasing number of boaters, as shown in her case book entries from April to August 1936. Some boaters presenting with long-standing, poorly managed but non-urgent conditions, on the other hand the case book shows some boaters arrived who Sister Mary deemed *serious / urgent* cases, often following an accident or injury[366]. The first record of Sister Mary detaining a pair of boats occurred almost immediately after the surgery opened, when a Captain arrived with *Tonsillitis and Congestion of the lungs* and a *temperature of 102.4 and a pulse of 100*. She immediately detained the boats for seven days during which Sister Mary visited the boat twice daily, only allowing the Captain to leave a week later when his temperature was recorded as normal.

It wasn't long before Sister Mary had cause to write to a boaters employer, the first letter was to Mr Richards at the Ovaltine Works in Kings Langley, which she sent as a result of an accident to one of the company's boaters children, a young boy who acquired an injury on the boat. On numerous occasions Sister Mary wrote to toll clerk Mr Ernest Veater at Hawkesbury Junction[367], who early in 1936 was offered a job by the Grand Union Canal Carrying Company, running their Hawkesbury office as Midland District Representative, which he accepted in February that year, effectively the company poached Mr Veater from the Oxford Canal Company. This was the same year the 1936 Public Health Act came into force, Part X Canal Boats, Section 251: repealed the Canal Boats Act of 1877 and 1884, thus commenced a new era of regulation[368].

As the first winter arrived when the surgery was open, the winter weather brought with it some serious respiratory conditions for boaters, as one case study illustrates in Table 27. Sister Mary was called to a boat that arrived in Stoke Bruerne late on a Sunday evening. The Captain had acute bronchitis, a raised temperature and some difficulties breathing, the boats were detained and Sister Mary kept a close watch on the Captain. Next morning Sister Mary called for the Doctor from Roade who admitted the man to Northampton Infirmary with *patches of pneumonia.*

After 48 hours in hospital, and what the Captain believed was an improvement in his condition, he discharged himself as noted by Sister Mary *left hospital own accord*.

Table 27   Captain presenting with respiratory problems (Case book extract)

Nov 21	(Saturday)
	Called at 8.30pm to patient. Examined. Acute Bronchitis.
	Some tubular breathing.
	Temp 104. Pulse 66. Resp 48. ? pulse rate
	Administered Mist Brom. MXX.ag
	Ordered: Milk & water
	            Chicken broth
	            Soda water & milk
	            Water
	            Egg & Milk

Nov 22nd	(Sunday) PT. appears easier Respiration less laboureds Temp 99.2 Pulse 77. Resp. 26 Complains pain in head & back of neck. Also difficult to breathe. Called Dr. Wharton of Roade Northants Ex. Diagnosis = acute bronchitis, patches of pneumonia Ordered pt to hospital. 4.30 Pt hospital 5.10 arrives hospital … admitted Compton Ward … left fairly comfortable
Nov 23rd	PT. fairly comfortable. PM.
Nov 24th	PT. Left Hospital own accord

In 1937 Chas Ward was becoming established in the village, having been elected to the Parish Council in the march and by the October he was serving on the Rating Authority committee[369], as well as attended Roade Baptist Church Fireside Club[370]. Although Thomas Amos's health was failing and his eyesight deteriorating he would have seen the Grand Union Canal Carrying Company new boats as they passed through top lock with their improved design features[371], and their change of livery to Red, White and Blue for the coronation shown in Figure 87. Thomas would also have been pleased when the same year the Grand Union Canal Carrying Company in conjunction with the Transport and General Workers Union issued a *Constitution*[372] transcribed in Appendix 10, which aimed to secure improved relations between employer and employee, and certainly went some way towards improving boaters well-being.

A number of events occurred in Stoke Bruerne in 1937. An unknown writer (L.D.)[373] made a trip on the Grand Union Canal, in many way's similar to that of Hassell in 1819 and George Smith in 1880. The writer travelled on *The Thaethon* which had been loaded at Brentford with timber for Birmingham, the Master being William Fradley accompanied by his wife, we pick up the story as the family and their visitor near Stoke Bruerne …

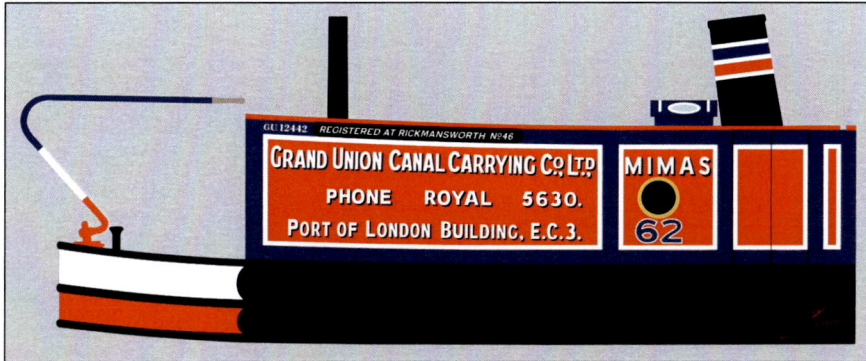

Figure 87   Grand Union Canal Carrying Company red, white and blue coronation livery
(Christopher M Jones)

We crossed the Tove – Towcester's river- which is siphoned underneath the canal … Came Stoke Bruerne with a glimpse of the busy Northampton-Stony Stratford road, a series of locks, and the long metal pipe line along the bank recalling the fierce drought of 1934, when water brought down by the locks had to be pumped back to the higher levels at a cost throughout the system of thousands of pounds.

At Stoke Bruerne we rise 52 feet in seven locks, Master Fradley taking his boats into some of the locks on the shorter stretches already locked side by side. They slide gently in, the distance judged to an inch. Bicycles are much in evidence. Every boat has one for its "advance guard". How the old hands must have shaken their heads at the appearance of the first towing path bicycle!

The women work as hard as the men on the canal and it came as no surprise to see sturdy bronzed girls cycling along the tow path with windlass slung behind them in leather belt, ready to work the next lock.

Picturesque Stoke Bruerne.

At the last of the Stoke Bruerne locks we see the bridge that once carried two streams of water, flowing through two lines of locks. One arch is now closed. Beneath the other sits young Northamptonshire, fascinated, as all boys are, by the passing barge. In front, Stoke Bruerne, poplars seemed higher than ever as we look up from the lower reach.

Once in the top lock we rise slowly to find ourselves level with the row of cottages in which that well-known Northamptonshire character, Mr T Amos, has carried on business for so many years. Many a stout rope has he turned out in the rope walk he once carried on there.

Swift on the charming old-world village of Stoke Bruerne, which lies half above and half below the canal, comes one of the most fascinating yet eerie experiences the Grand Union has to offer – Blisworth Tunnel whose dark and narrow shaft runs for a mile and three quarters through the earth. It is an unforgettable journey. Even when travelling at only five miles an hour one seems plunged into darkness within a few yards of entering.

In December a boater's wedding took place at Saint Mary's in Stoke Bruerne. The bride, young Mrs Sarah Franks, whose first husband fell from his boat and drowned at Slough a few years earlier, married Mr William Henry Blakeman, son of Walter and Mrs Blakeman who live canal-side at Stoke Bruerne. After the wedding the couple seen on the *good ship Coniston* in Figure 88, spent their honeymoon boating to Nuneaton *for a load of coal*[374].

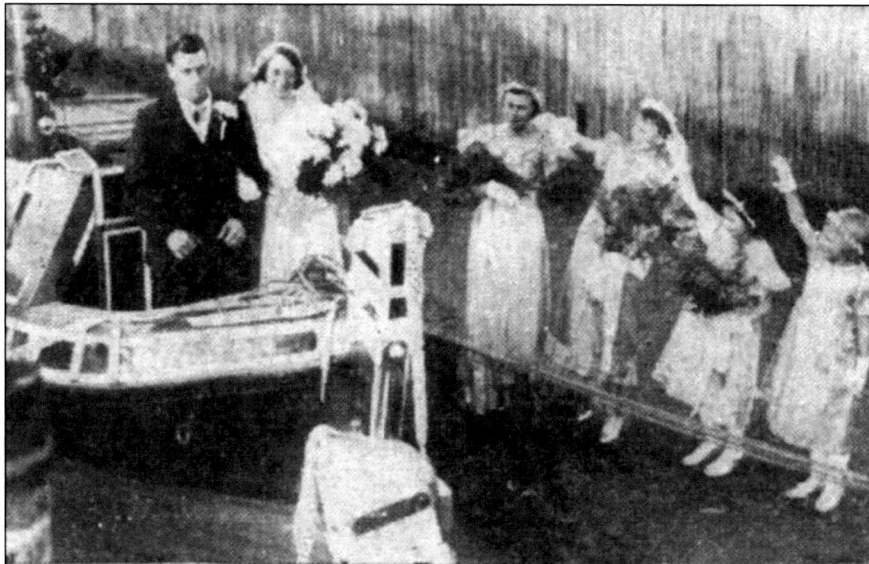

Figure 88   Bride and groom on *Coniston* with bridesmaids 1937 (Northampton Mercury)

Thomas Amos died in his canal-side home of almost 85 years on June 28th 1938. Son-in-law Chas Ward was by his side, the death was announced in the local paper[375];

> Mr Thomas Amos, a county magistrate, well-known in non-conformist and local government circles in Northamptonshire, died on Tuesday at his home at Stoke Bruerne. Aged 84, he had been ailing for some time. He was returned to the Northamptonshire County Council for the Blisworth division in 1919 and remained a member until he retired in January 1929, owing to ill-health and increasing age.

> For many years Mr. Amos carried on business as a rope and twine manufacturer at the canal side, Stoke Bruerne, where he was owner of cottages referred to by Mr A. P. Herbert in his novel, "Water Gypsies". He was an active leader in the Baptist Church, Roade, and a former president of the Blisworth and District Sunday School Union.

> He was a good tenor singer, and for nearly 60 years he was among the singers at the Blisworth and District Sunday School and Choir Union festival. He was formerly a rate collector for Stoke Bruerne and clerk to the parish council. At one period he was postmaster for the village. He was assistant overseer for the poor of Stoke Bruerne for many years and was a canal boat inspector under the Towcester Rural District Council.

The funeral was held at Roade Baptist Church *where he had been secretary and treasurer for over 50 years,* son-in-law Rev. A.E. Boyce of the Leysian Mission, London, assisted by the Rev. B. Reed (minister of Roade and Blisworth Baptist Church) and the Rev. A.W. Bagnall (superintendent of Towcester Methodist Circuit) officiated. The funeral was attended by family mourners from all over the country and *a representative of the Mayor of Northampton, Councillor W. H. Percival, in his capacity as clerk to Towcester Bench[376].* Probate was settled on March 6th 1939, Thomas's effects of £522 10s 11d were shared equally between his three son-in-laws; Francis Campbell Grant, Salesman; Arthur Ernest Boyce, Dissenting Minister; and Charles William Ward, shopkeeper.

The Amos's canal-side shop was according to Tom Rolt open when he passed through Stoke Bruerne during his journey along the Grand Union Canal. Tom Rolt must have visited the shop because he provided a first-hand account of it in *Narrow Boat* …

Interesting and unique though the Buckby shop undoubtedly is, it does not compare in attraction or variety of stock with another canal shop I knew of at Stoke Bruerne, sixteen miles south. It was one of a row of thatched stone cottages along the tow path, and its' cool, stone-flagged interior boasted so varied a stock as to call to mind the proud boast of Fleckers' Merchant Grocer at the Gate of the Moon:

We have rose-candy, we have spikenard,
Mastick and Terebinth and oil and spice
And such jams meticulously jarred
As God's own prophet eats in paradise

This shop specialised in ropes and lines. Coils of every thickness and quality, from coarsest manilla to finest white cotton, lay piled on the floor or hung from the low, whitewashed rafters of the ceiling. Yet this was only the principal item of a stock that catered for the boat family's every need. Here was a great basket full of crusty cottages loaves, there shelves of tea, jams and other groceries were crowded between piles of crockery, fat earthenware teapots and pendant festoons of hurricane lamps, kettles and saucepans.

For the ailing there were herbal remedics, salves, liniments and pills a-plenty; clay pipes, shag tobacco, braces and boots for the menfolk; aprons, buttons, hairpins and combs for their wives; while for the children there were liquorice bootlaces, sherbet suckers and great glass jars filled with enticing, gaudy-coloured sweets, bulls-eyes, aniseed balls and gob-stoppers. In the heyday of the horse-boat the shop was well placed, for the southern entrance of Blisworth Tunnel was visible from the threshold, and the tunnel tug had a well-chosen mooring before the door of the inn opposite[377]

At some point Chas Ward moved the Amos business to a building next to Lock 15, formerly occupied by Mr Cakebread the village stonemason, the move allowed Sister Mary to expand the surgery as one boat woman recalled …

Her husband moved the shop down to just below Top-Lock and they turned their front room into a spotless surgery where we could go to her for free and have treatment. For years she looked after us out of her own pocket. Later the Grand Union made her 'Sister' Mary and helped out with cost of materials[378] …

After the death of her father Sister Mary expanded the boatman's surgery. Sister Mary was by now in contact with a significant number of boaters,although from the beginning of opening her canal side service she was keen to acknowledge how resourceful boaters were in managing their own care in times off need, as demonstrated by a boat woman interviewed by Sheila Stewart who recounted an example of the floating populations resourcefulness in times of need, which Sister Mary endorsed …

About ADA

[she] had a quiet strength about her that made you feel she knowed wat's best. It was Ada I turned to when my arm swelled black and blue with poison. She worked out a tiny bit of Zebo polish got into sore crack of thumb when blacki-leadin my range.

Lead travelled to a big lump under my arm. Ada drawed the poison by poulticin my thumb with bread and boiled sugar, over and over. Agony it was, but she made me bear it. It done the trick, saved my arm. She made me go to Mary Wards when we got to Stoke Bruin, just to make sure it was all cured. Mary said Ada had probably saved my life[379].

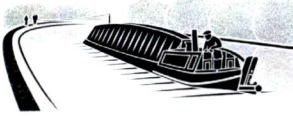

Sister Mary, World War II and boating on the Grand Union Canal

World War II commenced on September 3rd 1939, Stoke Bruerne was very different on this day than when the first World War began as indicated in a local trade directory; Rev., Newton was resident at Saint Mary the Blessed Virgin, Dr Clements from Blisworth held a surgery on Tuesday and Friday afternoons in the village, only two lock-keepers were employed by the Grand Union Canal Carrying Company (Reginald Fuller and Alfred Judge), there were two independent bakers (Willie Sarrington and Horace Ayres) and one grocer (Chas Smart). The post-mistress was Mrs Florence May Green[380], although the Boat Inn remained in the ownership of a member of the Woodward Family (Emily).

Stoke Bruerne prepared for war as did other villages and towns in England. A requirement of the Civil Defence Committee was for local councils to set up *Emergency Committees* with responsibility for three types of local First Aid Centres;

First Aid Points … to deal with simple First Aid and minor injuries, those expected to be treated here were able to get there themselves.

First Aid Posts … staffed by Doctors and one other medically qualified person, with facilities to treat people affected by gas. Ambulances delivered patients if they were not too seriously ill to go to hospital.

First Aid Depots … where ambulances and first aiders operated. *First Aid Parties* consisting of a driver and a group of first aiders.

Sister Mary with husband Chas set up a *First Aid Point* at their canalside home, installing the iconic red cross first aid point sign on the front of the house signifying the Ward's role in *planning for war* shown in Figure 89. Just after was broke out, South Northamptonshire suffered a severe storm bringing with it three

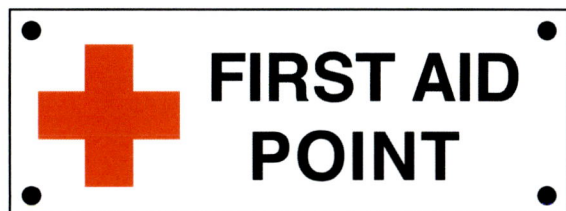

Figure 89   First Aid Point sign (Christopher M Jones)

161

inches of rain in 24 hours. Outside the Ward's home as the canal overflowed, water cascaded down the alley between the Ward's home and the rented cottages causing the cellar to flood. During the war Chas Ward served on Stoke Bruerne Parish Council, although for part of 1941 he was unable to attend meetings due to an accident[381]. In addition to providing the First Aid Point, Sister Mary organised the village youth into a team of firewatchers and auxiliary fire fighters[382]. On one occasion they had a serious *call to action* when the Rectory Roof caught fire, the event was recounted by Eric Smith a member of the firefighting team …

> I was about 15 years old and Sister Ward took up fire-fighting … it was during WWII she rounded up about a dozen village boys to form a volunteer fire brigade and once a week in her back garden taught us how to put out fires … We were called out when the rectory roof caught fire. It was a bit difficult because at the time the rectory was full of home guard ammunition. Sister Ward took charge in full uniform, directing operations from half way up a ladder. We soon got the fire out thanks to her[383].

The Ward's were also responsible for maintaining a number of inventories[384] throughout the war, extracts from these show each Stoke resident was allocated a number (1-79), with the numbers being used in each inventory to indicate who was allocated to specific roles in a number of Home Front groups, formed to manage the effects of war in the village. Table 28 shows members of the Stoke Bruerne Fire, Home Guard, First Aid and French Digging groups as of September 1942. The Ward's also maintained inventories related to the availability of *Transport Tools* and *General Equipment* in the village The transport tools inventory shown in Table 29 includes seven households with bicycles, the Tyrell family having four bicycles at their disposal, the village also had one motorcycle owned by Mr Parks. As well as monitoring transport tools, the Ward's kept a detailed inventory on the availability of more general equipment, ranging from blankets to wheelbarrows shown in Table 30.

Table 28   Inventory of Services **Stoke Bruerne September 1942**

Services: Stoke Bruerne
September 1942

FIRE		Home Guard Casualties etc		First Aid		French Digging	
1	Gardner	1	Gardner	2	Parke (Mrs)	2	Parke (Mr)
13	Bushel	2	Parke	12	Peppercorn Miss	44	Sturgess Charles
16	Tew Frank	4	Fuller	24	Miss King	53	Derry George
21	Valentine Edward	12	Newton Rev	42	Cooper (Mrs)	64	Ray Sow Thomas
29	Boffin John	16	Tew F	43	Hancock (Mrs)	77	Eyer Wm
59	Abbott William	17	Sturgess W	53	Derry (Mrs)	79	Stockwin P W
63	Smith Frank	35	Divey H	59	Abbott (Mrs)	79	Ward Peter
64	Ray Sow	42	Cooper	70	Wilcox (Mrs)	79	Stockwin C D

69	Cleaver Tom	43	Hancock	74	Jelly (Mrs)
77	Eyer William Jun	45	Dyke		Ayres
45	Dyke R S	58	Butler		Adkins
2	Parke	60	Johnson		Crofts
4	Fuller Reginald (Mrs)	69	Cleaver		Ward (Sister)
12	Hope (Miss)	72	Peabody		Wright
13	Bushel (Mrs)	77	Eyer	64	Ray Sow
16	Tew Frank (Mrs)		Ward		
17	Sturgess (Mrs)	79	Stockwin P W		
24	King (Miss)				
35	Divey H (Mrs)				
42	Cooper (Mrs)				
58	Butler (Mrs)				
60	Johnson (Mrs)				
60	Jackson (Miss)				
63	Smith Wm (Mrs)				
69	Cleaver Chas (Mrs)				
77	Eyer Wm (June) (Mrs)				
79	Stockwin (Gap) (Mrs)				

Table 29   Inventory of Transport Tools **available in Stoke Bruerne September 1942**

Transport Tools: Stoke Bruerne
September 1942

	Name	Cycle	Motor Cycle	Spade/ Shovel	Picks	Ladders	Axes	Buckets	Crowbar
2	Parks L G	3	1	3	1	1	1	3	1
8	Harris Harry					1	1	2	1
12	Newton Rev.			2	1	2	2	2	
13	Bushell H W			2	1	1	1	2	1
16	Tew Frank			1	1	1			
17	Sturgess W	1		1				2	
21	Valentin Frank			1	1			2	1
29	Boffin Victor			2	1		1		1
34	King Constance			1				2	

No.	Name								
35	Divey Kate (H)							1	
37	Woodward Emily			2		2			
42	Cooper Evelyn							3	
43	Hancock George							2	
45	Dyke Sudbury	2							
46	Tyrell Harry	4		3				2	
56	Butler R W	1							
63	Smith William			3		2	1	2	
69	Cleaver Charles	1		4			1	2	
72	Pebody Phyllis		1 Horse	1		2	1	2	
73	Lay Harry				1		1	1	
77	Eyer William	2		2	1	2		3	
83	Ward Charles W			3	1	3	4	6	2

Table 30   Inventory of General Equipment available in Stoke Bruerne September 1942

General Equipment: Stoke Bruerne
September 1942

	Name	Oil Stoves	Kettles	Blankets	Sheets	Pillows	Beds	Stirrup Pump	Wheelbarrow	Motor Car	Lamps
2	Parks L G	1	2	4	6						
8	Harris Harry		2								1
12	Newton Rev.	1	1	3	2	2	2	1	1	1	2
13	Bushell H W		1				1				1
16	Tew Frank		1					1			1
17	Sturgess W	1	1						1		
21	Valentin Frank								1		
29	Boffin Victor								1		
34	King Constance	1	1	2	2	2			1		1
35	Divey Kate (H)	1	1								1
37	Woodward Emily								1		
42	Cooper Evelyn	2	1	2		2	1				1
43	Hancock George								1		
45	Dyke Sudbury										
46	Tyrell Harry								1		

56	Butler R W			1		1	1		1		
63	Smith William		2						1		
69	Cleaver Charles								1	1	
72	Pebody Phyllis	1		4	4	4	2				
73	Lay Harry			2	4						
77	Eyer William	1	1						1		
83	Ward Charles W	3	4	4	4	4	2		1		

Sister Mary became Air Raid Precautions (A.R.P.) Warden, which required her to make sure everyone in the village followed the black-out rules, which she did by touring the village after dark, making sure no lights were visible. In October 1939 Towcester's general response to the *Defense Lighting Restrictions* were said to be good when the first two cases in breach of the restrictions were heard in the Division. One of the people brought before the bench was Phyllis Emma Peabody of Chapel-lane, Stoke Bruerne, during the hearing it came to light Mrs Peabody had been warned before of her breach of the restrictions. The bench found her guilty and imposed a fine of 10s, the Chairman intimating future fines would be more seriously dealt with[385]. From entries in Stoke Bruerne Primary School log book, Sister Mary's ARP role also included visiting the primary school *to inspect gas masks*[386].

The residents of Stoke Bruerne with those from the nearby hamlet Shutlanger formed the 13th Battalion of the Northamptonshire Home Guard, pictured in Figure 90 outside the rectory. Chas Ward joined the battalion at the age of 75, on *joining up* he was featured in uniform in the local newspaper shown in Figure 91, accompanied by the headline *oldest soldier in the British Army…*

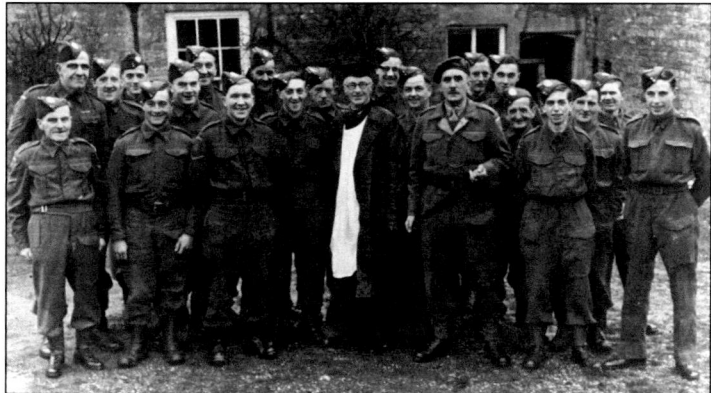

Figure 90   13th Battalion of the Home Guard (Christine Statham collection)

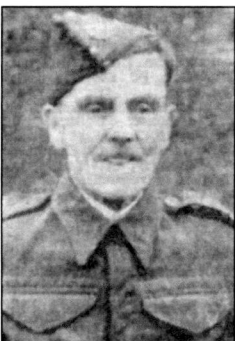

Because he is only five feet tall he was denied the ambition of his youth and early manhood of joining the Forces – until the Home Guard was merged into the Army. As Stoke Bruerne resident, he has performed orderly and clerical duties, first for the L.D.V. and then for the Home Guard[387].

Figure 91   Charles Ward. Oldest soldier in the British Army (Northampton Mercury)

The War and the Waterway's ...

On the outbreak of war railway-owned canals came immediately under the control of the Ministry of Transport, whilst independent canals remaining for the time being on their own.[388] For boaters working on the canals their role became a *reserve occupation*, although some boater's voluntarily *joined up* few were *called up* for military service. Some boaters left the canal as a result of the 1939-40 winter frost whilst others left to work in factories. The exodus of regular boaters meant canal carriers were beginning to be faced with an increasing shortage of experienced boatmen, creating a problem whereby their boats were lying idle at depots. Some canal companies tried to counteract this by commencing boat training schemes for men, a more detailed account of conditions related to boaters during the war is included in Appendix 11.

Wartime cargoes passing along the Grand Union Canal included coal to destinations in Hertfordshire and further south to Middlesex and West London, as well as ferrous and non-ferrous metals from London docks to the Midlands, and other metals like aluminium and spelter (a zinc alloy) needed to keep the government war machine going. Beer, notably Guinness was carried during the war from their brewery near London to Birmingham, as well as grain, cement, tubes, iron forgings, bricks, sugar and other foodstuffs like cocoa beans, and many other types of goods, including ordnance for the war effort. The general decline in canal carrying since World War One became more apparent in the early years of World War Two. The nationwide demand for coal created delays getting boats loaded at various collieries, which wasn't helped by antiquated loading facilities. This combined with the difficulty finding men to load and unload boats at their destinations, resulted in some canalside mills and factories not getting all their coal requirements by boat. Some tried to import fuel from other sources by rail or road at much greater cost, however not everyone could do this resulting in several firms closing down.

The war conditions specific to the canals meant bombing raids were sometimes successful at stopping traffic due to breaches in canal banks and damage to locks. At vulnerable points along the canal such as aqueducts and embankments, stop planks were inserted at certain times in case of bomb attacks, to preserve water supplies should they be hit, which inevitably delayed traffic. The risk of bombing was most acute in large cities such as Birmingham, Coventry and London, especially in the docks, and boaters with families aboard visiting those places were risking not only their own lives, but there children too. Boats also had to travel under blackout conditions like everyone else in Britain, which was not too much of a problem on a bright moonlit night, but the boaters skills were tested during dark nights and bad weather. At various places concrete Pill Boxes were constructed near the canal as a defensive measure in case of invasion[389].

The canal network was brought under government control on July 1st 1940, and a canal (defence) advisory committee was set up to advise the Ministry of Transport on the best use of inland waterways during the war, one of the difficulties they identified from the outset was *the inability of canal companies to work together.* At the beginning of November 1941 boatmen went on strike for a week, exacerbating the problem of keeping traffic moving. The following month 66 year old Brigadier-General Sir Henry Osborne Mance KBE, CB, CMG, DSO was appointed Director of Canals, his credentials included a distinguished background in international transport[390]. A Central Canal Committee with six regional canal committees was formed during the war, listed in Figure 92.

London: based on the Grand Union and the Lea, with its headquarters in London
North-East: based on the Aire and Calder system, with headquarters in Leeds.
North-West: based on the Leeds and Liverpool and Bridgewater Canals and the River Weaver, with headquarters at Manchester.
East Midlands: based on the Trent, with its headquarters at Nottingham.
West Midlands: based on the Birmingham Navigations, with its headquarters at Birmingham. and
South-Western: based on the Severn, with its headquarters at Gloucester.

Figure 92   Six regional Canal Committee's World War II

During the war fore-cabins continued to be used as dwellings on canal boats, Figure 94 shows a cut-a-way view of a typical narrow boat fore-cabin, inside is a bench for sleeping on and a stove, access was through a sliding hatch in the roof. The use of fore-cabins as places to sleep came to the forefront of towpath news in April 1941 when Mrs Beechy found her 13 year old daughter Susan Agnes dead, her other daughter Clara unconscious and the family dog dead in the fore-cabin of *Gifford,* a Thomas Clayton (Oldbury) Ltd boat. Sisters Agnes and Clara had been seen the night before on the towpath *laughing and full of life* by a number of boaters[391]. The Beechy's younger sons usually slept in the fore-cabin, but because the

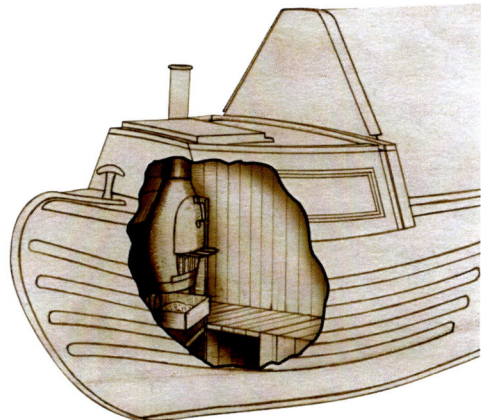

Figure 94   Fore-cabin with stove (Christopher M Jones)

family were due to move off early the next morning, the boys slept with their parents in the back cabin. It was a cold night when the girls went to bed so the stove was on and the *slide shut.* At the inquest it was announced Agnes died from *asphyxiation due to carbon monoxide poisoning from the forecabin stove,* her younger sister Clara survived. After the tragedy the family removed the fore-cabin stove and never used it again as a dwelling[392].

Agnes' death led to the Ministry of Health's Chief Inspector, Mr A M Legge to write to Colonel Forrester Clayton J.P., and Chairman of the National Association of Canal Carriers. The letter re-kindled discussion on the recommendations which had previously been distributed to canal companies etc. by the Ministry of Health on the use of fore-cabin's as dwellings …

Dear Colonel Clayton[393]

Arising out of the death of Agnes Beechy in April you were good enough to come and see some of us here who are concerned with living conditions on canal boats, and tell us about the condition and equipment of the boat "Gifford", and generally about the fitting of fore-cabins with stoves.

I should begin this letter by saying that there has been no suggestion that and Company or any individual was to blame for the occurrence or that the boat was otherwise than of standard type as registered and in proper order; and so far as we are able to discover no previous similar occurrence has been recorded or known with the exception of an apparently similar case at Stafford at the end of October last; also that we recognize the traditional habits and ways of boat folk. Nevertheless the incidents have caused us great concern and we think it very important that any lesson that is to be learnt from them should be studied and conveyed to both owners and masters so that any possibility of recurrence may be prevented. We feel sure that your Association and owners generally will agree.

It seems to us that your Association will prefer themselves in the first instance to consider the lessons that are to be drawn and the most effective precautions, and that we should best help by drawing attention to the dangerous combination of circumstances, although these are well enough known from comparable fatalities ashore. Where there is a fire burning (and a low fire is more dangerous than a blazing one) in a very small enclosed space with a minimum of ventilation and the minimum of draft given by a mere opening or a short funnel leading from a stove, dangerous conditions are produced.

I think that, although the considerations then in mind were different ones and the present times may be less appropriate to underline the point, I ought to put it on record that in a Memorandum prepared in 1935 and communicated to your Association it was observed that the Ministry had come to the conclusion that the fore-cabin had disadvantages as a sleeping cabin and that it was recommended that in designing new boats the fore-cabin should be replaced by a compartment for Stores.

> Yours sincerely,
>
> A.M. Legge.

In response to Mr Legge's letter Forrester Clayton agreed to raise the matter with the National Association of Canal Carriers, although in concluding his reply he stated … *I cannot agree your last paragraph with reference to the fore cabin*[394]. Mr Legge replied explaining his position …

Dear Colonel Clayton,

Thank you very much for your letter of 9th June with reference to the death of Agnes Beechy.

I may say that I did not really suppose that you would agree to the last paragraph about the forecabin, but we felt that when we were writing to you on this case we could hardly make reference to our previous considered opinion about the use of the forecabins for sleeping; we who saw you and concocted that letter were the remains of the Committee which considered canal boat conditions some years ago and evolved the suggestions set out in the 1936 memorandum. You will have noticed that in writing to you I was careful to say that previous opinion had nothing whatsoever to do with such a risk as this one from carbon monoxide poisoning, and, of course, I did not wish to imply that we were seeking to use this new lever to press you to accept the old recommendations.

As a matter of history that recommendation about the use of forecabins was just a recommendation. I think it is likely that if the War had not come we should have prepared a revision of the old Canal Boats Regulations (as indeed the Public Health Act, 1936, seems to require us to) and it might or might not have been that we should have put something in about forecabins. I cannot say whether we should have or not for it would obviously have had to be considered very carefully here, but in any case the Regulations in the draft stage would, no doubt, have been communicated to the Associations at any time, for their reactions following the usual practice of the Ministry.

This re-drafting question is certainly in cold storage for the duration, for I cannot conceive such a matter being taken up now. It seems too remote to envisage the possibility that if canal transport booms and is developed and expanded for was purposes to such an extent that new fleets of boats are created wholesale we might be reluctant to miss the opportunity of trying to effect any practicable modifications of canal boat design. Even the very mention of such a possibility is purely a personal and impromptu speculation of my own at the moment and has nothing whatever behind it.

I feel that this is a very long and probably unnecessary reply to your simple observation at the end of your letter, but I am very anxious that our passing reference to the former recommendation should not be taken for more than it was. We are now concerned with the prevention of similar fatalities. If, subsequently we were to feel justified in regulating the use of forecabins or even abolishing them as such, as I have said, we should first consider the matter very carefully before we altered the law and consult your Association and the other Association on the proposals.

Yours very truly,

A.M. Legge[395].

During the early war years 32 year old mother of two, Mrs Mollie Traill, daughter of retired Major General Harvey [RAMC] and wife of Commander Thomas Cathcart Traill, OBE, was *doing her bit for the war effort* cargo carrying on the Worcester and Birmingham Canal with Daphne March on the narrow boat *Heather Bell*[396]. Whilst crewing *Heather Bell* Mollie was working on a training scheme *whereby other girls could become canal boatwomen*[397], and most probably due to her "connections" she visited the Ministry of War Transport to discuss the scheme, which the

Ministry showed great interest in[398] In march 1941 Eily Gayford joined the *Heather Bell*, but due to being unwell towards the end of the summer Molly[399] left the boat to take a nursing job in Edinburgh.

Not long after Mollie left for Edinburgh, the first meeting of the Central Canal Committee took place (September 1941) at Berkley Square House, chaired by the Parliamentary Secretary Col the Rt Hon J J Llewellin from the Ministry of War Transport and attended by a range of officials shown in Figure 93.

Present :-

Col. The Rt.Hon. J.J. Llewellin, (Chairman)	Parliamentary Secretary, Ministry of War Transport.
Mr R.H. Hill	}Ministry of War Transport.
Mr S.W. Nelson	}
Mr H.B. Emley	Chairman, N.E. Regional Canal Committee.
Mr R. Davidson	Chairman, N.W. Regional Canal Committee.
Lt. Col. F. Rayner	Chairman, E.M. Regional Canal Committee.
Mr. P. Nadin	Chairman, W.M. Regional Canal Committee.
Mr. A.C. Lisle	Chairman, S.W. Regional Canal Committee.
Mr. S.R. Hobday	Chairman, London. Regional Canal Committee.
Mr. M. Kissane	Canal Association
Col. Forrester Clayton	}
Mr. J. Ironmonger	}National Association of Canal Carriers
Mr. J.C. Wood	}
Mr. F.G. Thomas (for Mr. Walley)	Ministry of Labour & National Service
Mr. D.W. Milford	Transport & General Workers' Union

(Mr. E.R. Batten – Secretary)

In Attendance :-

Mr. Frank Pick	}Ministry of War Transport.
}	
Mr. A.M. Rake	
Mr. A.J. Thurston	Ministry of Food
Dr W.A. Robson	Mines Department
Major R.L. Drage	Ministry of Supply
Mr. D.C.K. McCullouch	Railway Executive Committee

Figure 93   Officials present at the first Canal Control Committee

One of the first items the committee discussed was *Food For Canal Workers*, who alongside canal maintenance workers were experiencing *difficulties accessing adequate food*. The committee agreed to a number of points to deal with the difficulties[400]…

i.   Employers should be authorised to maintain shops or stores at suitable points, and to sell rationed and unrationed foods to their employees

    AGREED that application for authority will be made to local Food Committees by Employers where these facilities are desired and that Mr. Thurston will arrange for these Committees to be asked to give favourable consideration to such applications.

ii. Employers should be enabled to obtain "iron rations" (e.g. tinned meat and tinned milk) to be stocked in boats to meet cases of unforeseen enforced absence.

iii. The additional cheese ration (8oz. per week) should be made available for canal boatmen and maintenance men.

After Mollie Traill moved to Edinburgh, Sgt Nelson from the Ministry of War Transport wrote to Daphne March informing her that Mr Moll, the fleet manager for the Grand Union Canal Carrying Company was interested in Mrs Traill's women's training scheme, and made a request that *if you could train and recommend to them someone to act as a trainer of women on the Grand Union Canal, they would certainly like to give the thing a trial*[401]. Miss March in her reply indicated *the only two people [she knew] who could do this [were] Mrs Traill and [herself]*, Daphne also conveyed the information to Mollie[402]. Ten days later Mollie met Sgt Nelson, at the meeting she agreed to the scheme *after [she'd] served a certain time in her employment*[403]. Sgt Nelson confirmed this in writing to the GUCCCo, concluding his reply *I should imagine nursing was quite as hard work as canal barging*[404]. Mr Miller met with Daphne and Mollie and it was agreed in the new year Molly and Eily (Kit) would *do a trip with a pair of boats with regular boaters and learn the route and manage a pair*[405], due to bad weather the maiden trip was delayed till Monday 16th February.

Mollie and Kit were allocated to Mr and Mrs Sibley who crewed the Grand Union Canal Carrying Company pair *Edgware* and *Purley*, the Sibley's on *Purley* and the trainees crewing *Edgware*. Early into the trip they experienced 10 days when the *ice froze the cut,* once thawed they proceeded north to the seven uphill locks at Stoke Bruerne, on their arrival at top-lock they met Sister Mary for the first time …

    … we learnt from Ciss that it was a great landmark for the boaters as it was here that Sister Mary lived … Her house was right on the lock side, and on that day there were three pairs of boats tied up along the towpath … On one, someone was due to have a baby; in another, someone had a bad leg which needed frequent dressings; and the third was locked up as the boatman had had to go to hospital and his wife had gone to stay with her parents. We gathered that this Sister Mary was a great character and that the boaters thought the world of her. She apparently knew them all, and a lot of their mums and dads before them, so she had their complete confidence and trust[406].

Mollie and Kit despite *experienced bugs in the boat* returned to the GUCCCo depot, and immediately put it to Mr Wood they *needed a pair of boats of their own*, without dispute Mr Wood allocated *Bainton* and *Sulby* [sic], and on April 1st they set off with their first trainees Vivian and Rosheen. The boatwomen's training scheme with it's associated training documents developed by Mollie[407] was now up and running on the Grand Union Canal.

Sister Mary's canal-side surgery

Boater's went back and forth along the Grand Union Canal throughout the war years, many regularly stopping at Stoke Bruerne to visit Sister Mary. Although employed by the Grand Union Canal Carrying Company, Sister Mary did not confine her nursing services to the company crews, as the case books show she treated the Ovaltine Boat families , Fellows, Morton and Clayton crews as well as a number of independent carrier families. The surgery was at the start of war well established, and very well equipped as shown in Figure 95. On closer examination the image shows the *Pride of the Valley: First Aid Point* sign hanging above the dressing bench. *Pride of the Valley* was the name her mother gave to the temperance meeting place she set up in her first home after her marriage to Thomas. Sister Mary is

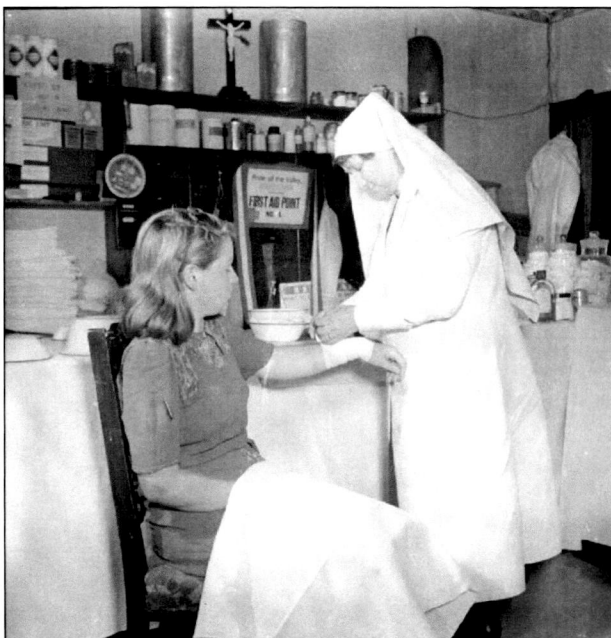

Figure 95   Sister Mary in her *Pride of the Valley* surgery

wearing a white starched full length coat as she treats Violet Wise, daughter of a canal boatman who crushed her arm when the family motor boat and butty entered a lock.

Sister Mary was well qualified to use the title *First Aid Point*, because she was an appointed lecturer for St. John Ambulance Nursing Division. Since November 1940 she had been teaching the children of Stoke Bruerne elementary school in preparation for their preliminary St John Ambulance examination. When all the children passed their exam a local celebration was held where the Rector presented each child with a certificate and a medal[408].

Boater's called at Sister Mary's surgery for many reasons, sometimes arriving in need of urgent treatment due to an acute illness, or following an accident, although on some occasions boater's *called in* after suffering from an illness or injury because they delayed seeking medical attention in preference for seeing Sister Mary. Some boater's had long-standing medical conditions and were on Sister Mary's books for a while, visiting the surgery regularly for either a check up or ongoing treatment, particularly wound care. The diversity of Sister Mary's nursing work with the floating population can be seen from her meticulously maintained Case Books, taking 1943, a mid World War II year shows the diversity and details of her work with boaters[409]. Although to get a complete picture of the first boater Sister Mary cared for in 1943, we need to wind back to the morning of Tuesday December 29th.

On the Tuesday morning of a typical week for Sister Mary a boat arrived in Stoke Bruerne, the captain visited the surgery and asked Sister Mary to see his seven month pregnant wife. She visited the boatwoman in the back-cabin, where she found her *very distressed, in shock and debilitated, pain in back and legs, pale and sweating profusely.* Sister Mary immediately detained the family and visited the woman morning and evening till new year's day. The woman had been assaulted at Fenny Stratford, as revealed from handwritten notes attached to a page of the case book where Sister Mary recorded her actions after visiting the boatwoman. The first note is a record of a telephone call to the police station reporting the incident to an officer … *two of your men boarded a boat […] at The Lock, Fenny Stratford on Monday Dec 28th 1942 without the permission of Mr […] Captain, that after questioning Mrs […], one of the men called […] examined this woman's breasts and abdomen.* At the end of the note Sister Mary recorded she asked the sergeant *Is this within the rights of a P.C. without a doctor present ?* The second document is a copy of a letter she sent to the Police Sergeant, and a clear example of Sister Mary's response to a social injustice to a boatwoman …

> please send this man [….] to me as soon as possible … I require an assurance such a thing will not happen again. Mrs […] is confined to bed suffering from shock as well as delaying an important cargo
>
> Mary E.H. Ward. Con Sister.

Boaters regularly sought care for *chest problems*; bronchitis, acute influenza, congestion of the lungs and pleurisy, common conditions in the boating population which had not gone unnoticed by the medical profession. Dr Dearden, Medical Officer for the Port of Manchester having noted *the weakness of the chests of people who lived-in* [boat cabins], he went on to acknowledged *the liability of the boatman to fatal accident … alone did not account for 'his extraordinarily high position' (above farm labourers and fisherman) in the mortality table,* which caused him to conclude *What really appears to carry him off is his liability to pneumonia and other respiratory diseases*[410].

In 1943 Sister Mary cared for many boaters with problems related to their teeth before and after dental extraction, often noting in the case book next to a boater's name; six teeth need extracting, four teeth extracted, treated boater for tonsillitis (due bad teeth), oral infection (poor state of teeth). There is nothing surprising about this aspect of Sister Mary's work because during World War II the labouring populations poor dental health was highlighted by the British Dental Association who found 97% of army recruits were *not meeting required dental standards,* furthermore greater than half of all mothers who required dental treatment only a quarter completed the treatment, with a further quarter refusing to attend a dentist[411].

Throughout 1943 Sister Mary detained boats in Stoke Bruerne. The length of stay ranged from overnight to an exceptional twenty seven days, the reason for *laying up* a boat family are outlined in Table 31, which shows two families were *laid up* on more than one occasion this year. The first was due to a Captain having *carbuncles,* which Sister Mary initially managed for five days, improving enough for the boats to be allowed to *move on.* One month later the boater visited the surgery again as the carbuncles had returned, requiring a further four days treatment in Stoke Bruerne. A more severe case arrived early in the morning on March 21st , after the boats tied up Sister Mary was called to see the boatwoman who she found had shingles and bronchitis, Sister Mary recorded her temperature at 104.4, pulse 120 and respirations 26, as all the observations were abnormal and the woman very unwell the family were immediately detained and the boatwoman ordered to *rest in bed.* Sister Mary visited the boatwoman on numerous occasions to administer medications and to check her observations, shown in Table 32, by day ten the observations were improved enough for Sister Mary to allow the family to proceed on their journey. One week later the family returned and the woman visited the surgery, Sister Mary recorded her observations as normal, and on examining the shingles scabs she noted *drying up and very itchy* she also made a note *naturally weak, continue with mixture.*

Table 31   Boats laid up in Stoke Bruerne for treatment by Sister Mary 1943

Days Laid-up	Month	Family Member	Reason
6	Dec-Jan	Wife	Weary and in shock due to an incident at Fenny Stratford
7	Jan	Wife	Acute influenza, swollen legs and anaemia. Elevated temperature and pulse
4	Jan	Wife	Rheumatism
		Son	Wound to hand
6	March	Wife	Influenza with bronchitis
		Child	Burn to leg
12	Mar-Apr	Wife	Shingles and Bronchitis
7	Nov-Dec	Captain and Wife	Bronchitis with complications
8	June	Wife	Accident with towing rope, also seven months pregnant
4	Sept	?	Acute influenza and constipation
5	July	Captain	Carbuncle Right axilla, swollen arm and chesty (wife wrongly dressed)
4	August	Captain	Return of carbuncles, very poorly
14	August	Captain	Carbuncle arm, excised and plugged
27	Aug-Sept	Wife	Thumb and arm inflamed and discharging pus, hospitalised for nine days
		Captain	Ulcerated legs

10	August	Captain	Acute tonsillitis and pain +++ in kidneys
10	Sept	Baby	Northampton Infirmary for an operation to remove a scalp nevus
		Wife	Tonsillitis and carbuncle face
		Captain	Bronchial catarrh, investigate for suspected tuberculosis (Northampton Infirmary)
5	Nov-Dec	Captain and Wife	Bronchitis due to influenza
		Wife	Ulcerated legs

Table 32   Observations of a woman laid up with Shingles and Bronchitis 1943

Day	Visit	Temperature	Pulse	Respirations
Sunday		104.4	120	26
Monday	am	102.2	116	22
Tuesday	am	103	118	24
	pm	103.2	116	22
Wednesday	am	100.6	110	20
	pm	101.4	114	20
Thursday	am	100	108	18
	pm	101.2	110	22
Friday	am	100	109	20
	pm	100.4	112	22
Saturday	am	99.2	106	20
	pm	100.2	112	18
Sunday	am	98.8	104	16
	pm	99.6	100	18
Monday	am	98.6	92	16
	pm	99.4	96	18
Tuesday	am	98.4	84	16
	pm	98.8	90	18
Wednesday	am	98.4	80	16

The boat family detained in Stoke Bruerne during August and September for 27 days (Table 31) was an exceptional case for Sister Mary. The boatwoman was early into her pregnancy and presented on August 6th with a *hard, swollen hand and arm and very sodden thumb,* the woman telling Sister Mary it was *due to a wood splinter.* Without delay Sister Mary called the Doctor who prescribed the *application of poultices,* which were very effective because the following day *foul smelling pus was pouring out of tip.* For the next four days twice daily wound care was given, by the fifth day the wound was ready for excision, and Sister Mary escorted the boatwoman to

Northampton Hospital where she underwent *surgery under gas*. The boatwoman was detained in hospital for eight days, Sister Mary visited every day but one. Whilst his wife was in hospital the Captain remained in Stoke Bruerne to allow Sister Mary to treat his *ulcerated leg*. On being discharged from hospital Sister Mary treated the Captain and his wife, only allowing them to move off on September 2nd after which they returned weekly for wound care.

Sister Mary regularly dealt with boaters as a result of accidents acquired during the course of their work, data related to boater's treated as a result of an accident in 1943 are shown in Table 33. The nature of boating accidents ranged from a child falling in the canal, to the most severe case seen in a boatwoman who arrived in Stoke Bruerne at 7.10 am Monday June 14th. On the previous day the boatwoman was *tangled with the towing rope* causing a *wound round thigh and leg (popliteal space), lacerations and burns to the leg* she was *in shock* and *seven months pregnant*. Sister Mary cleaned and dressed the wounds, and visited two more times that first morning, twice in the afternoon and again in the evening. The family were detained for seven days and on leaving Stoke Bruerne Sister Mary supplied the woman with enough dressings for seven days, instructions on how to dress the wound, and orders to revisit her on the return trip.

Table 33   Treatment of boaters as a result of accidents and injuries 1943

Injured Boater	Accident	Treatment
Daughter	Fallen in canal	Bed for three days
Woman	Severe strain of foot muscle	Advised needs an x ray Bandaged foot Foot somewhat deformed due to use before healed
Pregnant woman	Towing rope around thigh and leg (popliteal space) leg burned in several places, patient in shock and seven months pregnant.	Laid up for eight days. Dressings twice daily … then daily.
Child	Accident reported 1 week ago (Dr from Berkhampsted in attendance)	Wound care
Man	Patient fell from middle gangway plank into bottom of boat (plank rotten and broke right across)	Dressing Report to Hawkesbury Stop Instructed to have x ray Seen by Dr Baird
Woman	Wood splinter to thumb	Compress / poultice / dressings Seen by Doctor in Stoke Bruerne Hospital: Thumb incised under gas and a drainage plug fitted Laid up Dressings daily
Woman	Accident boats	Dressing

| Woman | Leg wound and bruising due crushed by boat | Dressing |
| Woman | Injury to patella | Dry dressing, padded, firmly bandaged |

During the war Susan Woolfit, one of the all women boat crews visited Sister Mary as a result of an injury …

> Sometime during that day I had pulled a muscle in my middle which worried me a bit. It caught me when I was pulling up the paddles … When I told Kit about the muscle … she exclaimed: Well, you have timed that beautifully! Now you can go and see Sister Mary: she lives at the top of Stoke … I was not at all sure that I wanted to be looked at by Sister Mary and asked anxiously who she was.
>
> She is the boaters' Nurse … she lives in a little cottage at the top here and anyone who is ill goes and asks her help. When the boaters' wives have their babies, they always tie up here so that Sister Mary can come to them and for ordinary illness they try to get up here before they have to knock off. If you see boats tied up here in the day-time you may be sure someone is ill, or else it's a baby.
>
> We had no sooner got into the top lock that Kit sent me off to Sister Mary, the first cottage on the right. Apprehensively I knocked. Come in, come in! I shan't be a moment, called a voice … walked into the cleanest room I have ever been in in my life. Everything seemed to be white; the chairs were draped in it, and the muslin curtains were tied up with bandages. All round the walls were hung First Aid charts and diagrams of the human body. At that moment in floated Sister Mary, I say "floated" because, with her white veil steaming behind, she did not look as if she was in need of any other form of propulsion. I was led next door into her sitting-room, which I took to be a mark of special favour, and a clean snowy sheet was spread on the sofa for me.
>
> But, Sister Mary, I can't lie on that…I'm filthy, I protested, but she would not listen and soon I was stretched in all my boat grease and dirt on that virgin surface. She prodded and pummelled me and finally announced that there was nothing the matter with me, nothing serious … only a pulled muscle. No paddles for three days, said Sister Mary firmly, and feet up whenever you can. Kit popped her head round the door at this point and caught the last remark. She was given minute instructions for seeing that I did as I was told and, with many thanks and a fond farewell on both sides … I saw Sister Mary on several later occasions, but I never needed to consult her again. If I had, I should have done so with perfect confidence. She knows her stuff all right and knew very well what kind of strains we were up against. The boat people trust her implicitly; I have often heard them say: I'll ask the nurse when we get to Stoke. She'll know, she'll tell me what to do[412].

At some point after the tragic death of his wife[413] Dr Joseph William Baird, who Sister Mary worked for prior to opening the canal-side surgery retired from his General Practice in Earls Barton and moved to a rented cottage in Stoke Bruerne. Figure 96 shows Dr Baird playing chess with Sister Mary in her front room. Sister Mary referred boaters to Doctor Baird and other medical practitioners for a range of reasons outlined in Table 34, sometimes this was because a boater had travelled a long distance with a serious medical problem to specifically see Sister Mary. Medical practitioners regularly conveyed information and instructions back to Sister Mary after seeing a boater which enabled her to ensure a boater's care was continued. On occasions boater's with severe medical conditions were transferred immediately to Northampton General Hospital, although on some occasions Sister

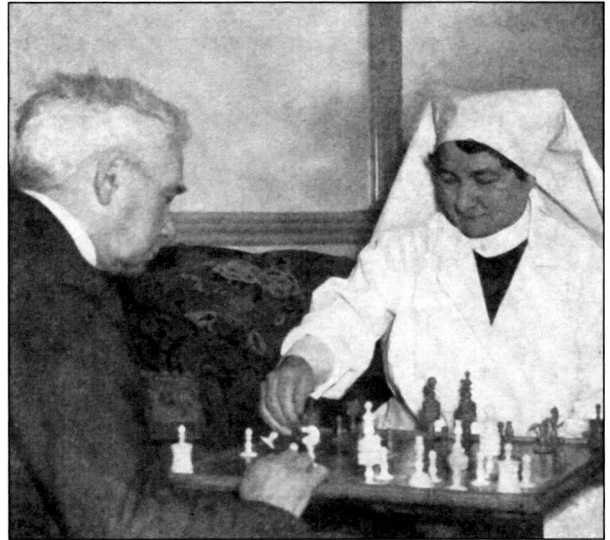

Figure 96   Sister Mary and Dr Joseph Baird playing chess (Della Sadler-Moore collection)

Mary's records show she advised *hospital case* next to a boater's name, the boater went against this advice by refusing admission, as can be seen in the case of one boatwoman. A pair of boats arrived in November 1943, the boatwoman visited Sister Mary who noted in red *? Ringworm*, she was advised of the need to see a dermatologist but refused. The boatwoman's condition worsened and later agreed to visit the skin hospital, where Ringworm was confirmed as *severe*. The dermatologist sent Sister Mary a detailed letter with instructions about *painting the affected areas, precautions for preventing spread to others in the family* and the *wearing of cotton gloves*, the consultant concluded by requesting Sister Mary provide him with *regular updates on the womans progress*.

Table 34   Referral of boaters to medical practitioners 1943

Patient	Reason for referral	Referral to	Outcome
Wife	5 months pregnant, sciatica.	Doctor	2 weeks later hospitalised
Woman	Pregnancy	Doctor and Nurse at Braunston	Arrange confinement
Woman	Suspected Ringworm	Skin hospital	Hospital confirmed suspected diagnosis.
Woman	Nervous debility due menopause	Doctor	
Wife	Boater poorly each time seen by Sister Mary (March to May) patient refuses hospital referral in april … Sister Mary reports this to doctor. June advised boater they should go to hospital … this continues.	Doctor Hospital	On-going patient deterioration. Hospitalised during September …

Woman	Accident	Doctor at Southall for certificate	Cared for at Stoke Bruerne
Man	Accident to foot	Dr Baird	
2 week old baby	Umbilical cord not off.		
Very tight	Midwife and Doctor		
Woman	Inflamed thumb, hand, arm	Doctor Hospital Doctor	Compress / poultice Excision under gas
Baby	Nevus of scalp	Hospital	Surgery
Man	Bronchial catarrh	Doctor	Refer for TB assessment Northampton Hospital
Woman	Pregnant – no dates given	Sent for assessment at Southall	Ante natal report conveyed to Sister Mary
Man	Leg discharging	Arranged hospital appointment	

Another boatwoman who Sister Mary had been monitoring and who had been seen by the Doctor in Stoke Bruerne on several occasions was advised by both she required *hospital treatment,* she refused and *boated on.* In July Sister Mary was *not satisfied with patients condition,* although she noted the woman *says much better.* The following month the boats arrived and on visiting the boatwoman Sister Mary immediately admitted her to Northampton General Hospital for *observation and surgical treatment,* the woman underwent surgery after which Sister Mary visited daily. On being discharged Sister Mary collected the woman by taxi and returned her to her *fathers home by the canal to recuperate,* on October 6th the boatwoman returned to the canal and on seeing the woman Sister Mary recorded *patient very cheerful.*

Children and babies were an integral part of the family boats, parents visiting Sister Mary due to their child being ill or injured, on some occasions mother's bought their children to have a *general check up.* Children were often seen when they were suffering with common childhood infectious diseases: a girl with measles, two girls with chickenpox and a boy with mumps. A small number of babies were seen who were teething, and a few children with tonsillitis. One small child had a *septic insect bite* which Sister Mary cleaned and dressed and supplied the parents with additional dressings. On one occasion a girl aged three years three month was brought to the surgery with a burnt leg, the family were detained for five days to allow Sister Mary to dress the wounds twice a day. The wounds were *healing well* before the boats were allowed to depart, upon which Sister Mary supplied the mother with dressings and instructions on wound care, they returned a fortnight later and *all well.* On one particular occasion Sister Mary was checking the wellbeing of a two week old baby and found the *umbilical cord not off and very tight* which was referred to the local Midwife and Doctor who both attended.

During the war Sister Mary's deep sense of compassion is seen in a letter to Isaac and Eliza Merchant, written after the loss of their daughter Brenda[414] …

Stoke Bruerne

Towcester

June 10 1944

My dear Mr & Mrs Merchant,

Will you please accept my deepest Sympathy --- you know how grieved I am to learn of our darling Brenda's passing, she was always an Angel, so sweet & lovely; no need to say I too loved her, but she was too beautiful for this world, 'God' Knew & he took her to be the little angel I had always called her, you I know will both be so lonely without her, but remember one day, none of us know how soon, you will meet Brenda again - no sin or trouble can ever hurt her now.

God bless you both & help you

Yours sincerely

Friend

Sister Ward

The management of wounds was by far the most regular aspect of Sister Mary's work, she assessed, cleansed and dressed many different kinds and severity of wounds; *long standing leg ulcers, burns, septic insect bites, lacerations, infected fingers and thumbs*, sometimes due to the severity of a boaters wound they were delayed in Stoke Bruerne to allow Sister Mary to *work her magic*. From a picture taken in the war of the interior of the boatman's surgery shown in Figure 97, Sister Mary's wound care procedures were performed using military precision. Sister Mary is working by paraffin lamp, dressed in a white coat, arranging sterilized kidney dishes on a dressing table covered with white cotton sheets, to the rear of the image are glass jars containing gauze and cotton wool swabs. Sister Mary is preparing to perform an aseptic (no touch) technique on a boaters wound, meticulous precautions which would prevent the spread of infection. The sterility of her surgical instruments and wound care products, alongside her meticulous aseptic dressing techniques were essential as antibiotics were not yet available to the general population[415].

Prime Minister Winston Churchill benefited from Penicillin in December 1943 when he visited the 8th army in North Africa. Churchill whilst in North Africa developed pneumonia, his

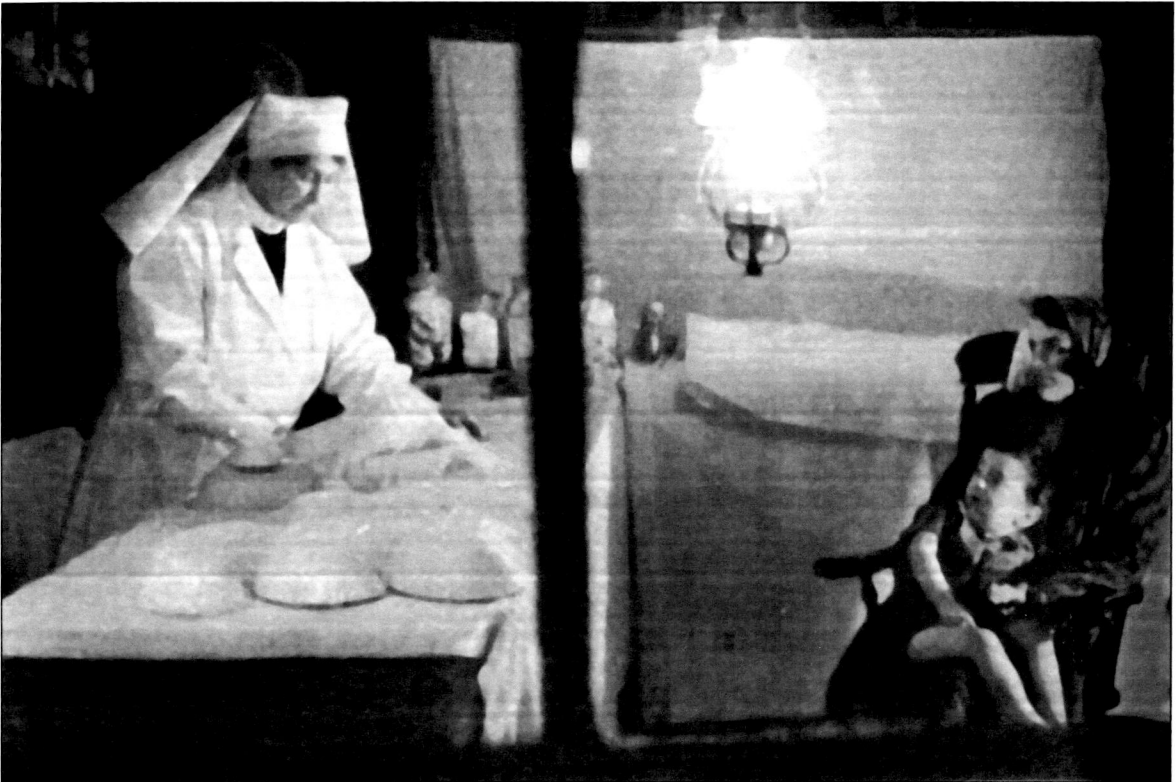

Figure 97   Military precision by paraffin lamp (Della Sadler-Moore collection)

recovery was attributed to the administration of penicillin, after which it was described as *positive proof the drug could work miracles*[416]. Penicillin subsequently became known as *the wonder drug*, due to the enormous beneficial effect on military personnels recovery and survival[417]. In 1943 the Ministry of Health sent a small supply of penicillin to hospitals across England for use with *such cases that it was thought to be lifesaving*. Just down the road from Sister Mary's surgery, Northampton General Hospital received it's supply of Penicillin, the medical board at the time decided to put this in the hand of the pathologist, with the honorary staff agreeing *that each should only use it with the consent of a colleague*. The pathologist was instructed it was only to be issued *against the signature of two members of the honorary staff*. One night the superintendent wanted some penicillin for a patient and ordered it from the pathologist who asked him to get a second signature, which he declined to obtain, *the pathologist refused to issue the penicillin and was subsequently dismissed*[418]. After a lengthy debate spanning numerous organisations and aired in the Northampton Chronicle and Echo *the decision stood regarding dismissal of the pathologist*. Penicillin became available as a prescription only drug in 1946.

Sister Mary often saw boatwomen who were *expecting*, although there are no records of a baby being born in Stoke Bruerne in 1943. It was not uncommon for women to seek help and advice as a result of pregnancy complications, particularly sickness and tiredness. During a boatwoman's pregnancy Sister Mary provided a range of care outlined in Table 35, including arranging a confinement at Braunston, and regularly advising women to *rest more*. On some occasions she wrote to the GUCCCo requesting the family be placed on a *shorter journey* as outlined in Table 36. Sister Mary's letters were written on her distinctive letter headed paper shown in Figure 98. A letter Sister Mary received from the GUCCCo fleet manager Mr Moll indicates the company were interested in knowing more about boater's pregnancies to enable the company to forward plan …

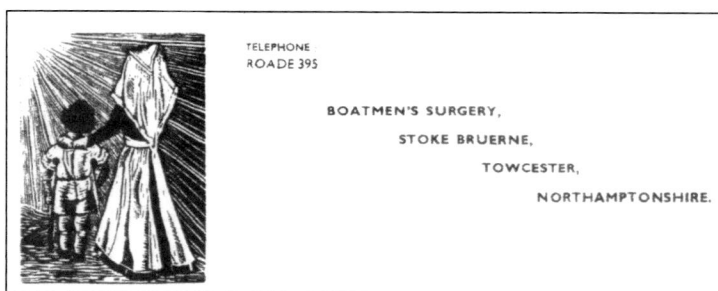

TELEPHONE
ROADE 395

BOATMEN'S SURGERY,
STOKE BRUERNE,
TOWCESTER,
NORTHAMPTONSHIRE.

Figure 98   Sister Mary's letter headed paper (David Blagrove Collection)

… With regard to maternity cases, I am wondering if it would be at all possible for you to assist us in avoiding delays to craft by letting us have as much forward notice as possible as to when the events are likely to take place. If you could let me have a note, say, six months ahead, it would be a great help to us in making forward traffic arrangements and avoiding delays to craft as far as possible. Perhaps you would let me have your comments on this suggestion[419].

Table 35   Pregnancy and suspected pregnancy 1943

Month	Woman's situation when seen by Sister Mary	Additional information
February	Pregnant	Sr Mary received phone call from Acocks Green re woman; if one month to go continue, if due shortly remain.
March	5 months Pregnant Sciatica	Called Doctor to examine. Two weeks later taken to Northampton Hospital.
February	5 months pregnant, collapsing frequently with cardiac disturbance.	Wrote to Mr Veater GUCCCo Hawkesbury Stop requesting shorter journeys Arranged confinement for Braunston with Doctor and Nurse
April	7 Months pregnant, fainting frequently, cardiac disturbance, fetus low, patient a high colour and breathless	Wrote to Mr Moll for shorter journeys to enable patient more rest.
March - October	Pregnant	Popped in to see Sister Mary once or twice a month during pregnancy
April	2 months pregnant	Seen on several occasions – headaches, backache, sickness
June	7 months pregnant, accident with towing rope	Laid up for for eight days … regularly seen after as passing through Stoke Bruerne for wound care.

September	3 months pregnant, vomiting	Seen five times from September to October … nothing to report
September	Reports pregnant, no dates given	Woman also has a 15 month old, born prematurely at 7 months. Sent woman to Southall for examination. Sister Mary received a comprehensive ante natal report from the Medical officer of Health at Southall

Table 36   Letters to canal companies 1943

Boater / Month	Reason for letter	Request by Sister Mary
Woman	5 months pregnant, frequent collapsing, cardiac disturbance. Needs more rest.	To Mr Veater. GUCCCo. Hawkesbury Stop. Shorter journeys.
Woman	7 months pregnant, fainting frequently, cardiac disturbance, foetus low, patient very highly coloured and breathless.	To Mr Mole. Shorter journeys to enable more rest.

Sister Mary replied informing Mr Moll she knew of seven boatwomen who were between 6 weeks and 5 months into their pregnancy. Mr Ernest Veater the GUCCCo representative at Hawkesbury Junction in a post war lecture briefly recounted his experiences of boaters and pregnancy …

Boatwomen invariably prefer that the event shall take place in their boat. Some of you may have heard a broadcast feature called "Midland Journey" in which a boatwoman was asked how they managed in maternity cases and she replied "We take the boats to back of Veater's shed" her description of my office. This stretch of water is popular for the occasion. Here they have telephone facilities for midwife and midwife can also communicate with Dr if required. The midwife understands boatwomen and threatens them with hospital if conditions in boats are not up to standard required. The spot is also very convenient to the local grocer (mentioned elsewhere) and their friends and relatives on passing boats are available with assistance or care of children in fact, they feel at home there.

The impending event is always announced to us by the husband who says:- "I don't want an order as I've got to tie up". We require a certificate from midwife who frequently says they are safe for further trips and we then arrange for short jobs according to case. Boats then remain until Midwife gives a clearance and meantime we give the boatmen suitable work where he can return at night. Following her confinement, we recently asked a boatwoman into the office for some telephoning on her behalf but she declined, saying I mustn't go in anywhere because I have not yet been churched – I am not able to say if this is peculiar to the canals. The new-borns are all christened before the boats move off again[420].

Sister Mary sometimes cared for a boater with long-term care needs as one case study illustrates. In 1943 Sister Mary visited a Captain and noted *Nephritic Oedema*, after which she regularly saw the boater over a number of years as the family passed through Stoke Bruerne. In 1946 the Captain arrived at the surgery with his wife, on this occasion Sister Mary immediately advised hospital admission, he agreed and a local resident took the Captain and Sister Mary to Northampton General where he was admitted to *Compton Ward* at 7.20pm. Sister Mary on her return noted *Captain very seriously ill …nephritis and cardiac collapse, oedema of face, legs and hands.* Sister Mary visited the captain the next four days during which he told her he was *very much more comfortable, glad to be in hospital,* although Sister Mary also recorded *condition not satisfactory.* Sister Mary continued to visit daily during May and into the middle of June, at the mid June visit she was informed *incurable / dying.* On returning to the surgery Sister Mary wrote to the boater's wife in Birmingham, informing her of his deteriorating condition, the family were *present when the captain collapsed and passed away.*

Mollie Traill, the Ministry and the floating populations wellbeing …

After the all women boat training scheme commenced on the Grand Union Canal the Ministry of Labour and the Ministry of War Transport played their parts in trying to recruit trainees. Sir Osborne Mance receiving a request from Hugh Beaver at the Ministry of Works and Planning (November 1942) to meet Mrs Buston, a woman who had previous experience of working with Daphne March[421]. At the meeting Mrs Buston suggested a number of *improvements to amenities on the boats … if women crews were to be recruited*[422] …

> we would be content with a lavatory and a basin (if space could be found) in the engine room and a very tiny cabin in the bow. This would give something to stand on as deck forward and not take so much cargo space as putting the lavatory and basin in separate compartment next to the engine room. A tank for water would also be a real blessing.

Would you be so kind as to let us know if you would give your authority for this to be done – after which I suppose we would approach the Grand Union Canal Company ? We would also like to pick our own boats as we know of one not in use which is free of bugs. Enclosed is a small sketch of our ideas for alterations to the barge (reproduced in Figure 99).

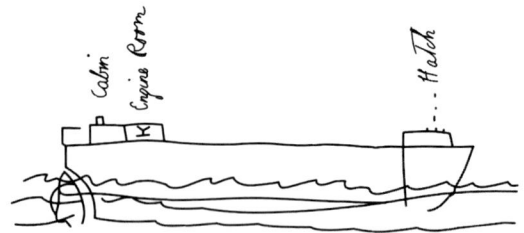

Figure 99   Mrs Bustons line drawing
(Christopher M Jones)

After Sir Osborne and Mrs Buston exchanged a number of letters, in which Mrs Buston insisted *conditions on canal boats needed fixing,* Sir Osborne inspected for himself a motor and a butty at the Grand Union Canal Carrying Company depot, after which he responded to Mrs Buston *other women had not complained*[423]. Recruitment to the women's training scheme was not going as well as expected, and after talking to Mollie Traill at the end of January 1943 Sir Osborne reported to the Canal Control Committee the scheme needed extending …

> … either by encouraging other companies to do what the Grand Union have successfully undertaken or by starting a government Training Establishment … Of the two, as at present advised, I prefer the second. If in fact this plan were adopted, I presume it would be done, as with other training establishments, under the auspices of the Ministry of Labour[424].

In march Mrs Traill met with the Parliamentary Secretary and Sir Osborne to notify them *six pairs of boats were manned by women, but due to sickness only five were currently in operation,* they also discussed how the scheme could be extended to a base in Birmingham[425]. Less than two months after the meeting Mrs Traill met with the Parliamentary Secretary to raise her concerns about *aspects of boaters lives she had experienced on the Grand Union Canal,* during the meeting Mollie suggested *government do more about them*[426]. The points Mollie raised with the Parliamentary Secretary were …

- the need for boarding-schools for canal boat children … with special curricula and post-school apprenticeships
- the removal of children from boats
- working pairs of boats two-handed
- improved rates of pay … for all crew including women
- abolish the system of fining boats when late running
- inspection of boats, including bed and cupboards etc
- the 'bug question'
- modified design

In his notes after the meeting the Parliamentary Secretary referred to the points Mollie raised as *Mrs Traill's premises,* counter-arguing these in the majority of cases even though Mrs Traill illustrated her concerns with detailed accounts of specific cases. The Parliamentary Secretary noted …

> The specific cases are, of course, bad. Presumably they are exceptions. I dare say they resemble similar cases on shore but there is the snag that the boats are not attached to any particular local authority, e.g. health, which could keep an eye on the family as on shore … in all this we are handicapped by war preoccupations and by not knowing what is to be our post-war canal policy. In the present conditions we are not likely to get much assistance from the canal undertakings and carriers[427].

A month later Mollie informed the Parliamentary Secretary and Sir Osborne[428] *the number of pairs manned by women crews had increased to eight, and one more would be ready in two weeks,* she also stressed the increasing number of boats awaiting repairs, as well as expanding on some of the points she raised with the Parliamentary Secretary a month earlier. All seemed to be going well until Mollie sent a handwritten letter to Sir Osborne expressing concerns regarding boat families, in particular women and children, as transcribed below

"Dodona"

Unloading at Tyseley

June 21st

Dear Sir Oswald

I wrote to you when leaving Leamington, but on arrival at Birmingham, I felt I must add to this. The reason being Mrs. Bob Hunt, her son was born a fortnight ago, full time & weighed only 4 pounds. The doctor says it is down to malnutrition and the baby is in hospital unlikely to live. They are one of our cleanest families and hard workers. Can nothing be done for these women? It takes 20 years to make a man.

I was disappointed with the result of our conversation. I suggested that you should find out the number of persons over the age of eighteen who were capable of taking our boats and who were now forming part of a family crew. My reason for suggesting this was one only. To insure pay for men & women who are now working 14-18 hours a day - the men getting their food & insurance & £2.10.0 a trip and the women nothing.

Often the captain steers the boat while his young children do all the heavy work for none or little pay. I still insist that some rigorous ruling should be made to prevent children of under 14 being allowed to touch the boats or the locks, as you say you can make no effort to have them sent to school. The fact that they work at all and have little schooling is illegal and I do not understand how it is allowed to go on.

The argument that the majority of the boats would be left idle does not hold now at all could be manned from dividing the existing crews and there are plenty of applicants to be trained for the work. Both men and women. In fact we will shortly need more boats built.

I do not exaggerate the conditions and the cases I stated were not isolated they were amongst my company except for one, it is well known that conditions on the Fellows & Morton boats are worse. Ovaltines are almost perfect. Their bed cupboards & --- cabins are inspected regularly.

Yours faithfully

F. M. Traill[429].

In fact Mollie was correct in her observations of the Ovaltine Boats *being maintained exceptionally well,* as the family crews were proud to be part of the Wanderer Company, always doing their best to keep a very high standard of cleanliness and neatness. Captain Arthur Stokes and his wife Ellen Stokes (nee Littlemore) worked a pair of Ovaltine Boats and won the cup for the *best pair* at the first Inland Waterways Association rally held at Market Harbough in August 1950, Ellen was known as *Queen of the Cut*[430] shown in Figure 100.

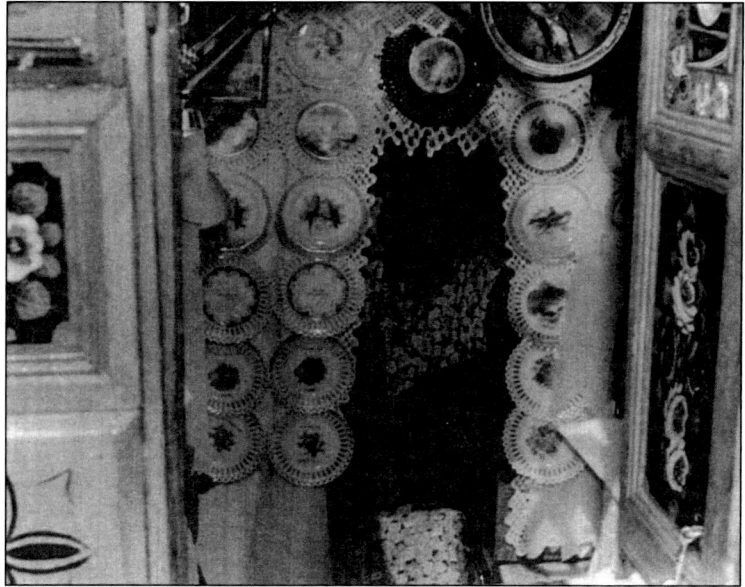

Figure 100   Queen of the Cut (Lorna York collection)

After Mollie's letter was received at the Ministry she met with Sir Osborne, during which his secretary recorded seven points *touched upon* during the meeting[431], one point related to the *outlook of the training scheme* which Mollie feared *would terminate very shortly*, and the following two referred to boaters health and wellbeing …

Point 6:   Lavatories and rest rooms are wanted at Birmingham, Leicester, Braunston and Hawkesbury, as well as at Bulls Bridge.

Point 7.   The wives of boatmen are not insured and lack proper medical attention. Mrs Traill thinks that a Doctor should attend at Bulls Bridge … at least one day every week in order to give medical information and attention to women and their families on canal boats. In her opinion regular medical inspection is long overdue and she thinks that this should be provided at the expense of the Canal Undertakings. Ante-natal care is missing and some arrangements should be made for looking after the families of boatwomen. So far as she knows the only case of regular inspection is carried out in connection with the Ovaltine employees. She will find out exactly the details of their scheme.

One small point was that the Ovaltine boats were painted white inside the cupboards and whilst, in the first instance, the Grand Union Company had agreed to use white paint they took advantage of her absence from Bulls Bridge to revert to the old brown grain colour.

Between May and July 1943 Molly Traill raised concerns about boaters on the Grand Union Canal to both the Parliamentary Secretary and the Director of Canals, mysteriously that summer Mollie left the canal. There are two accounts regarding her sudden departure, first is from Kit Gayford who wrote *Mollie went with two trainees to Fellows, Morton and Clayton to start a boatwomen's training scheme in Birmingham*[432]. The second is from Mollie's grand-son[433], who has the letter his grand-mother received from Philip Noel Baker, Parliamentary Secretary to the Ministry of War Transport[434] in which he *sadly has to dispense with her services*. Mollie's grand-sons interpretation of the letter is that it *seems to imply she made herself unpopular with canal company's,* also according to her grand-son Mollie *left the canal on a sour note, leaving behind the many schemes she had worked hard to set up. She was always strong minded … she effectively [was] sacked for being a troublemaker*[435]. Although Mollie was no longer on the canal, in response to the concerns she raised Sir Osborne Mance wrote to the Ministry of Health …

> Dear Reid
>
> The Director of Canals, Sir Osborne Mance, is concerned about the well-being of the crews of canal boats and is anxious to discuss with representatives of your Ministry the whole question of medical treatment amenities for those persons who, as you will be aware, comprise adults and children of both sexes. The main difficulty is to ensure that medical services may be available to crews wherever they may happen to be at a particular time. In the course of their employment the crews (who live on the boats) are seldom located at one spot for more than a few days at any time although, generally speaking, their journeys take them constantly over the same routes. A round trip may take from 14 to 21 days and cover some 250 miles of canal. I understand that you have a Departmental Committee who deal with such questions and Sir Osborne would much appreciate a discussion with one or more members of the committee at a mutually agreed date[436] …

The letter stimulated a lot of activity at the Ministry of Health, causing officials to exchange copious amounts of information about the floating population, with one official writing on the bottom of an internal report *Sir Osborne being some new broom at work*[437], on the other hand the same official reported unearthing the fact that the most recent reports by the Ministry of Health on canal boats were by Mr Owen Llewellyn on his retirement.

The meeting requested by Sir Osborne Mance took place at the Ministry of War Transport in September with four representatives from the Ministry of Health. Sir Osborne Mance opened the meeting with the statement *he was concerned about reports which had reached him that the families forming the crews of narrow canal boats lacked proper medical attention.* After much discussion the meeting concluded with a request from Sir Osborne Mance that Local Authorities attention might be drawn to …

> … the peculiar position of the canal boat people and that steps might be taken to ensure that the latter were made aware of the existing facilities and benefits of which they could take advantage. It seems appropriate that such advices should [be} issued from the Ministry

of Health and it was agreed that a formal approach should be made by the Ministry of War Transport on the matter[438].

The content of the meeting was written up by Ministry of Health officials, from which it can be gleened some of the points discussed at the meeting caused the officials concern, as the following extracts demonstrates …

It became clear that his mind was moving on a high plane; no less than that he was contemplating the present wartime Government co-ordination of national transport of all kinds being perpetuated after the war, of course by his own department, with the consequence that there would be a Department of State actively and permanently concerned with canal transport and the machinery and personnel of it in perpetuity…

All this and more is obviously very high policy and not for our discussion: but it was necessary to extract what was in his mind so as to get an idea of why he was not prepared to accept the experience of the past 70 years up to date that the social and economic conditions of canal boats in fact worked and were satisfactory to the population concerned …

He kept saying that the canal industry … was greatly neglected and that it was necessary to take comprehensive and long view of what had to be done. His trouble was that he had (unread) a copy of the Chamberlain Committee of 1921. His concern from the health aspect was that the population did not take or did not use doctors when they were ill or when their wives had babies; that there was no routine medical supervision or examination of the health of the canal population as such. My colleagues dealt with this so far as the Chamberlain Report did not do so.

He was clearly ready to maintain that some proportion of the canal population were the worse for this neglect, and he made a great deal of their being infested. It appeared that his information was that he was generalising from extremely slight evidence although he did not respond to my invitation to give us data as we offered to him ours; he told us that a certain number of voluntary trainees had been drafted to the canals who were women of enterprise and education and experience of a kind entirely different from that of the normal canal boat population [presumably he was referring to the women trainees]; and that these people told him things …

… the natural interest that comment from this fresh angle gives, scarcely, however, excuses the Ministry of Transport for apparently having failed to inform themselves of the evidence that we could have put before them, as for example our two annual reports, information about health, maternity benefits and so on. On all these subjects he was just ignorant.

… one current topic of some interest was mentioned; the question of food for the travelling population and particularly for expectant mothers and others entitlements to extra food. It appeared to be well known that food was a bit of a problem. This apparently would be due essentially to the fact that this was rather a hungry occupation involving days of long hours and that the women could not get to the shops at the best of times.

Nevertheless, it was generally agreed that a provision was made under the Ministry of Food's system for this, like any other, moving population and that the expectant mothers could get their extra rations and no doubt would. It might well be, of course, as elsewhere, that they do not consume them themselves, but give them to their children.

The typed report concluded we *headed Sir Osborne off to issue a circular of his own,* at the bottom of the report is a handwritten note *Sir Osborne Mance to be a retired officer ... from the Boar war[439].*

After the meeting Sir Osborne Manse sent a letter to the Ministry of Health *to explain the interest of his department in this matter,* in which he outlined his and the Ministry's concerns and responsibilities regarding boater's obtaining; *proper medical attention, continuity of medical advice, National Insurance and vouchers for travellers ... I welcome the offer of a Circular,* the letter concludes with a reference to his awareness of Sister Mary's clinic at Stoke Bruerne ...

The Grand Union Canal has endeavoured to mitigate the position by appointing a nurse at Stoke Bruerne, and whilst this arrangement is useful, it is restricted in character. So far as I know, similar arrangements do not exist elsewhere.

We are told that the boat people suffer from false modesty, and rather than seek medical aid, carry on when they ought to receive medical attention. A certain number of specific cases has been brought to our notice, and in at least one case, malnutrition was alleged.

As most of the complaints come to us in confidence, we find some difficulty in passing them on for investigation, but we admit to feeling uneasy in the matter. I think we agree that in the first place at any rate the matter might be dealt with on a broader plane[440].

As no response was received by the Director of Canals from by the Ministry of Health his secretary made a further request for a *copy of the circular,* this persistent interest in the boaters wellbeing un-doubtably *rattled cages* at the Ministry of Health, who set in motion an investigation into boater's health and welfare, after convening an internal meeting where officials identified four key points for action[441] ...

1. The need to probe more to see if we are doing everything [for boaters]

2. We could increase awareness to boaters via existing bodies

3. To allocated Miss Puxley to make notes of benefits and facilities [for boaters]

4. To allocated Mr Howell James to arrange and direct a general investigation [into boaters health and well-being][442]

The wheels were now in motion and the gaze was about to focus again on the floating population at a national level, although Sir Osborne Mance was unaware of this because on

November 20th his secretary sent a further letter stating *Sir Osborne Mance wants to know when circular issued*. In January 1944 visits were made by the Ministry of health to Brentford, Southall, Wolverhampton, Stoke Bruerne and Paddington, and interviews were conducted by Ministry officials with Directors of the Grand Union Canal Carrying Company (and Fellows, Morton and Clayton). On concluding their investigations a ten page internal report was issued on 31st January 1944[443], the content of which gives a remarkable insight into boaters on the Grand Union Canal during the war years.

After interviewing Directors and Depot managers from the GUCCCo the Ministry reported *[the GUCCCo are] interested in the welfare of their employees*, senior managers having reported to officials about their employees [the boating families] and the facilities the employer provided for boat crews, the officials reported the canal company in a favourable manner …

> The majority [of boaters] are aware of the facilities provided for mothers and children at the local clinic, and say that though many of them cannot read and write, they are pretty quick to take advantage of facilities … and pass the news from one to the other; at the same time, they state that they are in a privileged position to spread the light as the Ministry of Information show films to the canal boat population in a big hall at the depot. These films are well patronised, and the Company are willing to throw on the screen any information as to the facilities available to expectant mothers or mothers with young children, and would distribute any circulars dealing with maternity and Child Welfare Services … in addition they would be willing to give a talk on the loud speaker on the subject, and with regard to the circulars they would undertake to explain the contents to any who were interested …

The visit to Hayes Road, Southall revealed the GUCCCo depot had been extended and modernised to include a canteen, although managers reported *the canteen is not patronised by them … they prefer to have their meals on board*. The depot had no baths or washing facilities for crews but did have W.C.'s which were also noted as *rarely used, as the majority seem to prefer the more primitive amenities of the countryside*. A few years ago *the company supplied Elson Chemical Closets placed in the engine rooms* but crews *did not like them, and about 90% were discarded by them*. The depot had *benches with a roof to enable the women to do their family washing*, company representatives informing officials *cold water is laid on, and a boiler with a coal fire is kept burning to supply the hot water*. The director of the company was keen to point out 90% of their boats were fitted with electric light *powered by a battery supplied free of charge to the boaters, but captains have to supply their own electric light bulbs*, even so, *some of the crews still prefer to use the oil lamp*.

At Brentford officials visited a modern up-to-date clinic run by two trained Nurse's and a Health Visitor, situated five to ten minutes walk from the canal and open to canal boat people, the visitors met with Nurse Broughton who informed them …

> [she] does visit the boat when she knows there is a baby on board, and thereafter visits when possible … that many mothers or expectant mothers attending the clinic will take the hip or other fruit juices, but they cannot be persuaded to take the Cod Liver Oil …

does not think that the canal boat women ever take supplies of vitamins with them on their travels, and says that these women are apt to regard these facilities as new-fangled.

The GUCCCo were singled out for good practice in supplying food for their crews, as they had a scheme which allowed *crews to supplement rations by purchasing packaged food (a meat pie, or its equivalent, tea and sugar)* at the Southall Depot and at lock-keepers premises one day's journey apart on the Grand Union Canal, officials reporting the GUCCCo to be the only carrying company to have such a scheme[444].

Further insight into boater's accessibility to food and the type of diet consumed during World War II was reported by Mr Bucknell after a visit to Bulls Bridge at the end of December 1943, which concluded with an account of his observations regarding boaters diet …

> Milk: No fresh milk appears to be used by the canal boat population, presumably because of the difficulty in registering with any one firm; also, storage facilities are limited. All use evaporated milk, obtainable at certain retailers on the canal route by arrangement with the Food Office on Form S.A.4. The evaporated milk seen in use was all of the same brand, 'Pet', a full cream variety containing 7.9 butter fat and 25.9 total solids. It is described on the tin as having the vitamin D content increased. Very little Household Milk is used and it was spoken of with dislike …
>
> Eggs: The families visited do not appear to have received any allocation of fresh eggs. It was interesting to note, however, that dried eggs are much used and appreciated.
>
> Dietary: The boaters have good cooking facilities and all the families seem to manage at least one cooked meal per day. I noticed that potatoes were being very thickly peeled, and saw no green vegetables in preparation, though the values of these seem to be known … Dinners can be obtained in the Yard's canteen, but, at 1/3d. per head, they are rather beyond the purse of the average canal boat population. The strenuous open air life produces keen appetites, and all the families complained that they found it difficult to manage on the ordinary rations. A scheme is afoot to provide packed lunches by the firm for their canal boat employees, these will be over and above rationed foods, and no doubt they will form a very helpful addition to the diet.

Ministry officials visited *boaters at Stoke Bruerne*, where they obtained an insight into boat families experiences of rationing, shopping and medical care …

> We formed the impression that they [the canal boat people] were not the complaining sort, but they did tell us that the rationing came rather hard on them … under the present scheme they find it difficult to obtain even the ration they are entitled to as the regular customers of local butchers get preference when there is any suggestion of shortage of supplies. They also feel the shortage of tea and sugar as they are great tea drinkers …

I think it may be taken as a fact that cows' milk is practically never obtained, nor is it obtainable as these 'birds of passage' cannot be registered as regular customers; it does appear to be in general, however, to use 'Pet' full-cream milk. And most of the women seem able to get two tins a week. I understand that a tin of milk will make, when watered down, a pint and a half of milk as good as cows' milk …

Regarding shopping, crews were described as *managing fairly well on the whole as they are entitled to make purchases after shop hours,* but it was pointed out boaters on tidal waters were able to obtain additional points (normal ration 5 points, 14 points for tidal crew members) and 3/9d worth of meat as against a civilians ration of 1/2d, they noted these special facilities were not extended to canal boat crews whose rations were exactly the same rations as civilians. Boaters confirming they were issued with *emergency travellers cards for use anywhere*, reporting *this usually works well except for meat*, with some exceptions as a boater at Brentford re-called …

A man of about 16 stone told the Missionary at Brentford that in two months the only meat he had been able to get was two breasts of mutton. He tried through the Local Food Officer to obtain more without result, but when he sought advice of the Local Police, he was able to get the ration of meat he was entitled to through the good offices of a constable who accompanied him to the local butcher's shop.

With regard to medical care, boaters were issued with *travelling medical vouchers* under the National Health Insurance Scheme, and had no problem seeing a *panel practitioner* when needed, with some captains disclosing they paid regularly into hospital savings schemes. Although in summing up officials concluded …

I am not satisfied that the canal boat people always obtain the medical services available to them, as I have heard quite recently of the crews of three boats whose skippers have said that they applied for travelling medical cards … but have not received them, and so pay for medical attention when they want it, and presumably do not receive any National Insurance Benefit when sick. My enquiries cannot be considered exhaustive, and I feel that there is much that could be done to help these people.

Mr Bucknell made a final note which seemed to indicate the floating population had been somewhat forgotten and neglected since the retirement of Owen Llewellyn, *there seems to be no doubt that owing to pressure of other work, public health activities among the canal boat population have been allowed to elapse, though they appear never to have been very satisfactory.*

Sir Osborne Mance was never sent a copy of the Ministry of Health ten page report, and it was not until over a year after he made what seemed to be a simple request for a *circular to be sent out to raise awareness to boaters regarding their entitlements* that the Ministry of Health drew the matter to a close. In November 1944 the Ministry of Health issued a letter to Regional Joint Committees (with a copy to the Ministry of War Transport) requesting the availability of medical and welfare services and the extra facilities during the war *be brought to the notice of the boaters orally or visually in whatever way is thought practicable at the depots and elsewhere*[445]*,* enclosed with the letter was a Public Health pamphlet on *entitlements for mother and children.*

The Bigger Picture and Sister Mary …

Unknown to the Ministry of Health and to the floating population, Sir Osborne Mance during his time as Director of Canals was seeing the **bigger picture**. Between March and June 1944 Sir Osborne Mance was working *in the background* on a strategic change which would affect all transport workers because with some of his parliamentary colleagues they had identified loopholes in existing Acts of Parliament which did not cover transport workers. Sir Osborne Mance referred to the loopholes as *the fringe of a major problem …*

> … unlike most other industrial workers who are covered by codes laid down in the Factory Acts, the Mines Acts and the Shops Act, transport workers, in general, are not protected by any peace time code designed to promote their welfare; there are exceptions to this, particularly in repair shops, etc. where the factory acts apply, and individual transport undertakings have carried out a number of First Aid and other welfare arrangements, either voluntarily or under war time regulations.

> There may however, be strong pressure after the war to introduce a welfare code for transport workers who are not covered, and this pressure may be irresistible if it cannot be shown that the Department has taken steps to ensure the adoption of appropriate standards which are at least equivalent to those applying to other industrial workers[446].

At the initial informal meeting convened between parties interested in the loophole, Sir Osborne Mance identified two issues which needed addressing; first, the expansion of training in *Industrial First Aid* for transport workers, and second, the need for clarification of *departmental responsibility for industrial welfare and safety* in relation to each of the transport sectors (Road, Rail, Port and Inland Waterway's). After this exploratory meeting a formal group was set up with representatives from all transport sectors[447].

Sister Mary's canal side surgery was singled out by Ministry of Health officials in several of their investigations during World War II[448]. A visit by officials to Sister Mary's surgery being specially requested by Mr. Moll of the GUCCo. The officials noting in their report *[Mr Moll] takes a great interest in it, and he told me that it was the only one of its kind in England; he spoke very highly of the work of Sister Ward and said that his company paid her a small honorarium weekly.* After the officials visit the report contained a brief account of the Boatman's Surgery and the service Sister Mary was providing …

> Whilst on the subject of clinics I should like to mention the Clinic or Dispensary, to give it it's proper name, which is run entirely by Sister Mary Ward who has been running it single-handed for about fifteen years at Stoke Bruerne, about three miles from Blisworth. The Dispensary is in the private house of Sister Mary Ward, who is about 60, and who lives with her husband who is over 80. It is a big, old-fashioned house, facing the canal and adjoining the tow-path. Three of the downstairs rooms are used for the Dispensary, Surgery and Waiting-room. The Dispensary is spotlessly clean and very well equipped.

However the officials were incorrect regarding her husband's age because Chas would have been 75 at the time of their visit. From their assessment the officials also noted …

> It is difficult to understand how Sister Mary is able to carry on as she is only paid £2 per week by the Grand Union Canal Carrying Company and nothing from other canal boat proprietors whose crews take advantage of her good offices. Sister ward provides all her own instruments, drugs, bandages, disinfectants etc. and has to pay two shillings a week for the carriage of fresh drinking water to be provided for the Dispensary as the whole village is dependent on well water.

> Another draw-back is that there is no gas or electric light supply and paraffin lamps have to be depended upon. Sister Ward is entitled to charge a fee for any services rendered to her, but she finds that very few of her patients are in a position to pay anything as when the boats are laid up their pay ceases, and apparently very few of them have saved any money for 'rainy days'.

They also passed comment on the medical support Sister Mary received …

> … there is a Doctor at Blisworth, about four miles away … he is old and shaky, and she finds it difficult to get in touch with him when necessary as she has had to give up the telephone on account of the expense. At the present time, however, a retired doctor is living in Stoke Bruerne who is interested in the canal boat people and attends when necessary for a purely nominal fee.

The Doctor at Blisworth would have been Dr Clements, and in Stoke Bruerne Dr Baird shown earlier in Figure 95 playing chess with Sister Mary. A final extract from the report suggested *Sister Mary is performing all the duties of a trained nurse, and in practice seems to perform many duties which should be performed by a medical man.* Sister Mary is shown in Figure 102 with Evelyn Hunt[449] sitting on the balance beam outside her home and surgery, after what looks like a shopping trip to Northampton.

A copy of the Ministry of Health's report titled *Canal Boaters* dated January 1944 was sent to Mr Saunders, head of Civil Defence at Birmingham. In his reply to the Ministry of Health in February 1944 Mr Saunders said he found the report *extremely interesting.* As an afterthought on signing the letter, he made a note before posting his reply to the Ministry of Health …

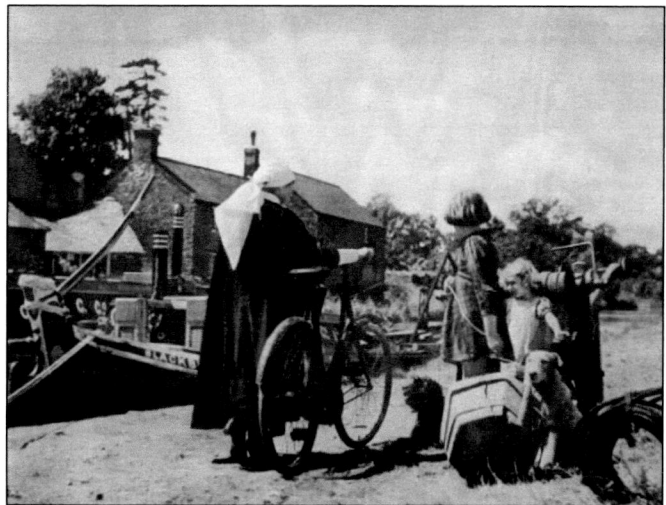

Figure 102   *Painted Boats.* Sister Mary with bicycle (Della Sadler-Moore collection)

It strikes me that Sister Mary Ward is self deserving of an honour for her devoted labours; but there is the decided snag that she appears to encroach on the medical side, which the ministry are fond to discountenance[450]

During the war years Ealing Studio began shooting a film in Stoke Bruerne in conjunction with the Ministry of War Transport[451] *depicting the life of the people of the canals, with their two-centuries-old traditions. The medium is a story of two families, one progressive and the other empiric. Interwoven is a love story —and something else.* According to the local reporter who went on location with the film crew Stoke Bruerne was chosen because …

> … it was an ideal setting of sylvan beauty, road winding up the hill over the bridge by the lock tavern on the lock-side, and the picturesque village itself. All combining to give just the right atmosphere for a film of simple charm.

The film named *Painted Boats* had Bob Griffith as the leading man, who was invalided out of the army after serving in France, with Jennie Laird as the female lead, *and diminutive, flaxen-haired four year-old Sarah Ann Wenlock as the darling of the film cast, the daughter of a bargee who with her father and mother, Enoch and Lucretia Wenlock proved a real discovery for the production team.* Also in the film were two Northampton children Marion (age 10) and Michael Ponting (age 5), with their dog GYP, discoveries of the film unit manager and Assistant Director Billy Russell, a one time music hall star. Sister Mary had a short appearance in the film but was featured in the promotional literature with her bicycle Figure 102. Regarding the film Mr Veater wrote about the boater's reaction to it in his 1948 lecture[452] …

> **Film "Painted Boats".**
>
> When showing at "Empire" Coventry we had a number of the boatmen who appeared in the picture, arrive in district for loading. I telephoned the Manager of "Empire" – result was his invitation for them to go along and some of them after being given tea went on stage – including the Wenlocks – and Enoch played his accordion – same tune as he played in the Public House depicted in the picture.
>
> "Painted Boats" reaction of boatmen was annoyance. They disliked the theme – their own moral standard is strict. The women objected to the pillows shewn with the bare tick, no pillow cases. The boatmen criticised the coal-lade boat north-bound towards the collieries. The tunnel legging scene – a relic of the dark ages – was performed by a boatman who was taking over a motor-boat (Clash of periods).

Eily Gayford was awarded an MBE in January 1945, but why was Molly Traill not recognised for her creation and initial implementation of the boatwomen's training scheme?[453]. The end of World War II was declared on May 8th 1945.

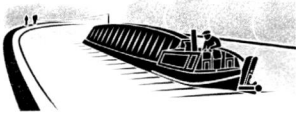

Sister Mary Post-War

Post-War Sister Mary continued to provide first aid and continuing care to boaters on the Grand Union Canal as they passed through Stoke Bruerne, although she did find time to pursue her passion for playing the piano as shown in Figure 103. Doctor Baird remained in the village and continued to see boaters at Sister Mary's request, he rented a cottage from the Wakefield Estate at an annual tenants rate of £15. 12. 0d.[454] Just after VE day Sister Mary was called to see a Captain who had *abdominal pain* and was *feeling sick,* after noting the Captains temperature, pulse and respiratory rates were all abnormal, she detained the boats and advised hospital admission, the Captain *declined*, Sister Mary making a note in her case book S*erious Case, Carcinoma?*, under these circumstances she advised a *milk diet and boiled water.* During the next 48 hours Sister Mary regularly visited the Captain, each time checking his observations and on each occasion he reported *pain not so severe,* at 11am on the third day Sister Mary called for an ambulance and the Captain was admitted to Northampton General

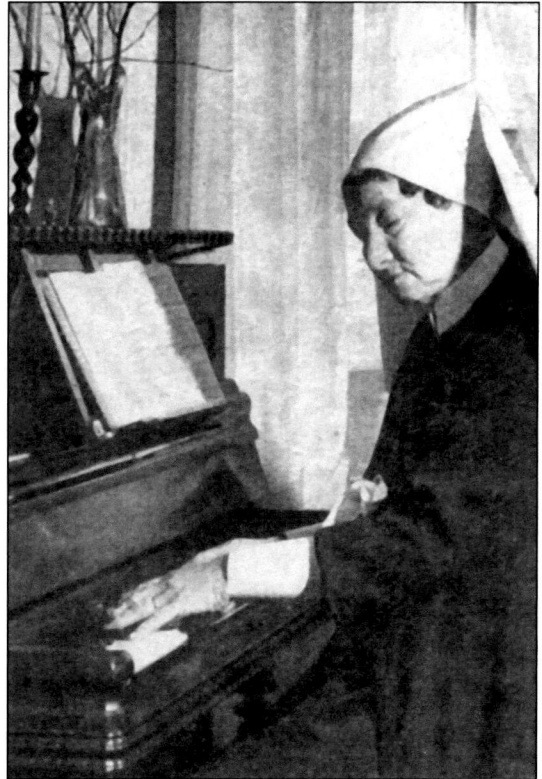

Figure 103   Sister Mary playing the piano
(Della Sadler-Moore collection)

Infirmary. On the same day Sister Mary admitted the Captain to hospital, another boat arrived with a three year old who on the previous day badly scalded both feet. Sister Mary examined the child and found *large broken blisters* and a *normal temperature*, after detaining the family she dressed the wounds twice daily for five days, the child was also seen by a Doctor on a number of occasions. Sister Mary also wrote to Mr Moll of the Grand Union Canal Carrying Company informing him about the incident.

Post-war Stoke Bruerne community activities continued, including monthly *Womens Institute* (WI) meetings and *Help for Hospitals* fundraising, both well attended and popular with the villagers, although behind the scenes in this rural idyllic community Stoke villagers were less than calm about their ongoing *lack of piped water*. The situation came to a head when the Northampton Mercury placed on the front page an account of the water situation, with the headline *Water, Water everywhere, but not a tap to turn*[455]. The front page included the pictures shown in Figure 104, with the caption … *The source of supply [of water] depends on the need. Cleaning water comes from the canal, and drinking water from a street pump which contrasts strangely with the modern council houses in the back ground.* If I am not mistaken, the small picture in the corner of Figure 104 shows Sister Mary second in line to fill her water bucket in Chapel Lane. The article commenced with the question *How many people know the village where there's water but no water?* Sister Mary's surgery being referred to as *the epitomy of plenty in the midst of little …*

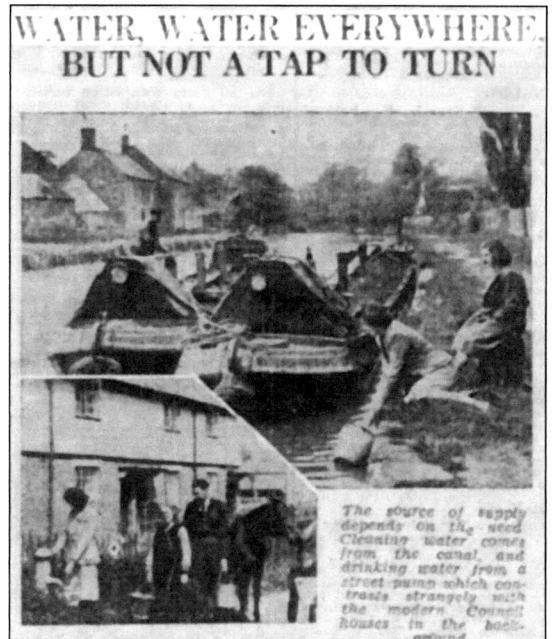

Figure 104   Water, no water in Stoke Bruerne (Northampton Mercury)

> Thus the irony of the well equipped surgery of Sister Mary E H Ward, consultant sister to the Grand Union Canal Carrying Company and associated companies. It has everything from various types of forceps, down to a fine range of coloured liquid that makes Col. Chinstrap shudder. She knows all the boatmen who pass- they are her patients and in her case-books they are listed for the complaints for which they seek her service when they pass her door. She attends 250-300 a month.

The residents of Stoke Bruerne, including Sister Mary and the only shopkeeper in the village Mrs Ursula Tyrrell, felt so strongly about the problem they told the reporter of their need for *piped water, as opposed to having to go 50-100 yards to a stand-pipe.* Mrs Pebody also reported *she had to pay a special water rate of 30s every year … but had refused to pay it and expected to go to prison!*. The paper also suggested *women in the village get their washing water from the canal into which the boat people tip everything … and the same village women tip rubbish.*

The Captain Sister Mary admitted to hospital returned to the canal in July after which Sister Mary recommenced his care, from the case book entries transcribed in Table 37 the hospital discharged the Captain with a note for Sister Mary, the report indicated the Captain had an *inoperable growth.*

Table 37   **Extract from Case Book July 1945-January 1946**

1945		*Mr [...]* *Motor Boat [...]*
		Brought forward. *Ledger No 55. Ovaltine*
July	*7*	*Saturday 11am returned from ... to motor boat xxxx left Stoke Bruerne*
		(Report Hospital Carcinoma Pelvis and Liver operation unsuccessful as regards removing growth)
	8	*Visit Patient more comfortable*
	10	*" " " "*
	12	*" " continues to rest better, still condition Serious*
	14	*" no possibility of curing disease, too advanced !*
	19	*" Patient bright & certain of recovery*
		Very thoughtful patient.
		Take patient to General Hospital for Radiotherapy when required
Oct	*9*	*Visit Hospital, treatment given Radiotherapy*
Oct	*16*	*Visit Hospital, treatment given, " "*
	23	*" " " " " "*
	30	*" " " " " " PT. Very Weak*
Nov	*4*	*" " " " " " but grateful*
	18	*" " " " " " for everything.*
Dec	*2*	*" " " " " " PT. Collapsed*
	11	*" " " " " " PT. not satisfactory*
		Patient transferred to St Edmunds Hospital
		Northampton. Not satisfactory condition.
Dec	*12*	*Visit St Edmonds*
	13	*" " " no improvement*
	14	*" " " " "*
	15	*" " " " "*
	16	*" " " " "*
	18	*Visit*
	20	*Visit*
	22	*Visit*
	24	*Visit*
	27	*Visit*
	30	*Visit*
Jan	*2*	*Visit*

	5	*Weaker*
	8	"
	11	"
	14	*Unconscious*
	17	*Passed away midday*
		Write Ovaltine works
		Sir Harry Hague helped (wife) after receiving my letter.

During the following months the Captain continued boating, but visited Sister Mary regularly, during which she escorted him to radiotherapy sessions at Northampton General Hospital. By December the Captain was so poorly his care was transferred to St Edmunds, Sister Mary visiting regularly until his death in January 1946. The Captain worked a pair of Ovaltine boats for *A Wanderer Ltd,* manufacturing chemist, Kings Langley. Sister Mary's last entry in her case book regarding the Captain is a note about a letter she sent to the

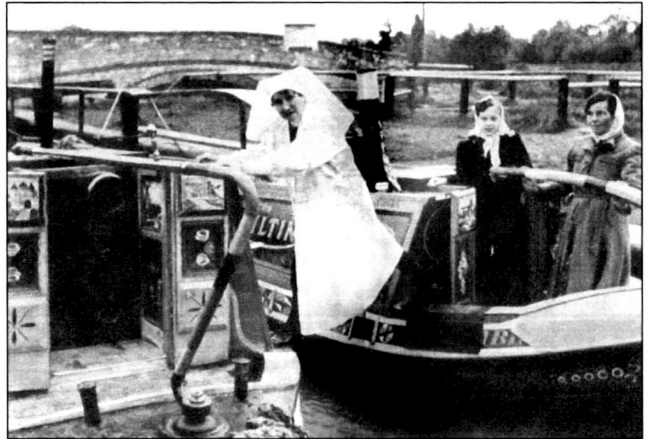

Figure 105   Sister Mary moving between a pair of Ovaltine Boats (Northampton Central Library)

company's Managing Director, Sir Harry Hague, after the entry she noted Sir Hague *helped the wife*. Sister Mary regularly saw Ovaltine Boat families as seen in Figure 105, where she is moving from the butty to the motor boat whilst the boats are in top-lock outside her home and surgery. Sister Mary regularly had contact with Mr Soar of the Welfare Department at A. Wander Limited, as shown in the response she received from Mr Soar after a boatwoman sustained a hand injury in Blisworth Tunnel …

Dear Sister Ward,

Thank you so much for clear report re Mrs […], motor boat […] I took the matter straight to the cashier. Now Mrs […] has received compensation up-to-date, she is quite happy about it. They do appreciate all you do for them.

I hope some day we shall meet, you may have off duty to spend this way and I would be pleased to have you.

Yours Sincerely

E. A. Soar

Post-War Sister Mary changed the format of her case book entries, moving to a daily log of boaters attending the surgery, as opposed to individual family records, from these it can be seen she treated 174 boaters in May 1946. A brief look at the entries for the first week of May, transcribed in Table 38, shows the scope of her work to be very varied with the boating families.

Table 38   Extract from Case Book May 1946

May 1946	Total per day	Boater	Sister Mary Comments
1st		Adult Female	Catarrh of Liver
		Adult Male	Severe Chill
		Adult Male	Chronic Gastritis
		Adult Female	Abscess of Ear
		Adult Male	Dyspepsia
		Adult Female	Rheumatism
		Adult Male	Nephritis
		Adult Female	Prolapse Uterus
		Adult Female	Varicose Veins of Legs
		Adult Female	Goitre
		Adult Female	Gynaecological
	11		
2nd		Adult Female	Uterus ?
		Adult Male	Bronchitis
		Adult Male	Carbuncle
		Adult Male	Accident to Hand
	4		
3rd		Adult Male	Treat Thumb & Report to Company
		Adult Female	Debility following childbirth
		Adult Male	Accident to thumb - redressed
		Adult Female	Gynaecological
		Adult Female	Catarrh Liver
	5		

4th		Adult Male	Catarrh throat and nose
		Adult Male	Fractured Clavice 2 weeks ago . Birmingham Hospital - redressed
		Adult Female	Gynaecological
		Adult Female	Due for confinement May 22nd
		Child	Bronchitis
		Child	Bronchitis
	6		
5th		Adult Female	Gynaecological
		Adult Male	Nil
		Son 7	Whooping Cough
		Son 5	Whooping Cough
		Daughter 3	Whooping Cough
		Baby 1 Month	Fine
		Adult Female	Adult Female
	7		
6th		Adult Female	Nephritis
		Adult Male	Nil
		Adult Female	Urine, Ulcerated Legs
		Adult Male	Consultation
		Adult Male	Letter re Compensation
		Adult Male	Letter re Wife
		?	Better
		Adult Male	Letter re Compensation
		Adult Female	Gynaecological
		Adult Female	Cards for Mrs X to Post-office
	10		
7th		Adult Female	Dyspepsia
		Adult Male	Disordered Action of Heart
		Adult Female	Debility. Anaemia.
		Adult Female	Gynaecological
		Baby	Well now
	5		

In September 1946 Sister Mary's husband Chas Ward visited his daughter, son-in-law and grand-son in London, a trip arranged so Chas could take his *small grandson to see the Beefeaters at the Tower of London.* Grand-father and grand-son toured the Tower of London on Saturday 28th September, the visit ended in tragedy …

> A mishap occurred after he had taken his small grandson to see the Beefeaters at the Tower of London was responsible for the death recently of 81-year-old Mr. Charles William Ward, of The Surgery Stoke Bruerne, who was Britain's oldest member of the Home Guard. Brought up within the sound of gun-fire at Aldershot. Mr. Ward was denied service in the Army owing to his small stature … Owing to injuries received in a car smash when he was of middle age. Mr Ward was unable to perform active duties and was given the rank of corporal in a secretarial position.

> It had always been his youthful ambition to join the forces, and it was after taking his grandson to see the Army, to which he had always wanted to belong; that he met his death. Turning round with his grandson to "wave good-bye to the Beefeaters and the Tower", he slipped, fell, and opened up old wounds. He died shortly afterwards in hospital.

Charles William Shepherd Perry Ward, age 81, retired secretary of Stoke Bruerne, died in Hendon Cottage Hospital, the inquest was held at Hendon Town Hall where it was reported Chas died from *General peritonitis following rupture of intestine following fall in street*[456], the coroner recorded a verdict of accidental death[457]. The death certificate gave Chas's age as 81, he was in fact 77, and as one boater recalled *canal folk didn't say a word when Sister Mary's husband died. They just left flowers on the doorstep.*

The same year Chas died the Littlemore's, a long standing Grand Union boating family and good friends with Sister Mary, posed for a national newspaper. One picture was published in The Daily Mirror[458] shown in Figure 106, Sister Mary is seen here tending 10 year old Rose Littlemore who is sitting in the chair opposite her mother, Ada Littlemore (nee Mellor), 8 year old Sylvia is standing beside the chair and Ada's youngest daughter Jenny is in her mother's arms. The article accompanying the picture was titled *The Lady of the Lamp – 1946 style,* the caption reads …

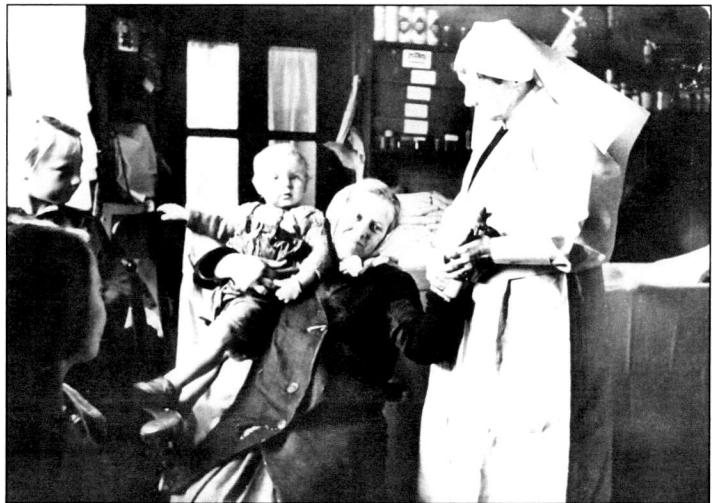

Figure 106   Ada Littlemore and her daughters visiting Sister Mary (Waterway's Archive)

Sister Mary Ward is *"The Lady with the Hurricane Lamp"* on the towpaths of Northants. Where there is sickness or an accident, whatever the hour, they send for her. Her surgery at the locks near Stoke Bruerne is *"the doctors"* for all the Grand Union Canal folk. She is tenderness itself, and little Rosie Ellen Littlemore, 8, here in the chair, with "something wrong with her heart" has a faith in her that ought to work miracles[459].

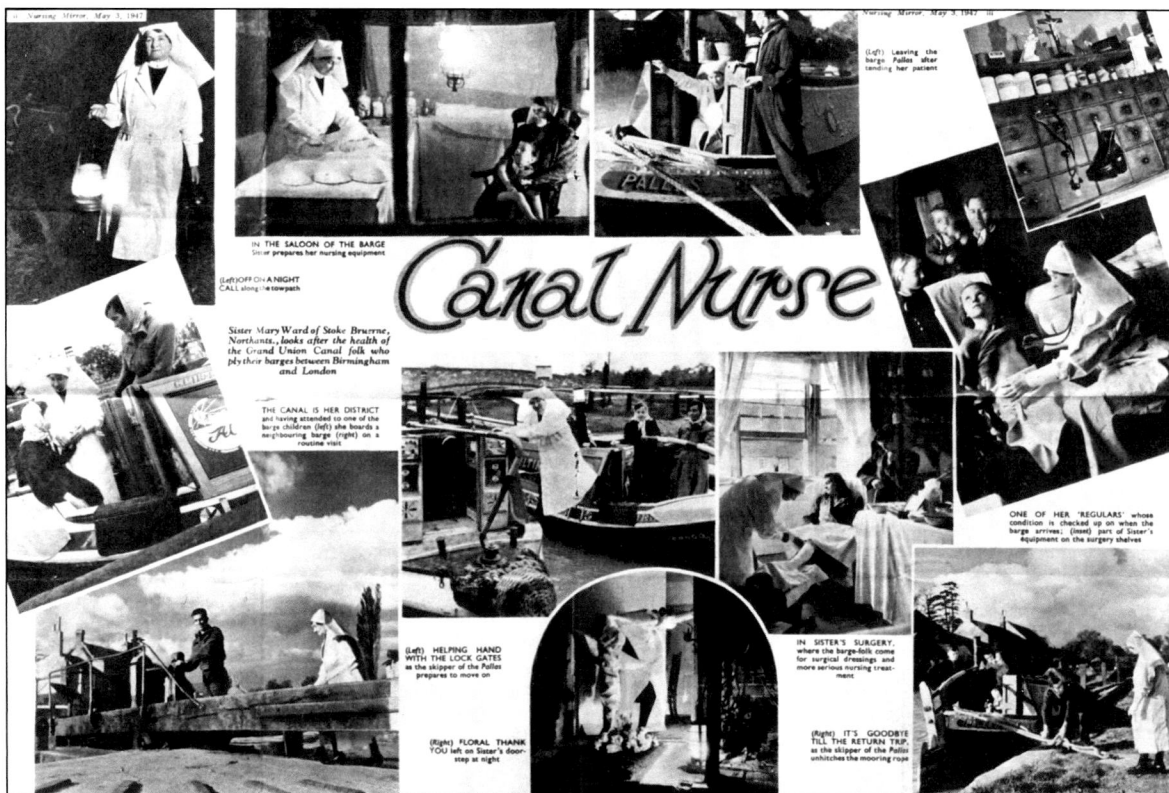

Figure 107   Canal Nurse (Della Sadler-Moore collection)

Sister Mary was also landlady to the canal-side terraced cottages, her tenants included tunnel tug driver Richard Dyke, and retired lock-keeper Jack James who around 1947 began to display his canalware outside the cottage, Jack eventually purchased the cottage from Sister Mary. In 1947 Sister Mary was captured in the nursing press for the first time, in a double page article titled *Canal Nurse*[460] (Figure 107). The picture in the top left hand corner of the article has been enlarged to show Sister Mary performing her *night duties* (Figure 108), the article marked the beginning of what was to become a regular media interest in her work.

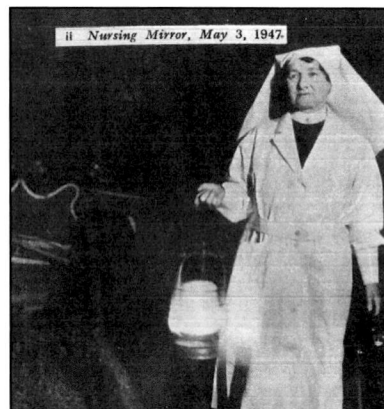

Figure 108   Night Duty (Della Sadler-Moore collection)

The same year the Littlemore's picture was published the post-war labour government brought into being The NHS Act (c81) which established a comprehensive health service to *secure improvement in the physical and mental health of people of England and Wales and prevention, diagnosis and treatment of illness … free of charge … except where the act expressly provides for charges*[461], legislation which applied equally to the floating population as it did to those living on the bank. A further government act saw agreement to the nationalization of the canals, railways and long distance haulage. At midnight on December 31st 1947 the Grand Union Canal Company and its subsidiaries ceased to own the Grand Union Canal, the boats and the associated property, on the dawn of the new year (1948) the British Transport Commission came into being.

Sister Mary adapts to change …

Post-nationalization the British Transport Commission devolved canal operations to the Docks and Inland Waterways Executive (D.&I.W.E.), who strategically created four Inland Waterways Divisions shown in Figure 109, Stoke Bruerne being in the South East (SE) Division. After nationalization Fellows, Morton & Clayton (FMC) started making a loss on its carrying, as a result they called a shareholders meeting in September 1948 at which point they decided to liquidate the company and release its assets. Following a later meeting with the new nationalised body running the canals, the British Transport Commission bought FMC's property and boats, absorbing these into the nationalised fleet[462].

Following nationalization Sister Mary's employment was taken over by the Docks and Inland Waterways Executive who produced a monthly house magazine *Lock and Quay*. In the second edition Sister Mary was the first to feature in a series titled *Lock and Quay Encounters*[463], the article carried with it a drawing of Sister Mary by artist Kathleen Shackleton shown in Figure 110, signed in the bottom left hand corner by Mary E H Ward. The portrait was accompanied by the following account …

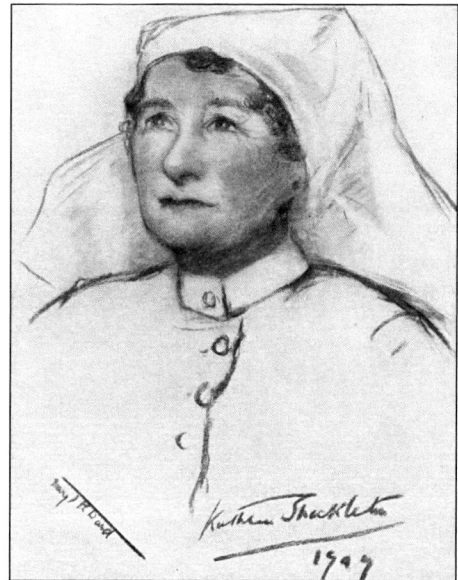

Figure 110   Line drawing of Sister Mary (Waterway's Archive)

> A picturesque though practical personality of our inland waterways is Sister Mary of Stoke Bruerne, Northamptonshire. She is consultant Sister to the boat people carrying traffic between London and Birmingham in the South Eastern Division. Her spotless surgery is in a nine-roomed house by the canal-side, not far from Blisworth tunnel, and incidentally it is the house where she was born.

Her cheery, bronzed face, sparkling eyes and neat figure, with white flowing veil and scarlet cloak, are a welcome sight to any sick boater in need of medical or surgical attention. Her

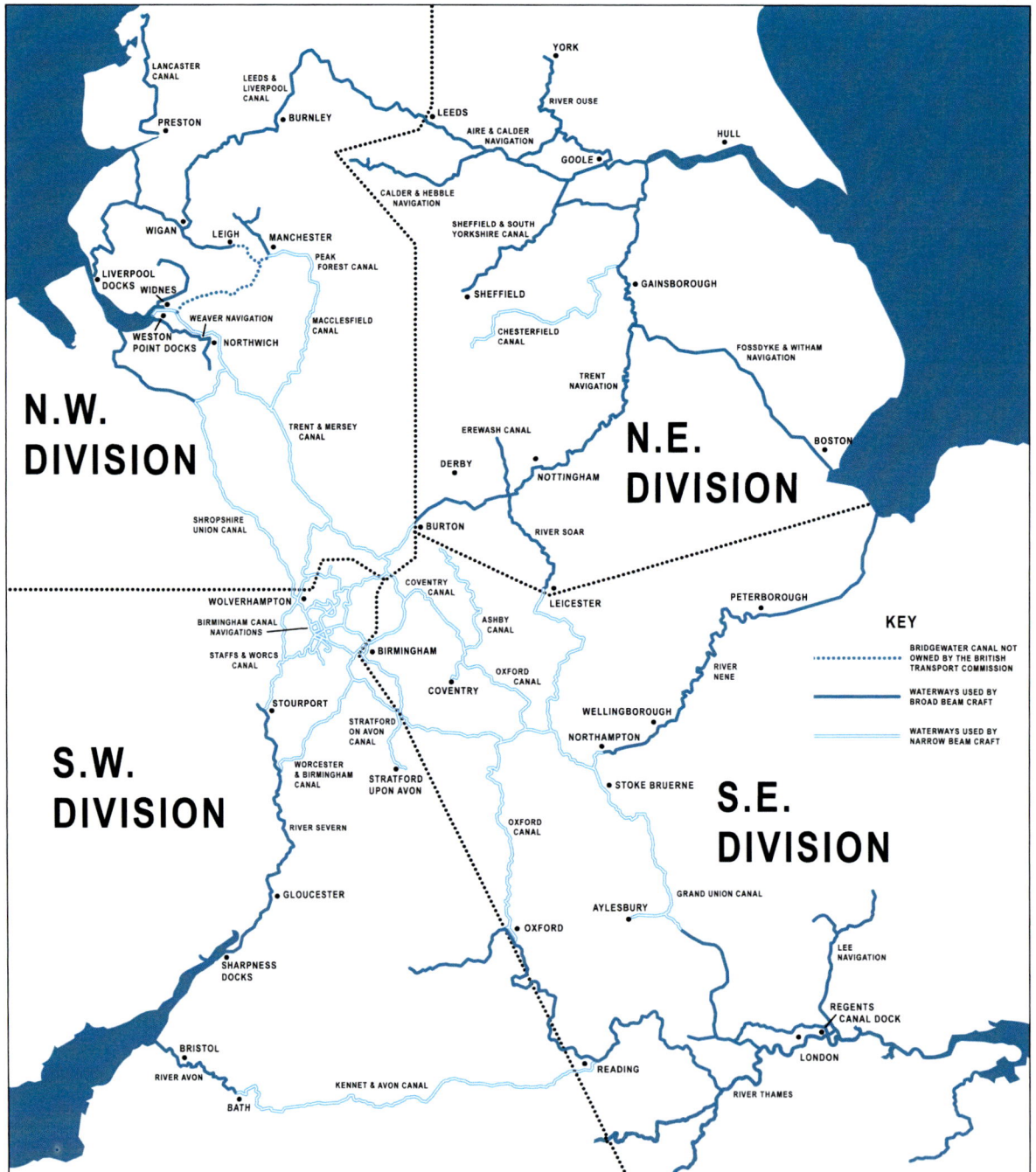

Figure 109   Inland Waterway's four divisions (Christopher M Jones)

present job started in this way. After employment as a nurse for twenty years … later she was called home to nurse her father and it was during his illness that she began attending to the boat people. This happy association thus started with them led the Grand Union Canal Company engaging her permanently. Sister Mary considers that her canal work has been the most romantic part of her … nursing career. She has a deep affection for the boat people. *They are brave and lovable folk,* she says. *unusual in their outlook on life, but when understood, loyal and true friends – it is a joy to serve them.*

Stoke Bruerne became a regular source of material for *Lock and Quay.* The following edition carried a report on the D&IWE first *Care and Maintenance competition [for] the best kept locks, cottages and gardens.* In the South Eastern Division Mr Jack James was awarded 2nd place for maintenance of the lock outside Sister Mary's house[464], this was a big event for Mr James as the local newspaper captured the prize being presented by a member of the executive[465]. Sister Mary began to write letters to the magazine, her first in response to a somewhat outdated picture of the village printed in an earlier edition …

> Sister Mary Ward … pleasingly tells us of the monthly interest and enjoyment which the Magazine brings to her, has drawn our attention to the picture of Stoke Bruerne Locks … of the January issue. This picture features Sister Mary's own cottage, and she reminds us that although the camera never lies, the picture is a little different now, only one poplar tree remains in the background, and the sunblind at the lounge bay window of her cottage has had its day-mostly her father's day. She now allows the sun to fade the carpets![466]

As the 1940's drew to a close electricity finally arrived at Stoke Bruerne and Sister Mary was the subject of a British Pathe film titled *Bargee Doctor[467]*, Sister Mary also remained on call for the village primary school, and on one occasion she was called to an emergency …

> At about 10.30 this morning many children complained of headaches and feeling sick. The children were sent out of school into the playground where two children lost consciousness. This was due to fumes from the coke stove. After first aid given by Miss King (manager) and Sister Ward the children were sent home[468].

Welfare arrangements for boater's was by all accounts well established at Bull's Bridge as the D & IWE were keen to announce in February 1950. In Lock and Quay the company reported they *maintain stocks of additional foods for mothers and young children, such as orange juice, cod liver oil and vitamin tablets,* which the company distribute to the boat families *to save them the journey to the local Food Office or Clinic.* The distribution service had the previous December been viewed by the local alderman and mayor *who witnessed the distribution of orange juice and other foods to the boaters[469]* .

Mr Ernest Veater who since 1936 worked as midland representative at the Grand Union Canal Carrying Company Sutton Stop boat control office[470] retired in June 1950, seen in Figure 111 with his colleagues at his retirement party[471]. Before his retirement Mr Veater delivered a lecture on his experiences of working within the boating community[472], due to *human interest and curiosity*

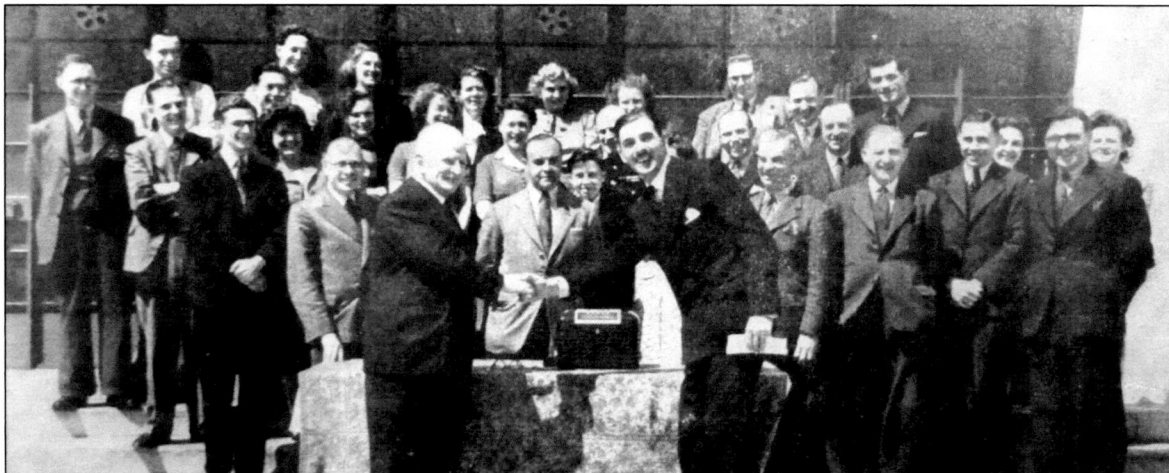

Figure 111   Mr Veater retirement (Waterway's Archive)

regarding canal folk the lecture has been transcribed in full (Appendix 12), it's content gives a remarkable insight into canal culture and traditions. In the opening to the lecture Mr Veater suggesting the subject matter to be just a matter of daily routine …

> I have been employed in various capacities for 24 years regarding canals which gives me some knowledge of the commercial side as well as an intimate view of the canal boatmen and family. I take it to be the latter or human side is the one which you would prefer to listen to and discuss …

Following the announcement of Mr Veater's retirement Sister Mary wrote again to Lock & Quay to tell readers about how proud she was of the canal beauty spot by her home …

> During the war years, the lock-side at Stoke Bruerne, Northamptonshire, naturally was somewhat neglected. Lock-keeper Mr. J. James, dissatisfied with the general appearance of it, set to work. Week after week he toiled, getting rubble, ashes and earth, filling in all the holes, until some sort of order was obtained. His next effort was to prepare flower beds to brighten the outlook of the towing path- Mr. James had been a boatman, like his father, and well knew the love of the canal folk for beauty and gardens.
>
> Today this part of the canal is a picture of neatness and loveliness, a wonder to the many visitors who come to Stoke Bruerne. The flower beds are now brilliant with blooms of wallflowers, tulips, forget-me-nots and many beautiful border plants; rambler roses are planted here and there and soon will be giving joy to the passers-by. I do wish every lock-keeper could see the lock-side and be encouraged to bring beauty to the towing path. Good luck to all lock-keepers on our canals[473].

Sister Mary continued to own three of the four canal-side cottages, renting two of them to Richard Sudbury Dyke[474] and George Hancock, on paying their rent Sister Mary recorded this in a ledger, Table 39 gives an extract from the records which on closer examination shows a periodic rent rise. George Hancock also rented from Sister Mary a *shelter for the car*. Both of Sister Mary's tenants left their canal-side homes (c1955-57) to take up residence in the newly built council houses in the village, Mr Dyke went to Wentworth Road and Mr Hancock to Shutlanger Road, leaving Sister Mary with empty cottages and no rental income.

Table 39   Mr Dyke's rent, including rent rise

1949/1950			£	s	d	Signature
December	19	2 weeks @ 4/6		9	-	MEHW
January	2	2 Weeks " "		9	-	MEHW
	16	2 Weeks " "		9	-	MEHW
Jan / February	30	2 " " "		9	-	MEHW
Feb	13	2 Weeks		9	-	MEHW
		etc etc				
1953						
July	27	2 Weeks Extra 1/8		10	8	MEHW
		etc etc				
1954						
July	12	2 Weeks rent 5/7		11	2	MEHW

Five years post-war and Sister Mary's surgery remained as busy as ever. In March 1950 she treated 359 patients, an overview of the numbers treated daily is transcribed in Table 40, which shows the surgery was open every day but one, on that day Sister Mary visited London, she was seeing between 5 -33 patients per day.

Table 40   Number of cases seen daily by Sister Mary March 1950

Date	Number of cases	Date	Number of cases	Date	Number of cases
1st	18	12th	23	23rd	12
2nd	8 Left for London	13th	10	24th	9
3rd	London	14th	5	25th	11
4th	Returned from London 8	15th	14	26th	15
5th	11	16th	14	27th	21
6th	11	17th	19	28th	8

7th	13	18th	10	29th	11
8th	3	19th	11	30th	11
9th	8	20th	3	31st	8
10th	7	21st	33		
11th	16	22nd	18		

The following January Sister Mary was awarded the British Empire Medal (BEM) by Lord Lieutenant, William Thomas Brownlow Cecil, 5th Marquis of Exeter, the landmark was celebrated in the local newspaper[475] and a national nursing magazine[476]. The Northampton Mercury reporting …

> The British Empire Medal has been awarded to Sister Mary Ellen Hollowell Ward., who lives at The Surgery, Stoke Bruerne. Officially bearing the designation "Consultant Sister to Long Distance Boatmen and Families British Canals", Mrs Ward gives expert nursing services to barge crews who make their way from London to Birmingham or vice versa, on the Grand Union Canal.
>
> She was born at the same house she now "reigns" as Sister, and where her father, Mr. Thomas Amos, was a rope-maker who became one of the leading public men in the county – county councillor and justice of the peace … her surgery is open all hours of the day, and she attends between 200 and 400 cases a month, dealing with anything from a broken leg to double pneumonia. Among the first letters of congratulations on her honour was one from Gilmore Jenkins, Permanent Secretary to the Ministry of Transport[477].

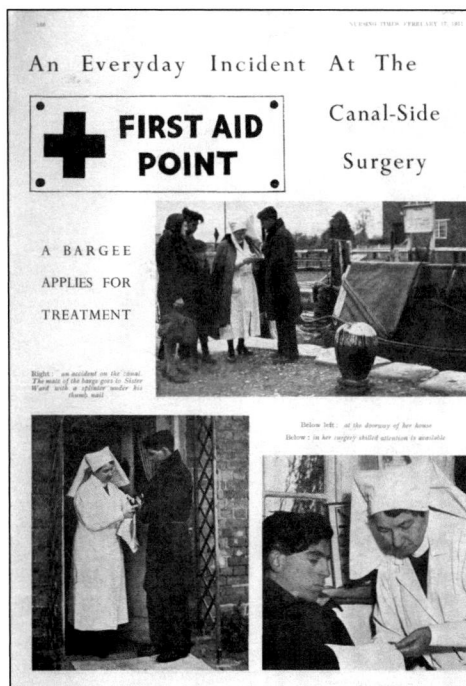

In recognition of the award of the BEM the Nursing Times ran a double page article on Sister Mary's work with boaters[478], the front page shown in Figure 112 included the following account …

… for many years she has been caring for the families in England who go up and down the canals. The watermen are reserved and independent, but they have come to know Miss Ward. They bring her all their difficulties, but it is particularly their health problems for which she is responsible; she is officially known as Consultant Sister to the Docks and Inland Waterways Executive. She has a surgery in her own house for minor ailments and serious cases are sent to the hospital at Northampton. The children on the barges receive her special attention … The parents are grateful that their health needs can be supervised

Figure 112   Sister Mary's First Aid Point (Della Sadler-Moore collection)

by Miss Ward, who is a family adviser and friend to countless waterfolk. In recognition of all her work, Miss Ward was awarded the British Empire Medal …

The canal and Stoke Bruerne were changing in the early 1950's, a subject which stimulated Jack James to give an interview on the subject[479] …

There have been many changes in canal life during the 56 years that Mr. John James, prizewinner last Saturday in the best-kept lock gardens competition, has been part of it. The colourful dress of the old-time boat families has been replaced by clothing more suitable for scrambling over cargoes and leaping from boat to lock to help open gates. To some extent, however, the women of the boats still retain the old style of dress. Skirts are still long; shawls are still thrown over their shoulders.

Life is easier now

But what has changed are the conditions under which the canal families work. To-day, according to Mr. James, life is "easier" on the canals. Once two men used to "leg" a boat through a tunnel – lying on their backs and propelling the boat by "walking" along the tunnel's roof. The modern motor boat does away with this "hard labour". And under nationalisation, too, pay is better. Hours are more controlled, and there are educational facilities for the children.

The Grand Union Canal at Stoke Bruerne was also used for a number of charitable activities. On one occasion a boat trip was organised in aid of a *Flood Relief Fund*, Sister Mary shown in Figure 113 went on the trip and recorded the event for others to enjoy …

Everyone has been shocked by the recent flood disasters here and abroad and throughout the country relief funds have been opened to help those so sadly affected by the storm havoc.

One unusual way in which the villagers of Stoke Bruerne helped to raise money was a canal trip. The idea started with

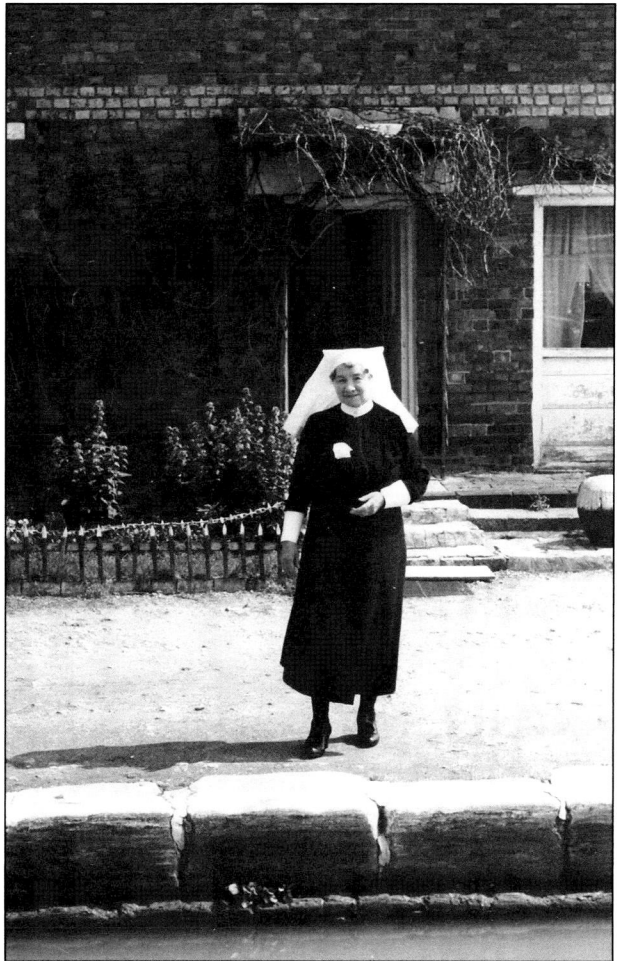

Figure 113   Sister Mary outside her home in the 1950's (Waterway's Archive)

Mr. John James, captain of the boat *Jason*, which has been anchored during the winter at the Top-Lock, Stoke Bruerne. He arranged a boating party for February 15. On that day the snow lay thick on towing path and fields, but the people of this small village, nothing daunted, and determined to make this effort a success, muffled themselves up and faced the icy north-east winds.

At 2.30 p.m. the *Jason*, well loaded, set off from Stoke Bruerne to Gayton and return, a journey which meant twice through the tunnel. For most of the passengers, it was their first glimpse of the interior of Stoke tunnel, and for many, as the Jason entered the black depths of it to travel below ground for 1 ¾ miles, it was a somewhat disturbing experience. Soon, however, the powerful rays of the *Jason's* headlights dispersed the gloom and the passengers were able to view the wonderfully phosphorescent walls of the tunnel, caused by the constant dripping of water- they were a grand sight, as the light revealed their many and varied colours, gold, green and grey predominating. The symmetrical building of the walls reminded one of those early canal engineers who, as far back as the 18th century, performed such fine workmanship that even to-day, in the 20th century, it remains still in good condition.

Suddenly a gleam of light heralded one of the many ventilating shafts which are at various points along the tunnel, the deepest one being 140 ft. As the *Jason* passed each shaft, water dripped on the heads and shoulders of the laughing people aboard. Also in the tunnel we met three pairs of loaded boats. The *Jason* slowed down to allow plenty of room, and all called to the passing boatmen and exchanged cheery greetings. After leaving the tunnel, we journeyed along to Gayton, then, turning the *Jason*, headed for home. We arrived at Top Lock, Stoke Bruerne at 5 p.m., after an enjoyable and unforgettable journey[480].

Jack James's son, art student John James and owner of the narrow boat *Jason* was also changing with the times, when John left Stoke Bruerne on *Jason* he was heading for London *to make his fortune*. On the first leg of the journey John took with him a number of passengers, including Sister Mary and a local reporter[481]…

On Saturday, artist John James … left his native Stoke Bruerne for London. His immediate aim: to make money; his ultimate aim; to realise a boyhood ambition. He took, not brushes and canvas, but a 72-feet narrow boat and a roll of tickets. Sitting on the bunk in the comfortable cabin of his canal boat, Jason, before leaving, Mr. James said: *I hope to make money by running canal trips for London's Coronation visitors.*

Tall, bespectacled, and wearing the scarf of his London art college, he added: *If I punch enough tickets, I shall do what I have always wanted to do- paint my way round Britain's inland waterway's.* John and his ambition were given a grand send-off by Stoke Bruerne. Villagers stood on the bridge and around the locks to wave farewell. And a party of 35 invited guests travelled with the Jason down the Grand Union (sic) Canal as far as Old Wolverton.

Among the passengers were Lady Hesketh, Sister Mary Ward, consultant sister to long-distance boatmen and families, and 20 year old Joan Smith, Stoke Bruerne's Coronation

Queen. Speed note; it took nearly a hour to cover the first mile, because of a flight of seven locks.

John's optimistic outlook came to fruition, because it was later reported he was *making a living by running Festival Cruises in the heart of London, taking American Visitors for a one hour trip through Regent's Park and London Zoo*[482].

Post-war the circumstances surrounding the floating populations welfare never really went away from the gaze of government. In 1951 responsibilities for new regulations under section 251 of the *Public Health Act (1936) under a Transfer of Functions Order (1951)* became the responsibility of the Ministry of Housing and Local Government. After the act came into force the new minister asked the House of Commons if *revised regulations governing the conditions of sanitation and ventilation in canal boats were needed in the interests of Public Health standards*. The Parliamentary Secretary replied *he would be consulting the Local Authority Associations on the matter*. The following march he asked if revised regulations were necessary, in particular, whether they should provide for …

a)   Suitable sanitary accommodation on all narrow boats and barges, and facilities for bathing purposes;

b)   Greater air space per person;

c)   Increased storage of water required for all purposes

Eleven months after the question was posed the General Council of the Sanitary Association, replied[483] with what were referred to as *a set of brief observations* on sanitary accommodation, bathing facilities, water supply, space in cabin, ventilation and lighting for boaters. A more detailed account of these points and a set of recommendations as to regulatory changes were proffered in February of 1953[484] and submitted to the Minister the following month.

No further developments were reported until the publication of a *seminal article* by the Chief Sanitary Inspector for Heston and Islewoth A.B. Hauldren, whose patch *included a small stretch of the Grand Union Canal (2 miles), including Bulls Bridge*[485]. In the paper Hauldren gives a definitive resume of the *issues surrounding canal boats and sanitary inspection* in his words *seen through the eyes of the inspectorate*. Hauldren writing candidly about his experiences of boatmen and their families …

> The average boatman is courteous and amiable and willing to give any information required, particularly if rightly approached, and seldom nowadays does one come across the arrogant type.

> Cases of bug infestation, squalor and neglect of living conditions found in earlier years are now a rare occurrence. The overall cleanliness and pride in the boat portrays a change in the character of the personnel. This change may be due to the fact the motor is of some importance and requires the development of knowledge and responsibility. There is

a tendency for the men and women to dress up when frequenting the town establishments or shopping, and one of the major complaints received in my talks with the younger element is the lack of wardrobe space for their clothes. Surely the provision of such accommodation should be considered and self-respect fostered.

A boatman and his family usually control two boats – one motor and one butty. In the case of the larger families both boats are used for sleeping, whereas if manned by childless couples or just a crew of two, living quarters are usually confined to one boat. In my experience very little use, if any, is now made of the fore cabin for sleeping purposes and is more often than not utilized for the storage of miscellaneous articles, such as ropes, etc.

The boatman is responsible for the cargo from the time of shipment to discharge; the removal of bilge water by pumping at least every 24 hours; the keeping of the cabins in a cleanly and habitable state, and he must notify as soon as possible the occurrence of any serious illness or infectious disease to the proper sanitary authority and to the owner of the boat. The master also has a certain responsibility in connection with overcrowding and education of his children.

If required by the inspecting officer, the master must produce the certificate of registration. Refusal is deemed to amount to obstruction of the officer in the discharge of his duty and a person so obstructing is liable to be fined. The expression "Master" in relation to a canal boat means the person having for the time being command or charge of the boat.

In concluding Hauldren made two suggestions *which could improve the living conditions for boat families*; 1) the erection of more sanitary blocks, and 2) improving natural light by inserting in the cabin top a reinforced glass or perspex panel[486].

In the 1950's Stoke Bruerne began to see an increasing number of holiday boaters pass along the Grand Union Canal, which Sister Mary approved of as indicated in a letter to her friend …

you would enjoy being here this a.m, four holiday boats arrived last evening from London way … this morning all the guests aboard gathered inside and outside the surgery – some requiring treatment, mostly for sunburn, others just an excuse to visit, - but with the painted boats, the brilliant sunshine, it was indeed a picture of life and animation[487].

In 1954 the first *Hotel Boats* passed through the village, the *Floating Hotel* as it was referred to in a publication was captured on canvas and published on the front cover of John Bull shown in Figure 114. This new use of 'a pair of old canal boats' was such an attraction, it was reported in the local newspaper … *the Hotel was converted from two old barges – Nelson and Nancy, by Mr. Michael Streat of Braunston. One barge is a lounge, galley and dining-salon; the other has eight sleeping cabins*[488]. The same year the hotel boats passed through Stoke Bruerne *Willow Wren Canal Company* came into being on the Grand Union Canal, set up by the Inland Waterway Associations (IWA) honorary treasurer (banker) Vivian Bulkley-Johnson, with Mr Lesley Morton appointed General Manager of the fleet.

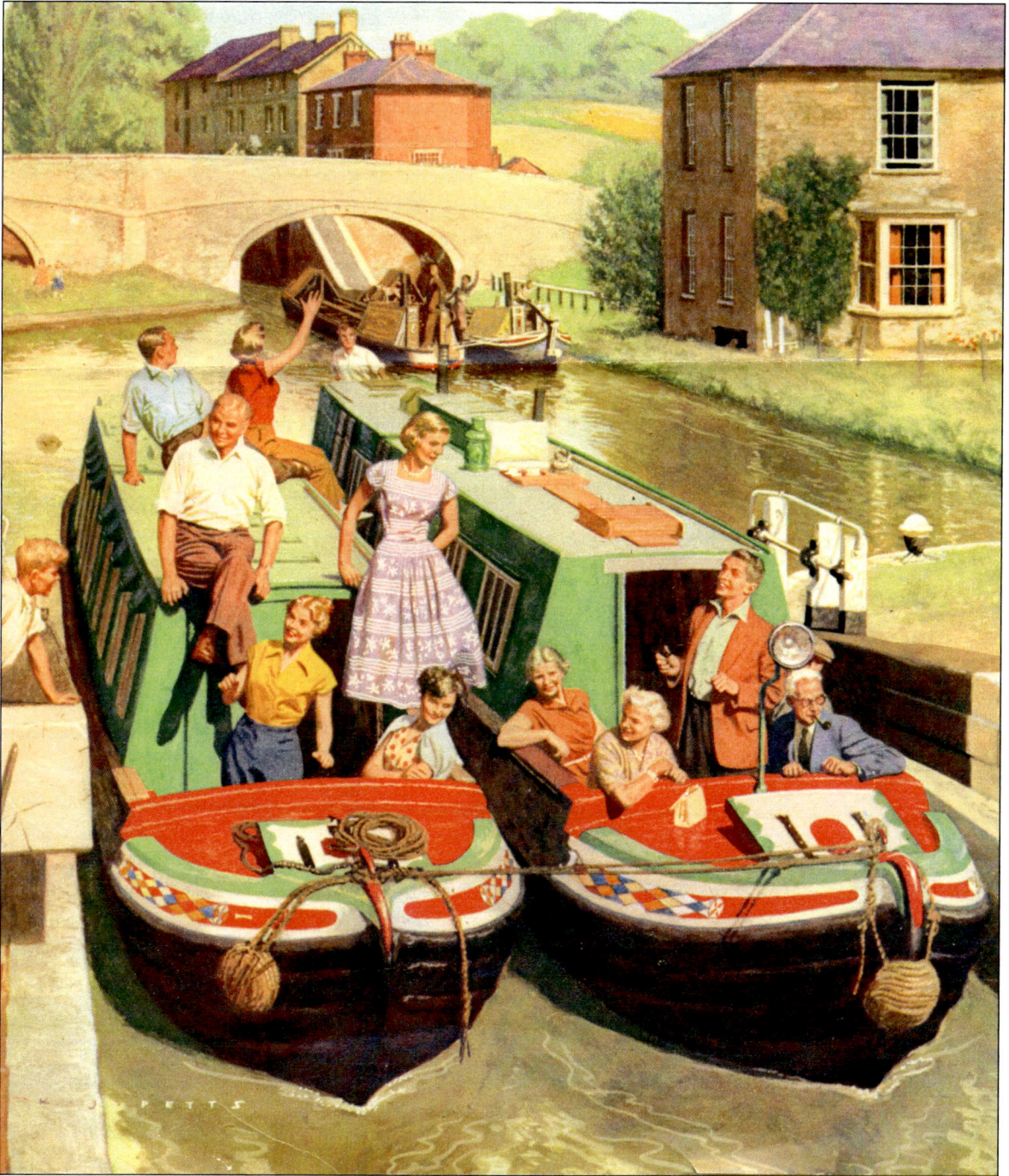

Figure 114   The *Floating Hotel* passing through Stoke Bruerne (Amoret Tanner / Alamy)

After the Willow Wren fleet became operational Mr Morton engaged the services of Sister Mary, after which she commenced a Willow Wren case book. From reviewing entries in the case book a key aspect of Sister Mary's role with Willow Wren boat families was to regularly keep Mr Morton up-to-date on the company employees health and wellbeing (via the telephone, letters and through Mr Morton visiting the surgery). Sister Mary made meticulous notes on each Willow Wren boat family, including when a boating family changed from one company boat to another, all Willow Wren being named after birds; Red Shank, Willow Warbler, Mallard, Quail, Teal, Sky Lark and Greenshank etc[489]. Willow Wren Company boaters presented to Sister Mary with conditions / ailments no different to other boaters; minor injuries, fractures, colds and respiratory conditions. What is more evident in her records is her *family health* role with boater's, where she reported she did a *check up,* or *boater seen ... no treatment necessary.* An aspect of Sister Mary's health promotion role with the Willow Wren boaters was dispensing batches of 100 Halibut Oil tablets, paid for by the company. In the case book there is evidence of one baby being born in Stoke Bruerne to a well known boating family, her report regarding this extraordinary event was *all well.*

Throughout the 1950's Sister Mary continued to be called to emergencies at Stoke Bruerne Primary School ...

> During the morning assembly Paul ... fainted and in doing so hit his chin violently against the teacher's desk, thereby rendering himself unconscious for some time and making a deep cut under the chin. Sister Mary Ward was called in and advised his attendance at the Outpatient Department of Northampton General Hospital as she thought there was a risk of a fractured jaw. He was taken there by the head teacher. The wound was stitched and he was thoroughly examined and sent home with instructions to see his own doctor the next day[490]

Sister Mary's *official retirement* from the Docks and Inland Waterway's Executive was on December 31st 1956, a party at the company's Southall depot was well attended as shown in Figure 115[491]. The write up accompanying the picture reads ...

> After having spent very many years looking after the well-being of narrow boat families, Sister Mary retired ....

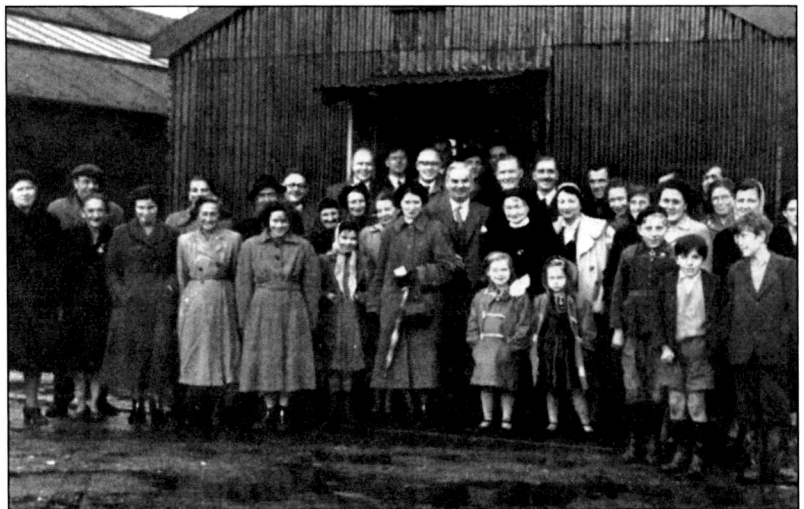

Figure 115   Sister Mary's retirement party at BW Southall Depot (Waterway's Archive)

From her surgery … she watched the present generation grow up from childhood and nursed them through many illnesses. In a lot of cases she cared for their parents before them.

On the last day of her service, Sister Mary travelled to Southall where she was entertained to lunch by the Divisional Manager. Afterwards there was a pleasing little ceremony in the canteen of Bulls Bridge where, in the presence of several officers of the Division and a number of boating families, C. A. Saywood, the Divisional Manager, on behalf of British Waterways, thanked Sister Mary for her long service. He presented her with a clock set in a model of a ship's wheel. F.J. Norris, the Staff & Establishment Officer, also thanked her on behalf of the General Manager who was unable to be present. Sister Mary was also presented with a silver teapot and tray by Mrs Hambridge, wife of Steerer W. Hambridge, on behalf of the boating families of the South Eastern Division. Sister Mary will be very much missed[492].

After official retirement …

Regardless of *Official Retirement* and a very small pension, Sister Mary continued to provide care to boaters from her surgery for a further six years, as seen in Figure 116 outside her home with Mrs Alf Best. Although now 'officially retired' and under no obligation to boaters or carriers

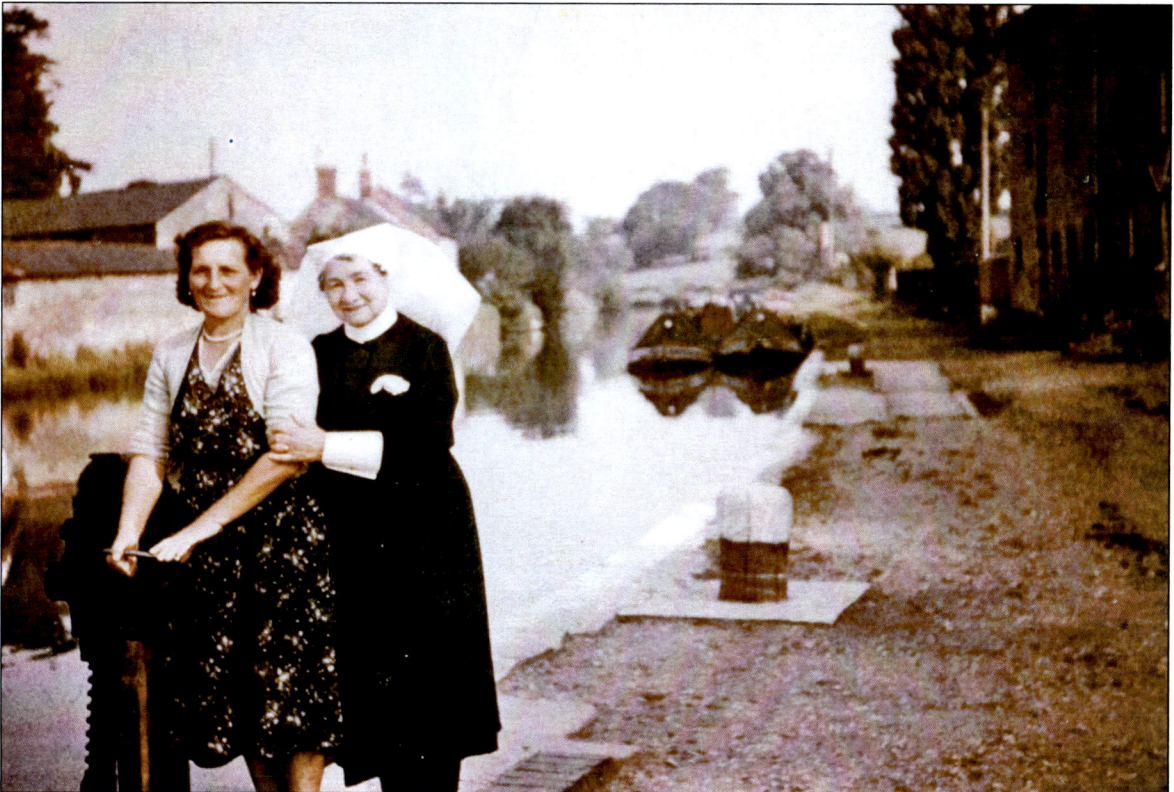

Figure 116   Mrs Alf Best with Sister Mary Ward (Unknown source)

she continued to maintain her case book entries although these are somewhat sparse[493]. It is evident from the records Sister Mary continued to write to canal officials to keep them up-to-date regarding a boater, as seen in a letter to Mr Campbell written after she treated Sam Higgins for a hand injury …

> The Surgery
> Stoke Bruerne
> Towcester
> Northamptonshire
> *April 30 1957*
> *Monday 10.42 P.M.*
>
> *Dear Mr Campbell,*
>
> *Regret to report, Sam Higgins, Steerer, had an accident to hand, thick steel wire was wrapped around blades, Sam tried to remove the same, which caused a nasty wound, I stitched wound, dressing of course, but as patient had lost rather a lot of blood - & naturally could not use right hand, I said, bed for some hours, therefore am afraid Boats will be somewhat delayed, - although I said they could continue journey, hence this note to you.*
>
> *Hope you and yours are well.*
>
> *Yours truly*
>
> *Sister Mary*[494]

A remarkable insight into Sister Mary's character was immortalised by John Thorpe[495]. John as a young lad met Sister Mary in may 1957 whilst on a family hire boat holiday, as the family passed through Stoke Bruerne John's father spoke to Sister Mary and she invited the family for a *cup of tea,* John recounts the meeting after the family tied up …

> There were two doors at the front and a light alongside the first of these seemed to indicate which should be knocked upon. Trim gardens fronted the house and foliage crept up the walls before spreading luxuriantly out over the porch to neatly encompass the main door upon which we knocked. Warmth flooded out to greet us as Sister Mary hurried us inside and we found ourselves standing in what was evidently the boatman's surgery. Everything was painted white and was spotlessly clean. In the centre of the room a medical bed occupied pride of place and glass-fronted cupboards were filled with bottles, bandages, and other medical paraphernalia. A bay-fronted window with a low wooden seat afforded an excellent view of the lock and adjacent towpath. I knew that Sister Mary had been ministering to the boatpeople's needs for very many years, that through a mixture of kindness and selfless devotion she had acquired their complete trust and loyalty, and that she was paid only a small sum by the carrying companies for her efforts.

After looking round the boatman's surgery, the Thorpe family were invited into Sister Mary's sitting room …

> We passed across a narrow passageway into a comfortable sitting room amply furnished with settee and armchairs with several small tables scattered about. Two bookcases lined

one wall and thick heavy curtains added to the atmosphere of old fashioned comfort. Photographs of family and friends, small ornaments and miscellaneous objects completed thye friendly and welcoming effect. A tray of cups, plates and biscuits stood on a low table in front of a pleasant fire.

Tea over, the Thorpe's made their way back to the boat John took an interest in the empty *rather dilapidated looking terraced cottages* next to Sister Mary's home. On the return journey John looked again at the *canal side tall cottages … with basements below canal level,* this time John asked Sister Mary about their ownership, she replying *they're mine (except Number 3).* John gathered from Sister Mary she was hoping to sell some of the property to fund her work with the boat people, although she told him *you can't give them away … that end one has been empty for two years, nobody wants it.* John and his mother looked more closely at number 4, the end cottage …

> A battered high brick step led up to a bright green front door with a brass knob, sadly in need of a clean. Sash windows were partially shrouded by an old climbing rose which also made its way across the top of the door and, Sister Mary assured us, gave beautiful deep red roses all summer. Similar sash windows opened out of bedrooms on the first floor and second floors and a steeply cobbled pathway, running between the cottages and Sister Mary's house, gave access to a cellar and wash-house at the rear of the property. It all looked rather sad and neglected but what a fabulous place to live:

Sister Mary informed the Thorpe's she wanted £150 for each cottage, a viewing was booked for the following weekend. On arriving, Sister Mary was leaning out of the Surgery window and after tea she produced *a large brass key* and the tour began, John meticulously recording every detail as transcribed in Appendix 12. The tour completed, John's parents looked at the *councils closing order* on the property, Mr Thorpe then emerged from Sister Mary's and a handshake sealed the deal, renovation commenced and by early September 1958 the Towcester council official *lifted the closing order, declaring the cottage fit for habitation.* During the renovation Sister Mary took John *under her wing,* frequently inviting him for mid-morning coffee and a biscuit, John recalled the meetings ….

> I learnt a good deal during those warm summer days chatting with Sister in the peace of her cosy little room. She was extremely unsentimental and realistic about the boatpeople to whom she had given such care and devotion, each family being treated individually with their foibles and idiosyncrasies accepted and understood. Rarely critical directly, she nevertheless understood the harsh nature of their working lives and the strict, almost Victorian, moral views that so many of them held. Sister gave them her unstinting support and always made herself available at whatever time their boat was passing. She knew that nearly all of them would make every effort to cope with their medical problems and families often travelled for several days to see Sister Mary rather than consult a local doctor. This could have its drawbacks. On occasions problems had become much worse before Sister Mary could begin to deal with them. The boatpeople were undaunted by this, her devotion and their unswerving trust formed the bedrock of a unique relationship.

From Sister Mary I learnt a good deal about the people of the boats who passed regularly up and down past the cottage during the course of the summer ...

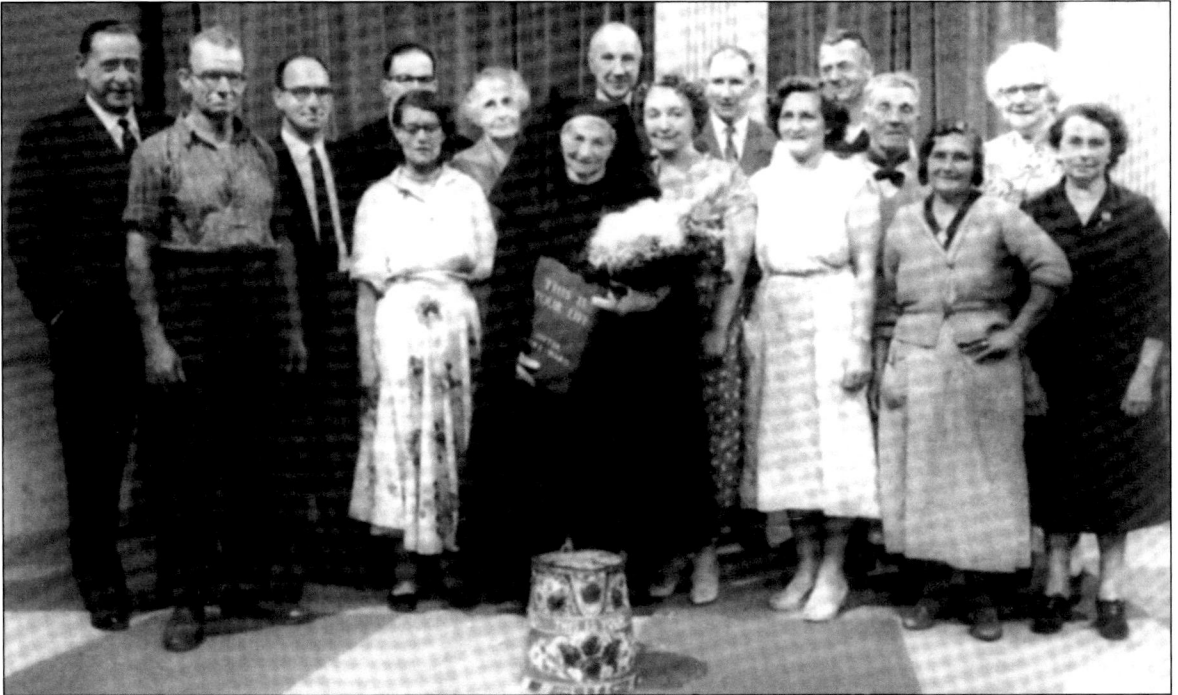

Figure 117   The whole entourage during Sister Mary's This is your life (David Blagrove collection)

Sister Mary was the guest of honour on Eamonn Andrews *This is your life* in 1958, at which many of her boating friends and colleagues were in attendance *shown in* Figure 117[496]. During the programme much was revealed about Sister Mary from her longstanding boat families, including an account by Mr Alf Best ...

> I remember once I was taken seriously ill with pneumonia, I reckoned I was at deaths door. But Sister Mary nursed me day and night for four days and pulled me through. I reckon she saved my life and I can honestly say she can't be praised too highly. There will never be another like her.

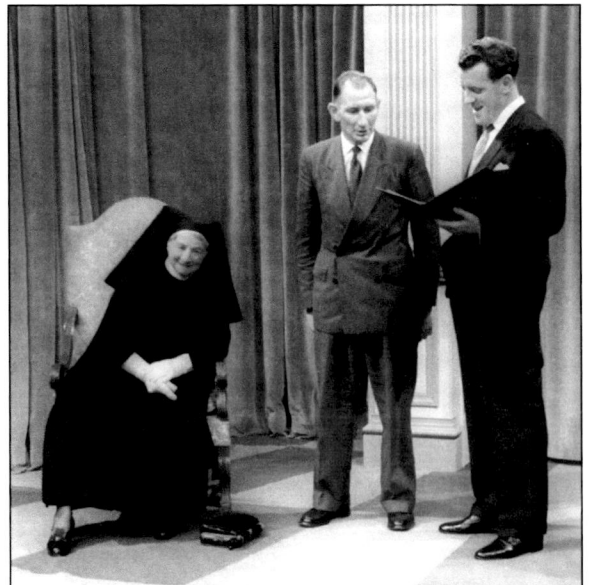

Figure 118   Sister Mary with Mr Eric Smith during This is your life (David Blagrove collection)

Also shown in Figure 118 is Eric Smith who recounted the amusing incident during World War II when Sister Mary organised the village firewatchers. Figure 119 shows the end of the programme where Eamonn Andrews presents Sister Mary with *The Book of Her Life* and a bunch of flowers, note on the floor is a specially painted *This is Your Life* water can. The final picture shows a close up of Sister Mary at the event (Figure 120).

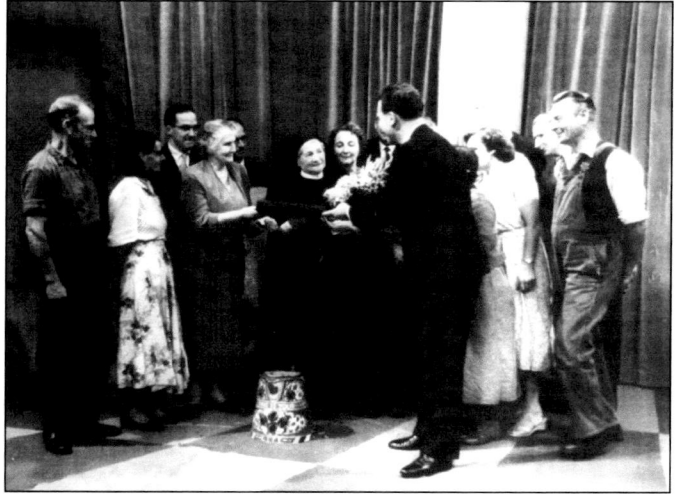

Figure 119   Sister Mary with friends at This is your life (Dennis Monk collection)

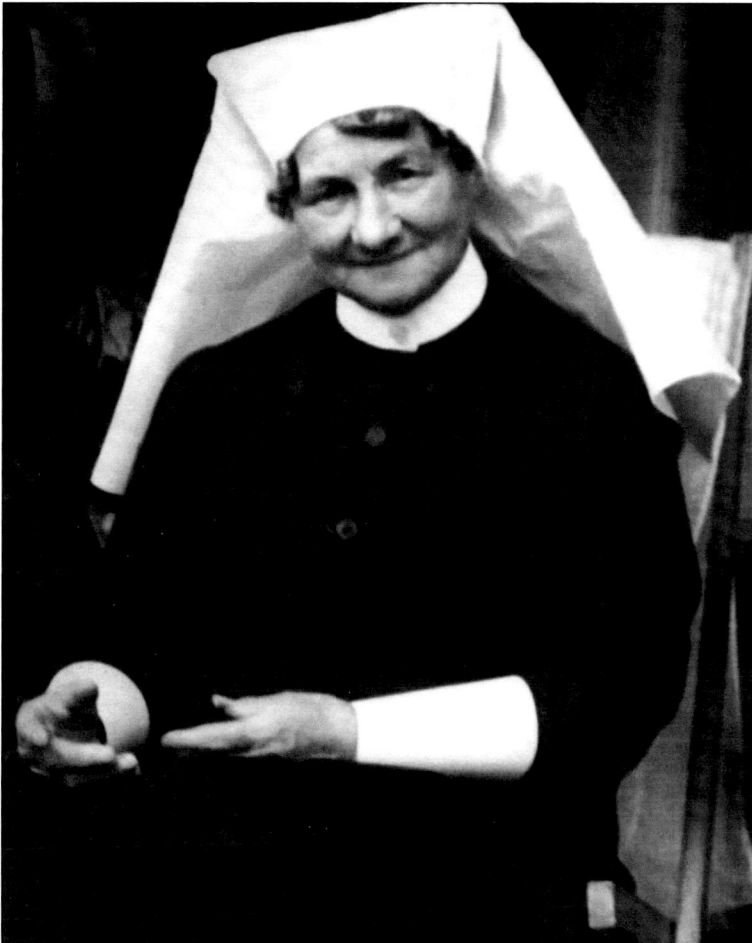

Figure 120   Close up of Sister Mary during This is your life (Waterway's Archive)

After appearing on *This is your life*, Sister Mary remained active in Stoke Bruerne, as she had done for 30 years providing care to the boat families. In the 1960's she was as busy as ever, particularly with Willow Wren families. Mr Morton continued to be in regular contact with Sister Mary and she with him., one letter found in a case book indicates she kept him up-to-date on a number of issues …

> *April 11th 1960*
> *Monday 8.10am*
>
> *Dear Mr Morton*
>
> *at 4.42 pm on Sunday, 10 inst [xxxx] came into Surgery, he was very angry, re no operation as arranged, - I suspect you are aware [xxxx] is unsettled & by the look of things, will soon leave us. Perhaps its better that way, trouble makers are most unsettling to the other crews. - Mr [xxxx] The [xxxx] & [xxxxx] arrived here at 5.50 PM, also on Sunday - but locks were fastened up for the night, so had to remain at Stoke for Sunday night, but was away at 6 AM today 11th inst, Mr {xxxx} & family all well & very loyal boat people.*
>
> *Yes as you said, - I did find also {xxxx} altered, but like the warmer days, will strengthen him, he tied up here for one night - & I listened to him coughing frequently during the night & again when he left, no wonder he's weak, must take hours to recover after such coughing. - I gave him Halibut Oil Capsules, & will give [sic] Bronchial Mixture when he returns, was out of it when [xxxx] was here, but ordered some & its just arrived & its wonderful - I do hope it will help, especially the morning cough.*
>
> *Hope all well, kindest regards*
>
> *Yours sincerely*
>
> *Sister Mary.*

For the majority of the floating population post nationalization their new employer's, British Waterway's, *reviewed progress towards the welfare of their boaters*. In the report arising from the investigation *Welfare and Amenities*[497] two issues were flagged up …

175.   Industrial modernisation is not just a matter of new tools and techniques. There are men involved, and on the waterways the dispersed nature of much of the work has militated against the provision of many of the welfare amenities today enjoyed by those in large factories and offices. On the narrow canals in particular, the historical development of a way of family life on the boats quite separate from that of the rest of the community has provided welfare problems not met elsewhere.

176.   These problems have been tackled energetically. For the narrow boat crews and their families, modern baths, wash-houses and lavatories have been installed at Hawkesbury (near Coventry), Broad Street (Wolverhampton) and Bulls Bridge (Southall). At the latter depot a surgery has also been set up with a trained nurse in attendance

Sister Mary was not the only celebrity residing in Stoke Bruerne at the beginning of the 1960's, her neighbour Mr Jack James won the competition for the *best-kept lock on British Waterways*, the achievement was celebrated on September 22nd 1960. A coach arrived in the village containing representatives of staff and management from British Waterway's who presented at the lock side the first prize *Ritchie Rose Bowl* to Mr John George James. Jack with his wife Emma James (nee Bray) are seen receiving the cup in Figure 121 after which Jack told the BW reporter about his lock and it's effect on The Boat Inn …

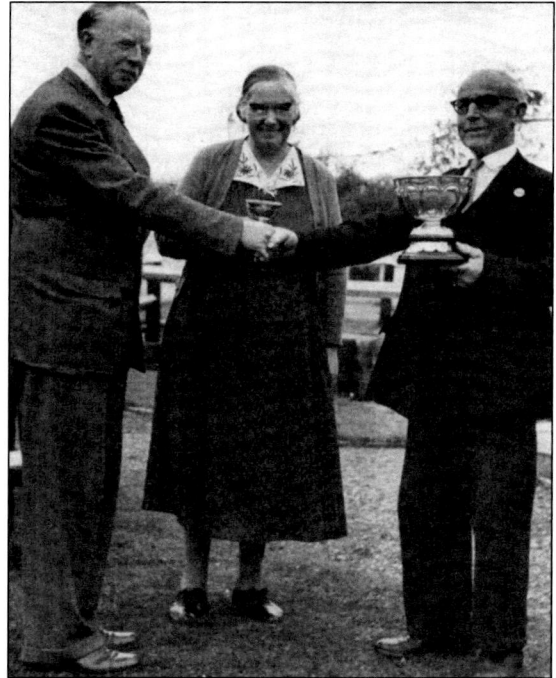

Figure 121   Jack James and wife Emma James (nee Bray): BW SE Division best kept lock (Waterway's Archive)

One of the centres of attraction in the area to tourists and sightseers, especially at weekends. People from far and wide enjoy sandwiches and perhaps a pint from the one and only pub – "The Boat" – which stands alongside the lock and is now being enlarged to cope with the extra business[498].

Jack maintained the lock in immaculate condition as shown being observed by Sister Mary in Figure 122. Whilst in Stoke Bruerne covering the prize giving the reporter observed Jack's display of canal ware …

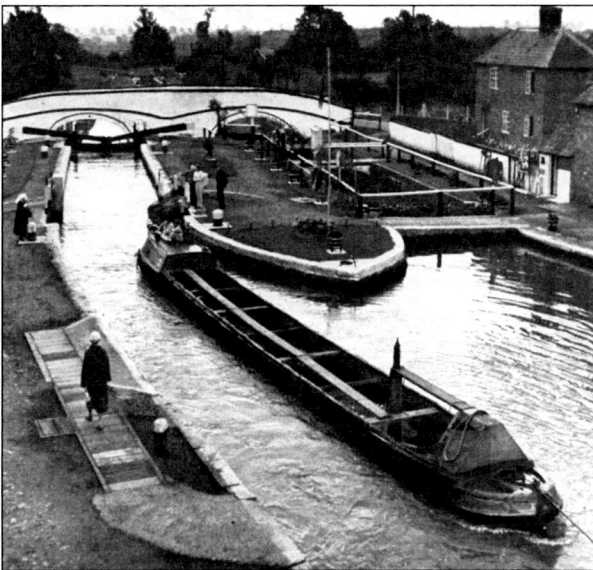

Figure 122   Sister Mary viewing the best kept lock in the SE Division (Waterway's Archive)

Jack's old tiller

The tiny office, is one of the most interesting parts of the lock. Here Jack has collected a few museum pieces and hopes to enlarge it if accommodation becomes available. The whole office gleams with highly polished brasswork. There is a barge table cupboard installed next to the fireplace; china cabin plates adorn the walls, together with a pair of crocheted horse earcaps, an old draught plate from the days of steam, and Jack's proudest possession, his own tiller handle which he used when a boatman. "Ah!" said Jack, looking round the walls, "waterways will always be a part of England."

The following year Mr James *did it again*[499], shown in Figure 123 with the first prize Richie Rose Bowl besides the runners up, note the painted cabin stool in the foreground. During the early 60's a young photography student Hugh McKnight lived for three days with the Harris family on their boat on the Grand Union Canal. On climbing the flight at Stoke Bruerne and arriving at top-lock Captain George Harris and the crew were greeted by Jack James, and as they were leaving *Sister Mary came sweeping out of her cottage in full regalia,* she asked if everyone was all right?. As the boat moved on *sufficiently far off, George shouted back that he'd messed his foot up a bit and he'd like her to look at it when they returned south.* The reason George gave for not telling Sister Mary earlier about his injury was probably a regular reason for a boater delaying treatment in view of their tight delivery schedule … *he knew only too well that she would insist on them lying idle for several days with consequent loss of time and money.*[500]

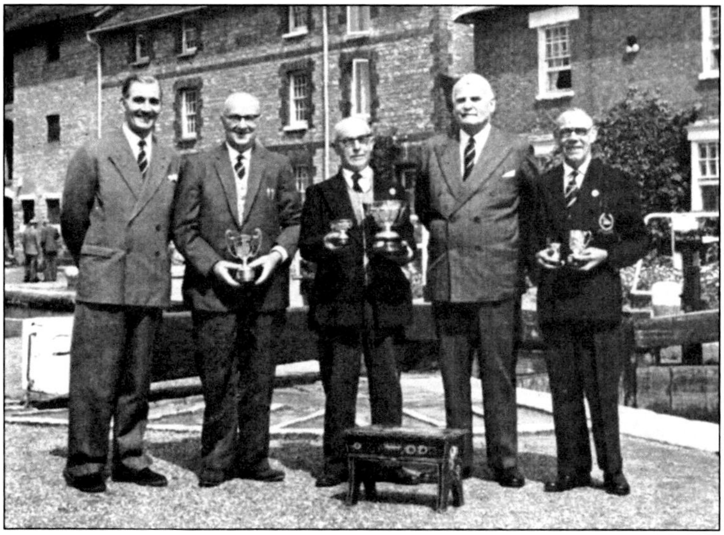

Figure 123   Best kept lock again: Jack James and Runners up (Waterway's Archive)

In the early 60's children continued to be an integral part of family boating, and Christmas was an opportunity for British Waterway's to celebrate with their employee's, as seen when they hosted Christmas parties at Brentford and Bulls Bridge. At Bull's Bridge depot canteen a Christmas party was provided for *fifty excited boat children* where they *enjoyed seeing Father Christmas,* shown in Figure 124 and Figure 125. Sister Mary also did her bit for the boat families during the Christmas period, the headline in the BW magazine said it all, *Mother Christmas at Stoke Bruerne…*

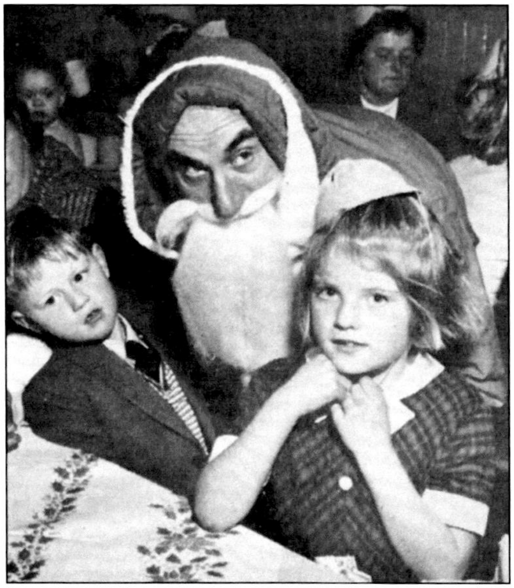

Father Christmas – or should it be "Mother Christmas" ? – was waiting at Stoke Bruerne, on the Grand Union Canal near Northampton, for the children of the narrow boat families as Christmas approached. As boats arrived at the canal lock, the children were invited into Sister Mary's cottage to pick a toy. Altogether, towards 400 children received gifts

Figure 124   Father Christmas at Bull's Bridge (Waterway's Archive)

Care on the CUT

The toys had been given by Inspector K. H. Cue of the NSPCC, Northampton, and formed part of the annual Christmas appeal. A decorated Christmas tree stood in Sister Mary's cottage; this was given by the students' association of Northampton College of Technology. Depot Superintendent L T Spracklen was the man-on-the-spot who sent in this story[501]

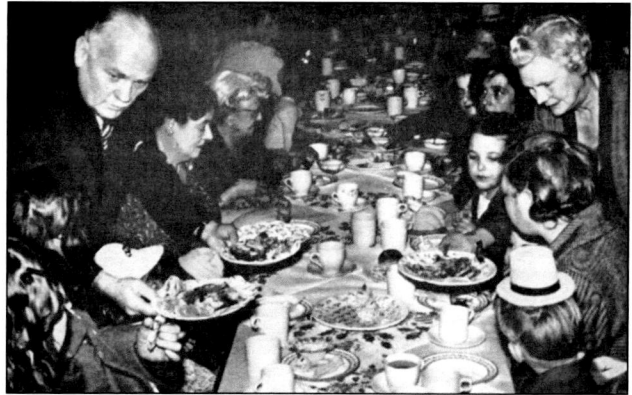

Figure 125　Bull's Bridge Christmas celebrations (Waterway's Archive)

In a staged picture shown in Figure 126 from The Times, the headline says *Sister Mary not deterred* she is seen handing out Christmas gifts, having trekked through snow drifts to the bottom-lock *on yet another stage of her traditional distribution of gifts to the boatmen's children*[502], note the swans have also come to have a look on this icy winters day.

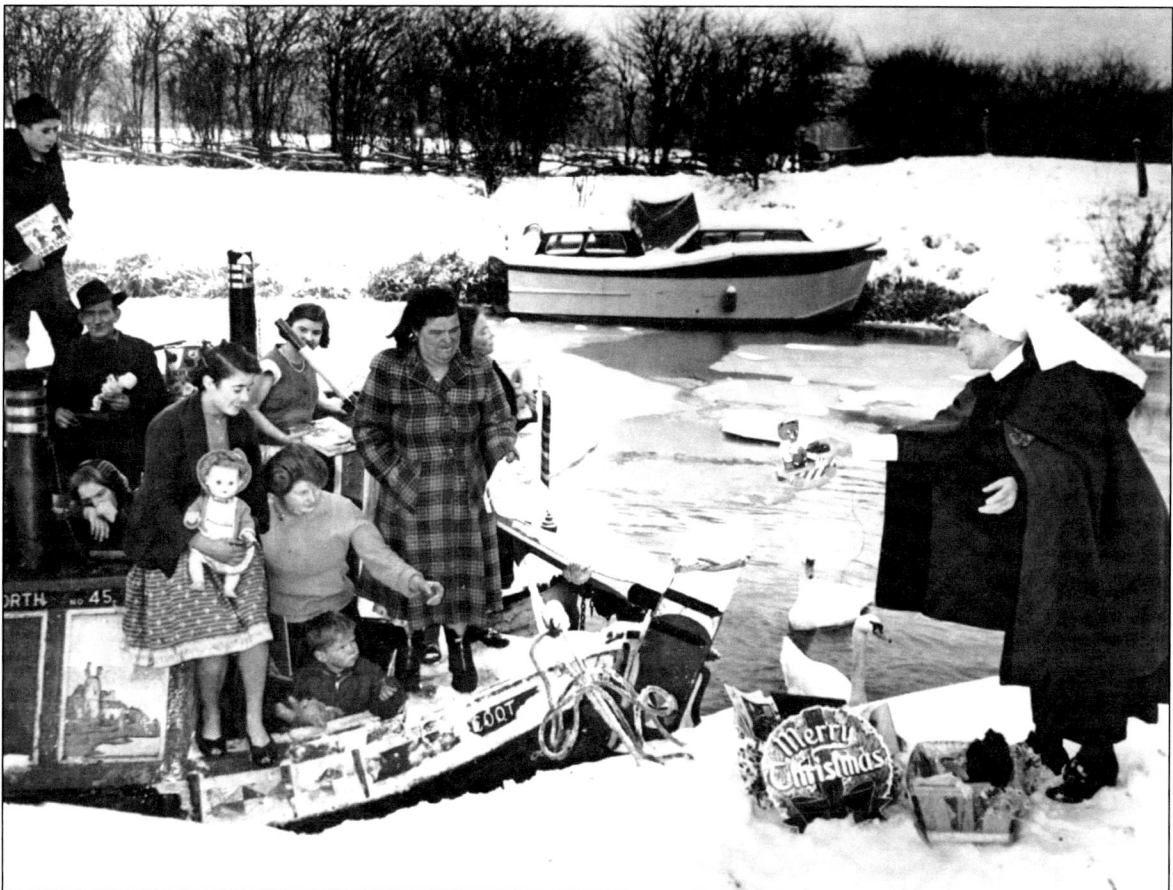

Figure 126　Sister Mary doing her Christmas deliveries (Northampton Central Library)

Sister Mary's final media interview was with Brian Vaughton from the BBC Midland Home Service. Brian approached Sister Mary and a number of boaters in 1962 to participate in the radio programme *Cry from the Cut*[503], the recording on Saturday 10th February was held at Studio 4, Broad Street, Birmingham, and the programme broadcast the following Tuesday, Sister Mary told the audience about her experiences of caring for boaters on the Grand Junction Canal. During the interview Sister Mary commented on her dislike of the new BW colours …

> …and personally I think it was the saddest thing – the British Waterways boats are ugly, blue and yellow. They don't tone with the landscape in any way – they jar on one's nerves.

Sister Mary listened to the live broadcast and was so impressed with the content she wrote to Brian Vaughton the following day, Valentines Day[504] …

> *Dear Mr Vaughton,*
>
> *A happy St. Valentine.*
>
> *Many congratulations. – Your broadcast was a great success – true to life, the very speech of your boat people, typical of the race; how you managed to get them to talk is marvellous, they appeared to forget themselves, unusual I can assure you, generally most self-conscious. Of course I approve of the final result, glad I did not ruin it, actually sounded happy – thanks to you for understanding your difficult task – well rewarded.*
>
> *God ever bless you.*
>
> *Yours Sincerely*
>
> *Sister Mary.*

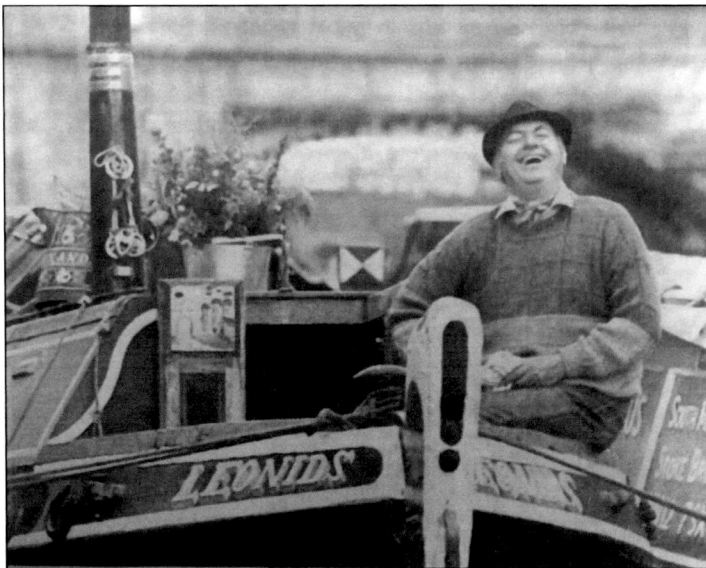

Figure 127   The Aspirin story and David Blagrove
(Della Sadler-Moore collection)

David Blagrove was boating through Stoke Bruerne the month after the Cry from the Cut broadcast (March 14th 1962), he recalls his only meeting with Sister Mary at top-lock where he told her he had a headache, she supplied David with two aspirins. The treatment went well as David is seen in Figure 127 on the stern of *Leonids* enjoying himself at one of the largest Inland Waterway's National Boat Rallies in Britain[505]

The Surgery closes …

In August 1962 *Sister Mary left the canal*, the departure was announced in the local newspaper as Stoke Bruerne will never be the same[506] …

> For the first time since she returned home nearly 30 years ago to nurse her sick father, Sister Mary Ward, who has been called *the Florence Nightingale of Canals*, has left her beloved waterways – *and for good,* she says. Ill health (a heart condition) forced the decision upon her and only a short while ago Sister Mary, winner of the B.E.M. and the subject of *This is your life*, sold the canal-side house that has been in her family for four generations and left for London.
>
> Sister Mary is staying at the flat of her daughter, Mrs Olive Drage, 35 Raffles Court, King's Drive, Edgware. Mrs Drage still has a cottage at Stoke Bruerne locks, but at the moment Sister Mary dare not even think about returning for a visit. *It would upset me too much*, she said. In an exclusive interview … Sister Mary told how the boat people wept at the news of her departure and pleaded with her to stay. *We'll look after you*, they promised.
>
> **Surgical Instruments**
>
> But now the familiar surgery, open to callers day and night for so long is closed. Sister Mary's furniture and belongings – including the surgical boot which she was able to cast off after overcoming a spinal deformity – are in storage. She took with her to London only clothing and a few possessions – including, of course, her surgical instruments. *Someone's always cutting themselves or something, my dear*, she said. Soon Sister Mary and her daughter will move into a house near the present flat in Edgware. Colonel Alfred Ritchie has bought the 15-room house at Stoke Bruerne. Sister Mary, who is 78, will be missed not only by the boat people but by the thousands who have seen the busy, uniformed figure on the lockside. Stoke Bruerne will never be the same.

The Amos family home was sold to recently retired Colonel A.J.P., Richie, although she did keep the two canal side terraced cottages. Colonel Richie after moving in purchased a redundant iceboat, from which he operated trips to and from the mouth of Blisworth Tunnel, Colonel Richie became a Director of Willow Wren Canal Transport Services. Sister Mary made a timely exit because that winter the canal froze from December 26th to March 6th, there was no boat movement for 12 weeks. John Thorpe whose family owned the cottage next to Colonel Richie recalled the canal scene at the time of this dreadful winter …

> The canal scene as 1962 drew to a close appeared largely unchanged. The three carrying companies still plied their trade, the boats still moved up and down as regularly as ever, although it was apparent that the British Waterway's fleet was slowly shrinking and the Barlow/Blue Line fleet numbers had halved … Willow Wren, to all outward appearances, was holding steady and still seeking fresh contracts, despite the occasional gloomy rumours that the company was losing money on its operations. A casual observer on the Stoke Bruerne canalside would have noticed less traffic than a few years before …

By December 23rd it had turned much colder and a heavy frost greeted the dawning of Christmas eve and a deep penetrating frost gripped the country as Christmas Day dawned. It was the beginning of the great freeze of 1962-1963 (Figure 128). Over the next few days ferocious blizzards swept across the country with the inevitable disruptions to road and rail links … a visit to Stoke revealed that, whilst all was well with the cottage, the canal was in dire straits. Ice stretched right across in the cutting up towards the tunnel and also in the lock ponds further down, although clear water was still visible by the cottages and the mill.

Boats were stranded up and down the cut and most people had contrived to put themselves in places where a long ice-up could be sat out in reasonable comfort … In fact things got worse. More heavy blizzards fell and the countryside groaned under the burden of week after week of unremitting frost. … For the cut there was no respite. The ice was anything up to three feet thick …

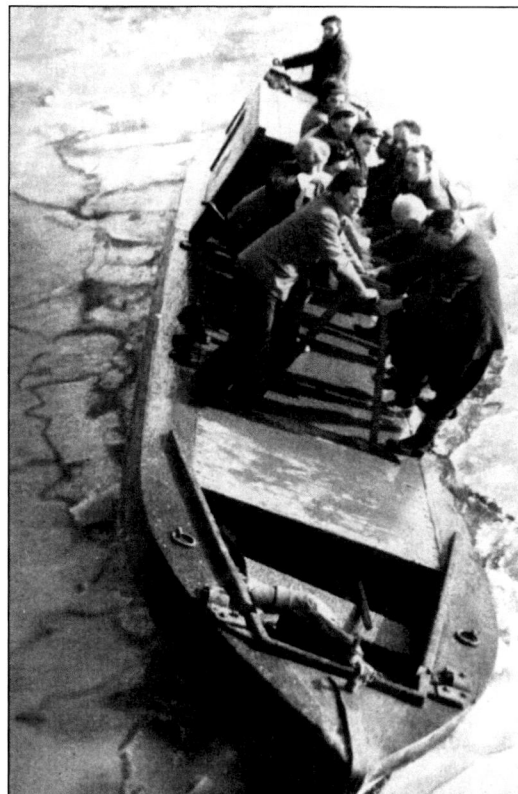

Figure 128   Ice breaking on the Grand Union Canal (Waterway's Archive)

On December 31st 1962 responsibility for canals was taken over by the British Waterway's Board (BWB), their remit being to develop the leisure potential of canals, British Waterways was formed on 1st January 1963 from the former British Transport Commission[507]. The hard winter was the final nail in the coffin for the nationalized canal system, in the Eastern Division the fleet of boats decreased to 40 pairs in April 1963. There were a number of factors which combined over several years to herald the decline of canal carrying by narrow boat. After the Second World War carriers found it increasingly difficult to find crews for their boats, and boat builders to repair them. Coal became a more dominant cargo for narrow boats on the Grand Union, but this actually contributed to their demise. After the passing of The Clean Air Act of 1956, and some collieries being closed down, coal started to be phased out both industrially and domestically, with a corresponding reduction in consumption. All this combined with the increased use of road transport and the opening of the first section of the M1 in 1959, made road transport more of a threat than it already was. Despite these problems, canal carriers tried to stay in business.

One person Sister Mary left behind in Stoke Bruerne was *Old Gibby,* who she *kept an eye on[508]. Old Gibbie,* or to give his full name, Edward Thomas Gibson lived at No 1 canalside as Sister Mary's tenant. 89 year old Mr Gibson's executor was Olive Mary Winifred Drage, and after his death on February 3rd 1963 at Danetree Hospital, Daventry Mrs Drage proved the will, witnessed by Retired Army Officer Colonel Ritchie. Probate was settled on June 17th 1963 the beneficiary of his estate £895. 15s being Mary Ellen Hollowell Ward.[509]

On this rather dismal backdrop *a dream came true in Stoke Bruerne for Jack James when the doors of the Waterway's museum opened for the first time to the public[510]* on Saturday May 4th 1963. Sister Mary returned for the occasion as shown in Figure 129 and Figure 130, holding a piece of white crochet as it drapes over the arm of the museums new exhibit of a boatwoman in traditional clothing.

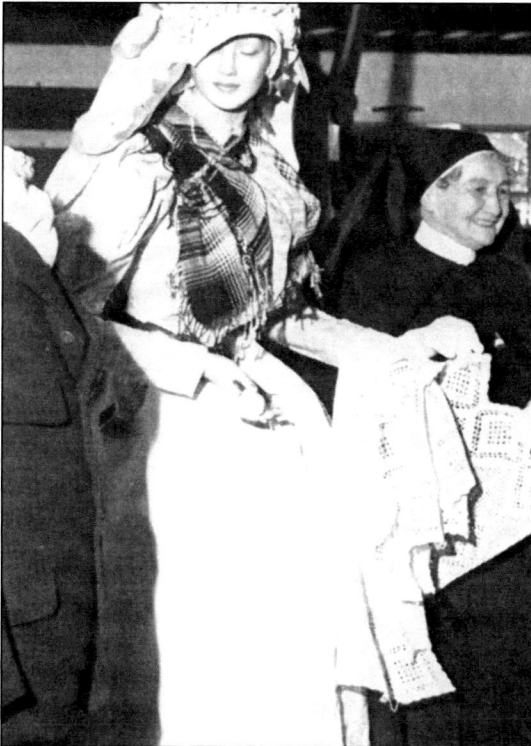

Figure 129   Sister Mary at the opening of the Canal Museum (Waterway's Archive)

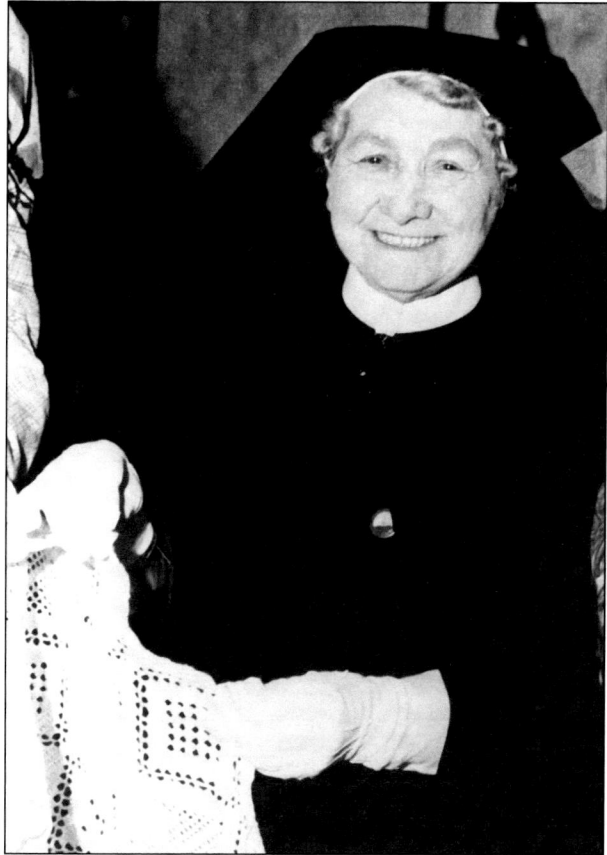

Figure 129   Sister Mary at the opening of the Canal Museum (Waterway's Archive)

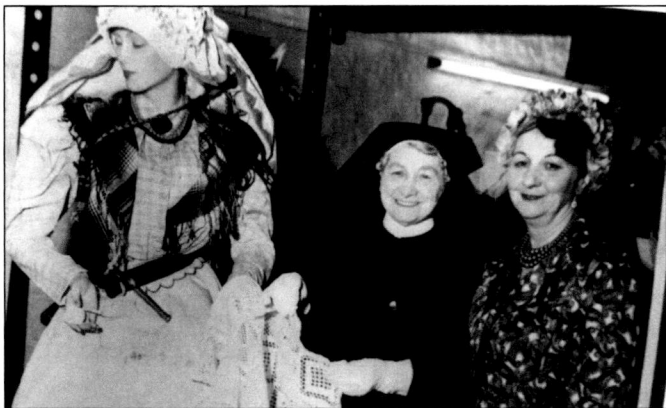

Figure 131   Sister Mary with daughter Olive at the opening of the
Canal Museum (Waterway's Archive)

Figure 131 shows a close up of Sister Mary and her daughter Mrs Olive Drage, standing beside the exhibit, on closer examination you can see a leather belt around the models waist containing a windlass for opening the locks, and just below the models neck is a brooch and a set of twister pearl, with a horse whip across the chest. The opening of the museum also featured retired lock-keeper

Mr Jack James seen in Figure 132 is standing alongside the re-created *Sunny Valley* back cabin. In Figure 133 is Mr Charles Hadlow the first Canal Museum Manager / Curator, seen holding a traditionally painted water can, on the wall is a painted table cupboard front and in the foreground a painted barrel.

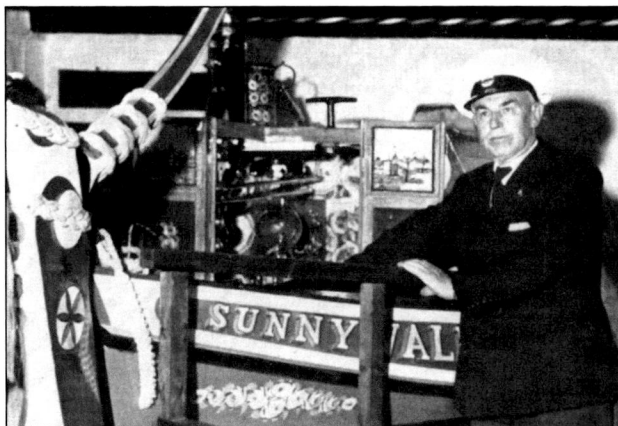

Figure 132   Jack James with *Sunny Valley* at the opening of the
canal museum (Waterway's Archive)

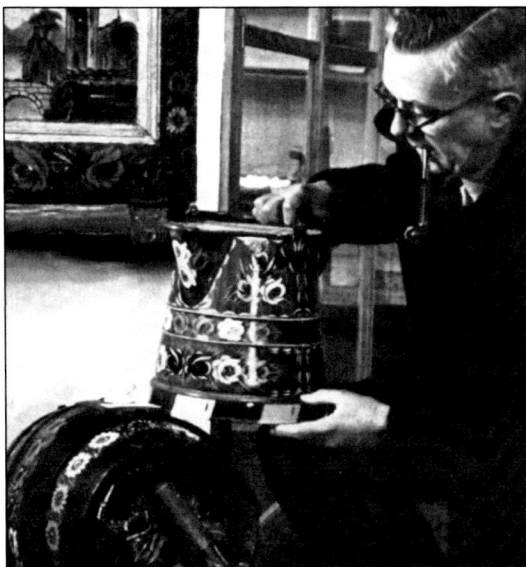

Figure 133   Charles Hadlow at the opening of the
Canal Museum (Waterway's Archive)

Throughout the London Year's Sister Mary lived with her daughter Olive and son-in-law Eric. Only one record of this period has come to light, a letter to Cousin Jamie written on a *little bit of Stoke Bruerne she took to London with her*, as shown from the letter head she named her new home *Bruerne ...*

BRUERNE
58 Stag Lane
Edgware
Middlesex
February 12 1966

Saturday 6.50 P.M.

My dear Jamie,

It was indeed a joy to receive again, a letter from you – to read of days, when we were young. I remember so well, of father telling my twin Sister Dolly, & myself about Uncle William Mitchell & uncle George Chalmers, the clever Scotsmen, who built the London North Western Railways & to let us walk for miles along the track with him, sometimes to scamper along, under the bridges & think of our uncles.

Your father & Uncle George Chalmers, used to spend Week Ends, at the old Home Canal Side, Stoke Bruerne, where both their dear Wives were born, auntie [xxxxx], whom father loved so dearly – I believe I wrote you, how they would often walk 20 miles to a concert, both so fond of music, <u>OUR</u> Grandpa (John Amos) would not allow a Horse out at night, that did not prevent them going anywhere, where good music could be heard, of course you must know, both your dear mother and my father could both sing gloriously – music was an open book to both, I still have many compositions, composed by dear father & our grandfather, – John Amos, both would train choirs & help music lovers to play any instrument to form bands. – The old house must still sing with that music, – everyone blessing the name of Amos, was a musician in those glad days, my mother also, like your mother, sang like a nightingale.

I've just remembered, whilst I was at Bristol I went down often to the Barry Docks, built by Uncle William & Uncle George. Did you know- ? the foreman of Works, filled the Docks, before quite ready & all had to be rebuilt, it was a great anxiety to your father, but he wow through it all Jamie dear, it is wonderful to hear how you manage alone, you must be very brave. I'm here with Olive & family, but I liked living alone in the old Home. Every room was precious, this house, is all right but not the same, still Dear, wherever I am, I must try to make others happy, all here are very kind to me & love me. I do understand how readily one tires at 80, never mind Jamie, "God" is ever present & will help us always, we are never alone. I shall be thinking of you so much & try to be brave like you are, I do miss my patients so much, but remembers all with gladness. – Its difficult to write now the one thing I loved so much, but sight fails, I really do not know what my writing looks like, but if you can read it. Alls well. I can see everything Jamie, but <u>everything</u> <u>is</u> <u>misty</u>; although I've fresh glasses, its difficult still.

Glad to hear about your daughter; don't laugh too much, when I say, will you be my Valentine Dear ? this should arrive on the 14th.

My dear love to you & your daughter. May "God" bless you and yours. With prayers always,

Your loving Cousin,

Mary.

Sister Mary's canal-side cottages in Stoke Bruerne were visited by her daughter and son-in-law in January 1969 during which a further tragedy befell Sister Mary, when her daughter Olive Mary Winifred Drage had a heart attack which she did not survive (age 59). Three years after the death of her only daughter Sister Mary passed away in Colindale Hospital Hendon, the cause of death recorded as Heart Failure[511], her usual address was 58, Stag Lane, Edgware. Sister Mary's death was immediately reported in Northampton as *Florence Nightingale of Canals dies*[512], the funeral was held at Roade Baptist Church and she was buried there alongside other members of her family.

Sister Mary's inspiration lives on

In June 2014 when the Sister Mary research was in full flow the authors attended the Braunston Canal Festival and during a walk along the *Towpath* two authors (LY and DSM) spoke to Jenny Glynn (nee Littlemore) about the research. During the lengthy chat Jenny told us about Sister Mary and an oil painting of her which hangs on the wall of her home, Jenny also told us the fascinating story about how the

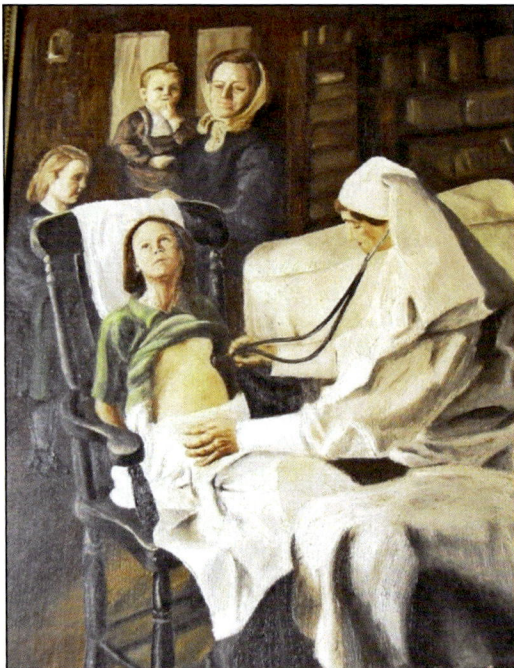

Figure 134   Oil Painting of Sister Mary with the Littlemore family (Jenny Glynn collection)

painting came to be in her possession. A picture of the oil painting as it hangs on the wall in Jenny's home today is shown in Figure 134 and thanks to Jenny's husband a close up is shown in Figure 135. The story behind the oil painting is one of inspiration and how *Sister Mary's inspiration went beyond the canal folk*, the story of the painting and how Jenny came to acquire it is re-counted here from our towpath chat and from Jenny's recent article in NarrowBoat[513] …

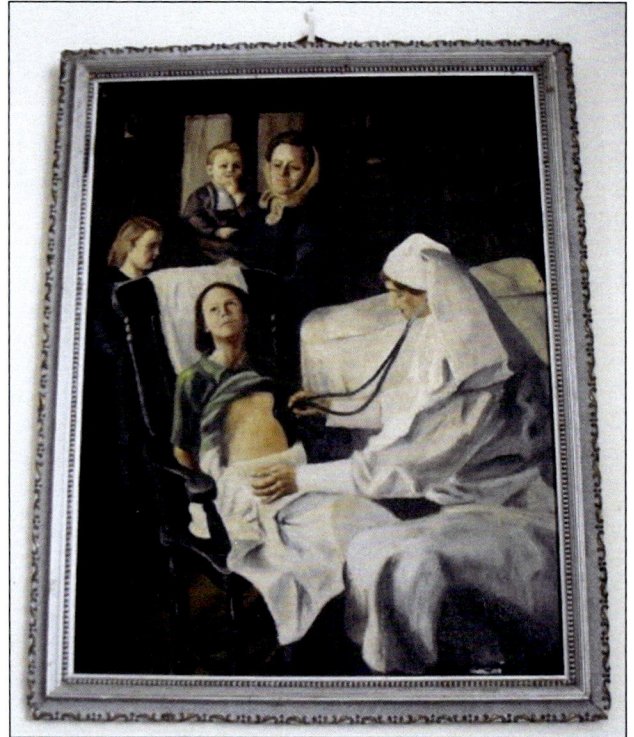

Figure 135   Close up of oil painting (Jenny Glynn collection)

It came about when my friend [a Community Nurse in Banbury] Mary Jarvis tended the needs of a Mr Grant. [Nurse Jarvis] noticed the picture on several occasions during her home visiting … and became increasingly convinced she had *seen it before* … so she asked Mr Grant about it. Mr Grant told her it was of the boat people and was copied from a photograph in the newspaper by a prisoner of war who had given it to him. He added, he had *always had a special interest and affection for canal boat people, but had never known the names of this particular group.*

Nurse Jarvis told Mr Grant she knew the family and *he was overjoyed and begged her to bring me [Jenny] to see him* … the visit was arranged and the friends arrived at the house, the housekeeper then informed us Mr Grant had passed away. BUT, before his death he had decided I should be given [the painting] as he was absolutely certain of who I was after the conversation with Nurse Jarvis.

Jenny's personal account of her boating heritage and of Sister Mary is very poignantly captured in her own words …

It is a firm reminder of where I come from, and the harsh realities of my former life as a canal boat child, growing up in a way so far removed from my experiences of children today as to be unbelievable … The kindness and concern shown to the boat people in Sister Mary's little canalside surgery was invaluable, and her interest in their children too was always appreciated as she ran to the lockside to see them if the boats were working through without stopping at Stoke Bruerne.

She was a welcome and familiar sight with starched collar and cuffs, a headdress that impressed a comforting confidence in her, and a ready, radiant smile, that expressed her warm friendliness. She was devoted to *her boat people*, and they in return loved and trusted her.

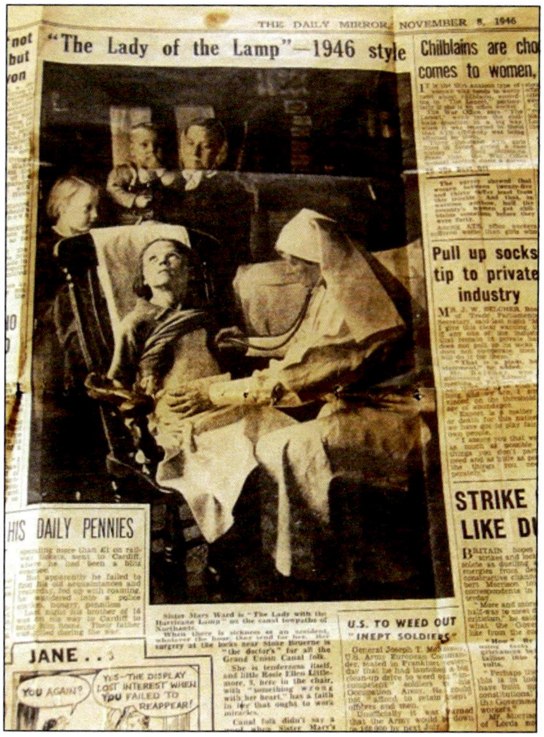

Two iconic pictures of Sister Mary delivering care in her surgery to a boat family were published just after World War II. The first you may remember has been discussed in an earlier chapter and is shown in Figure 106, when this picture was taken a second picture was also taken and published in The Daily Mirror and reproduced from the original article Jenny treasures to today shown in Figure 136. In Jenny's recent article she points out that *whenever the picture was featured in canal articles … it was never captioned with the family's names,*

Figure 136   Article from the Daily Mirror showing the Littlemore family with Sister Mary Ward (Jenny Glynn collection)

like so many others that lacked the names of boat people. There is a lesson to be learnt from Jenny's observation. In future when gazing at the remnants of the canal folk; pictures, water cans, painted ware or one of the many working boats that continue to ply our canals, ask yourself who was that man, woman or child on that boat?, What boating family do they belong to?, Whose water can was that?, Who painted it ?. By asking these questions and seeking answers you will be opened up to a whole new dimension of the social / family history of the canal boat people. The commercial carrying floating population weren't *just boaters*, they were individual's who were part of a large family. For those families who visited Sister Mary, she knew every one of them by name, every one of them she cared for professionally and respected as did they her. As one boatwoman concluded … *to the end of our boatworkin days she gave as all unstintin' of her time and comfort. Many a boat child owed its survival to Sister Mary*[514].

Appendices

Appendix 1

**Management of the Sister Mary
Case Books / Ledgers**

Initial mapping of the case books / ledger's content

Five Sister Mary's case books / ledgers were made available to two authors throughout the research project (DSM & LY). Initially each was reviewed to identify the content and scope of the material included. The case books content was then mapped in more detail and Table 1 constructed to summarise the content.

- Each book was given a Unique Name according to the front cover (Table 1: Column 1).
- A Unique Code was allocated (Table 1: Column 2).
- A brief account of the content of each book was noted (Table 1: Column 3),
- The years covered by entries in each case book were mapped (Table 1: Column 4).
- The number of pages in each book was identified (Table 1: Column 5), finally
- The section of the book Care on the Cut to which case book entries related to was identified (Table 1: Column 6).

Table 1: *Classification / Mapping the content* of surviving Sister Mary Case Books / Ledger's

Column 1	Column 2	Column 3	Column 4	Column 5	Column 6
Case Book / Ledger Classification	Unique Code	Overview of content	Years covered	Total Pages	Book Section
Red and Blue	**RB**	***Boat family entries*** family per page / several pages.	1942-1958 (Majority of entries 1943-1945 … some years missing)	1-127 Double pages (total 254)	World War II / Post-War
Deep Red	**DR**	***Rent records*** December 1949- March 1957	1946-1961 (Some years missing)	350	Post-War
		Boat family entries family per page / several pages.	Jan – May 1946		
		Cases visiting daily	May 1st 1946 – September 1950 – July 1961 (Some years missing)		
		Surgery Accounts	1958		

Willow Wren	**WW**	***Boat family entries*** family per page	September 1954 - December 1955	27	Post-War
Surgery Dressing Book	**SDB**	***Earls Barton*** *Care of patients * Special *black & red* diet *Carbohydrate diet *NDFS accounts *Surgery accounts	May 1932 - January 1935	1-155	Inter-War years
		Stoke Bruerne *Care of boaters	April 10th 1936 – Early 1937	1 56-184	Inter-War years
Red Indexed	**RX**	***Inventories*** **Stoke Bruerne** *Transport Tools *General Equipment **Shutlanger** *Transport Tools *General Equipment ***Services***	September 1942	50	World War II

Preamble:

From reviewing the content of each case book / ledger the initial concern was in regard to the data included in the case books as these related to individual boaters (and other patients cared for by Sister Mary) , medical diagnoses and treatment by Sister Mary, with the last entry being made in 1962. As the case book content is classified as medical data, current regulations require a 100 year embargo, therefore a protocol was devised to manage the case books shown in Figure 1.

- Two photocopies of each book (for D Sadler-Moore [DSM] and Lorna York [LY])
- After photocopying, return of original books to owners
- Creation of a framework and set of database's for data entry from case books
- Transcription of case book entries (DSM): Anonymised at the point of entering into database, password protected and no electronic transmission of databases
- No linking of Boat Name, Boater's Family Name or Individual Boater to a medical condition or treatment given by Sister Mary
- Reporting of data anonymously in publications and presentations

---

Figure 1: Protocol: Management of Sister Mary Case Books / Ledgers

Pilot analysis

Following the mapping exercise it was decided to undertake a pilot analysis of the case book data. Before the pilot could be conducted it was identified Sister Mary used ***two types*** of methods for entering data on patient care in her case books

1) Dedicated case book pages allocated to each Boating Family eg The Sadler-Moore family. Motor Boat (MB) *Hercules*. Carrying Company. Benson's (The same format as traditional patient records maintained by General Practitioners).

2) Daily entries of patients seen eg 21st May 1955: Baby Mary Smith 3 months. MB *Magpie*. Sore eye. Cleaned. Captain Jones. MB *Hawkeye*. Accident painful ribs. Examined and strapped up.

Two different pilot analysis frameworks were devised to manage the case book entries;

Pilot analysis - Type 1 entries.

A framework shown in Table 2 was developed to enable data entry and analysis of care delivered by Sister Mary to individual boaters (Type 1 entries), the aim being to put together a picture of Sister Mary's contact with boaters over a period of time.

Table 2: Framework for management of the Case Book data

Case Book: RB … 1943

Page(s): p.18

Date S/B Sr Mary	Boat Family 'Patient'	Sr Mary Assessment	Diagnosis	Treatment	Analysis Category
'Profile' from ledger:					

The pilot analysis was carried out on twelve boat families treated by Sister Mary during 1943. Data was transcribed from the Red and Blue (RB) case book and each boat families care was entered into a separate grid an example is shown in Table 3. The pilot was successful and all the 'family based' data was then transcribed.

Table 3. Example pilot analysis

Case Book: RB … 1943

Page(s): p.18

Date seen by Sr Mary	Boat Family 'Patient'	Sr Mary Assessment	Sr Mary Diagnosis	Sr Mary Treatment	Analysis Category
Jan 2nd	Wife	Consultation & examination			
Jan 13th	Wife	Consultation		Dressing to thigh	Wound Care
Jan 14th			Knee (fluid) Rheumatism		Orthopaedic
Jan 15th	?		Rheumatic Juspula	Bed 24 hours	Orthopaedic
Jan 16th	Child			Dressing to sons hand	Wound Care
March 1st	Wife		Rheumatic juspula	Mixture ac.cxx 8oz 3x daily for 8 days	Orthopaedic
	Son	Consultation	Tonislitis		Childhood illness / respiratory
March 14th	Daughter	Consultation - Fallen in canal	Shock complains giddy / faint following falling into canal	Bed 3 days	Accident

'Profile' from ledger:

December 1942 records indicate Wife diagnosed with septic legs … 3 dressings (cotton wool jaconet, Dettol) … also refers to child suffering from Mumps.

This approach enabled identification of the scope and details of her nursing work with the boating community.

Pilot analysis - Type 2 entries.

A framework shown in Table 4 was developed to enable data entry and analysis of care delivered by Sister Mary on a daily basis (Type 2 entries), the aim being to put together a picture of Sister Mary's contact with boaters over a defined period eg one day, one week, one month or one year.

Table 4. Framework for management of the Case Book data – daily entries format

Page	Code	Condition Treated	Male / Female	Number of visits / frequency	Additional Information
2	a	Eczema of arms (septic)	F	14	Initially seen daily, then every other day until discharged
	b	Cyst of scalp (septic / incised)	M	16	
	c	Fractured Radius	F	4	Saw after treated at hospital
	d	Fractured arm	F	4	Saw after treated at hospital
3	a				
	b				
	c				
	d				

This proved to be a further method for identifying the scope and detail of Sister Mary's work with the boating community.

Thomas Amos reports and correspondence to Towcester Rural Sanitary Committee

Date	Reference to Thomas Amos
January 1887	In respect of salary of Canal Boat Inspector it resolved Messrs Franklin, Savage and George form a committee to wait upon Mr Amos and after making inquiries as to duties and to report thereon to the authority.
1st March 1887	Mr George reported regarding committee appointed to consideration of Canal Boat Inspector salary. Considered that the remuneration of the Canal Boat Inspector was insufficient and that £10 per annum was not in their opinion too much. Proposed and seconded that £10 be paid in full – carried.
March 1887	Cheque for salary to Mr T Amos £2 10s.
May 1888	Clerk produced a letter from Mr Amos requesting the supply of stationery and stamps. Resolved nothing be done in the matter.
January 1890	Report from the canal boat inspector read for the year ending December 31st 1889. 'I have entered on the inspectors journal 36 boats for the year 1889, of which I find, 5 boats not registered in name of present owner, 8 without certificates of registration, 2 needing painting for cleaning. I have examined boats as follows for registration by your authority':

Date of examination	Name of boat	Owner	Address
January 17th	George	Edward King	Boatman no address
May 9th	Resolute	E J Brown	Gayton
May 13th	Victory	E J Brown	Gayton
July 12th	Liverpool	Greaves, Bull and Lakin	Stockton
August 6th	Lily	Thomas Simpson	S (Coventry)
August 13th	Laura Emma	John Lightbourne	Simpson Wharf
August 13th	Mary Jane	John Lightbourne	Simpson Wharf
October 13th	Two Sisters	Edward King	No address
October 17th	Our Daisy	Alfred Simpson	Berkhamstead

I met HM Chief Inspector at Towcester 4th July 1889 when he examined the books, forms etc. Have not been refused admittance to any boat.

I remain gentlemen

Your obedient servant

Thomas Amos

January 1891	Report of canal boat inspector for year ending December 31ˢᵗ 1890.
	Inspected and entered on journal 58 boats:
	8 Not registered as dwellings
	7 of these have been registered by your authority
	The other boat 'Shannon' belonging to FMC, Birmingham, at present time blocked by the ice at or near London is to be registered on return to Birmingham.
	I inspected a boat named 'Weedon' the master T. Smith had lost a child at Birmingham and one at London by Diphtheria – the boat had been disinfected.
	The girl named 'Annie Webb' whom your clerk instructed me to report on I have not at present been able to trace.
	There are a number of boats blocked in the ice at Stoke Bruerne locks with children on board who ought to be attending school.
	In conclusion I must state there is a great improvement in the habits of the boat people working on the Grand Junction Canal.
	I remain gentlemen
	Your obedient servant
	Thomas Amos. January 6ᵗʰ 1891.
26ᵗʰ January 1892	Report of canal boat inspector for year ending December 31ˢᵗ 1891.
	38 boats inspected and entered in journal.
	3 new boats without certificates registered by your authority.
	2 new boats changed owners and have been registered.
	On Wednesday 18ᵗʰ met J. Brydone. esq H M Chief Inspector.
	In June last Messrs FM&C of Birmingham sent out several boats in bad condition without certificate which were not fit to be used as dwellings. The captains in charge stated they did not sleep on the boats – but on notice being given the aforesaid company discontinued working these boats.
	In addition to the number of boats entered on journal. I have seen nearly all the boats working on the GJC.
	The boat people appear to better understand the requirements of the acts – hence they try to comply with them.
	I remain gentlemen
	Your obedient servant
	Thomas Amos. January 13ᵗʰ 1892.

January 1893	Report of the canal boat inspector.
	40 boats
	10 not registered as dwellings – which have now been
	1 case of improperly occupying – which has now been remedied
	1 needing painting and repairing.
	The total number for which the cabins were registered is 130, and the number occupying 90 … as shown in detail by the accompanying statistical report.
	There is great difficulty in tracing these boats from place to place, and I have been in communication with the inspectors of other authorities in reference to cases dealt with by them.
	I remain gentlemen
	Your obedient servant
	Thomas Amos.
January 1894	Canal boat report
	42 boats – infringments as follows:
	4 needed to be registered as dwellings
	6 needed re-registering by change of owners … all remedied
	2 needed repair (1 reminded)
	Total number of adults for which the cabins were registered is 126

Occupying Adult Males	50
Occupying adult females	17
School age children	6
Under school age	10
TOTAL	83

On july 3rd last several children almost suffocated in Blisworth tunnel by the smoke from the steam tug which plys through the tunnel 16 times a day. I made a report to Mr Brydone H M Chief Inspector and received a reply to say the GJCCo engineer had promised to remedy the complaint, but nothing to my knowledge has been done to prevent a similar occurrence.

The same complaint has come under my notice several times during the summer months; if your authority can make any suggestions the company's local engineer informs me he will lay the matter before the committee and endeavour to carry out the suggestion to remedy the evil.

In July I met Mr Brydone.

I remain gentlemen

Your obedient servant

Thomas Amos. January 8th 1894.

The clerk was directed to write to the Grand Junction Canal Company calling attention to the matter of the complaint alluded to in the above report.

January 1895	Canal boat inspectors report
	50 boats inspected
	15 needed to be registered as dwellings
	2 needed repair
	Number of persons occupying 106
	Occupying Adult Males 66 Occupying adult females 20 School age children 8 Under school age 12 TOTAL 106
	In the month of June another case of persons almost suffocated in GJC Tunnel caused by steam tug, a similar occurrence to one reported in year 1893.
	Then there was that unfortunate case of Small Pox, Mrs Humphries and her child (of which you have had reports from other sources) which was imported into my home on October 1st from the boat named 'Daisy' belonging to Messr FMC of Birmingham when it was contained on the 4th October the serious nature of the complaint. I at once took measures to trace the boat for disinfection, the boat was stopped on the return journey from London and again on arrival at Birmingham for disinfection, the isolation of this case undoubtably stopped further contagion along the canal route.
	There are always great difficulties in tracing canal boats, but as a rule the canal boat people are anxious to carry out the requirements of the acts which have done much to improve their social conditions. I can verify this having resided by the GJC for 40 years.
	Several children of school age belonging to boats registered by your authority I have not been able to trace.
	I remain gentlemen
	Your obedient servant
	Thomas Amos. January 5th 1895.
March 1899	A letter from Mr Amos was read tending his resignation of the office of Canal boat Inspector. After some discussion Mr Young gave notice that at the next meeting he would propose that Mr George S Phipps be appointed canal Boat Inspector at a salary of £10 per annum.
11th April 1899	Mr Phipps officially appointed.

Appendix 3

Caroline Yarnall death certificate (Great- great-grandmother of Lorna York)

CERTIFIED COPY   of an ENTRY
Pursuant to the Births and   Deaths Registration Act 1953

FC 125290

Registration District Berkhamsted								
1910. **Death in the Sub-district of** Berkhamsted					**in the** County of Hertford			
Columns:- 1	2	3	4	5	6	7	8	9
No.	When and where died	Name and surname	Sex	Age	Occupation	Cause of death	Signature, description and residence of informant	When registered	Signature of registrar
197	Eleventh December 1910 The Boat Portugal Lower Kings Rd Lock Berkhamsted UD	Caroline YARNALL	Female	81 Years	Widow of William YARNALL a Boatman	Diarrhoea Exhaustion Certified by Sidney A Bontor M D	X The mark of Joseph Yarnall Son Present at death The Boat Portugal Berkhamsted	Twelfth December 1910	Harry Holloway Registrar

Certified to be a true copy of an entry in a register in my custody.

.... *Superintendent Registrar*

Appendix 4

Account of boaters during World War II

(Christopher M Jones)

Having to apply for exemption by the 2nd March 1916, and perhaps attend a local Tribunal held near their place of work. Officially they were entitled without any formal hearing to an exemption certificate and so be protected from conscription provided they could show that boating was their principal and usual job on their application forms, otherwise signed statements from those who employed them giving details of their occupation were necessary if they were required to attend a Tribunal. Under the old instructions of 'reserved' or 'starred' occupations, in order for a boatman to be placed on the list, his employer put in a claim that he was individually indispensable to the business and therefore not to be called-up for military service. But under the Military Service Act a man should be granted exemption from military service on the grounds that his work was expedient to the national interest rather than to the needs of his employer. Also that he was employed in work which he was habitually engaged and on the grounds that the work was what he wanted to do whoever his employer may be, provided his job was on the list of certified and protected occupations.

The Government recognised that a man should be able to change his employer after he was protected just so long as he remained in his certified occupation. Local Tribunals were supposed to be aware that any man forced to remain with a particular employer amounted to what was called 'industrial compulsion', which was an abuse of the regulations. This did not stop some employers putting pressure on boatmen to stay with them and those unfamiliar with the regulations would give in to these threats, perhaps fearing they might lose their exempt status. This happened to owner-boatman Abel Skinner, who worked for the Oxford Portland Cement Co. Ltd. He wanted to leave and handed in his notice so he could go and work for the OCC Traffic Agency. It was the usual custom that a boatman gave one trip's notice to leave any employer, however Skinner gave up his attempt claiming the cement company would not allow him to leave and he could not do as he liked.

Both carriers and traders found it increasingly difficult to satisfy the demands for the transportation of coal and materials. With a dwindling population of boatmen and a shortage of boats, those ignorant of the finer details of the Military Service Act left themselves open to exploitation by those desperate to keep them. Boatmen employing any young men had to be careful regarding the Military Service Act. If they were found to be employing men who were liable for military service and were not exempt, the boatmen as their employers could face a fine of up to £20. Even if their men were vital to the running of their boats, ignorance of the law was seen as no excuse unless the boatmen could prove otherwise. A situation could arise where an owner-boatman was exempt but his mate refused exemption and then called-up. Because the boatman depended on his mate the help run his boats it could result in him tying them up for wont of a crew, and traders in turn suffered because their deliveries would cease forcing more trade onto the already congested railways. Owner-boatman Matthew Townsend of Abingdon applied for exemption for his son Alfred who worked as his mate, but his application was rejected. Matthew was in his mid-sixties and he could not manage without his son as crew.

To show how Tribunals' were out of touch with the demands of boating life it was not unknown that in a similar situation where a boatman said he needed his mate, that the Tribunal might suggest he take on a discharged ex-soldier instead. The owner-boatman would have the difficult task of trying to convince officials, who have no idea of the difficulties faced operating commercial canal boats, that men with no experience and also possibly recovering from injuries sustained at the front, were likely to be of limited use as boatmen, especially on river navigations. Some firms did employ discharged ex-service men as boatmen such as Kaye & Co., cement manufacturers of Southam and FMC was said to have employed Belgian and Polish men at some point. The OCC Traffic Agency employed one man from Huddersfield to work a hired boat but only lasted one trip before being dismissed, due to his ill treatment of the boathorse which had to be stabled for several weeks after to recover from the ordeal.

The Army trained personnel in the Transport Workers' Battalions to become canal workers, assisting with maintenance, loading and unloading, etc., but their contribution in the Midlands region appears to be very limited. Any person who felt aggrieved at a Tribunals decision could lodge an appeal within three days of the hearing which was held at a special appeals Tribunal, but Matthew Townsend had overrun this deadline. After hearing about this the OCC clerk advised Matthew to make a personal call upon the clerk of the Tribunal and plead ignorance to try and get an extension to lodge his appeal, which was successful and was extended another ten days. Matthew then engaged a solicitor with experience of getting exemption for a boatman and Alfred was allowed to continue working with Matthew for the time being at least. Over two years after the outbreak of war the Board of Trade eventually advised the Tribunals' boatmen should be kept on the canals against the aims of the military due to the chronic congestion on the railways. By then traders had suffered due to the lack of boatmen and some businesses were failing, and the dramatic reduction in tonnage carried meant a corresponding loss in toll revenues.

Because of the worsening state, Government took over responsibility for canals from March 1st 1917, setting up a Canal Control Committee (CCC) under the Board of Trade and dividing the network into local regions. The south Midlands became part of the Southern Sub-Committee based at the Grand Junction Canal Company the London offices. For boatmen remaining on the waterways they had their own problems to contend with; difficulties finding suitable boats for hire; cost of living increasing making repairs to their own boats difficult, and; persistent and lengthy delays when loading at collieries; all of which had a detrimental effect on their incomes and contributed to their demand for higher pay. By late 1917 reports were reaching thc CCC clerk that some local shopkeepers were refusing to serve boaters as they were not considered regular customers, they responded by ordering local food committees' to make temporary arrangements to ensure boaters received supplies without difficulty. To settle the matter once and for all the CCC clerk arranged with the Food Control Committee to distribute food cards to boatmen, and helped boatmen and some traders who employed them to complete the forms. Similar arrangements were made regarding the supply of horse feed, where boatmen were expected to register with a licensed hay merchant to receive a supply fixed by the Board of Trade.

Report of Deputation by NTWF Mr Ernest Bevan's speech 1919

Docks, Wharf, Riverside and General Workers' Union of Great Britain.

Registered Office: Effingham House, Arundel Street, Strand, London, W.C.2.

General Secretary - - - Ben Tillett, M.P.

CANAL WORKERS.

REPORT OF DEPUTATION.

A deputation from the National Transport Worker's Federation waited upon the President of the Board of Education, who was accompanied by a representative of the Ministry of Transport and the Ministry of Health, on Wednesday, November 12th.

The deputation was introduced by Mr. Harry Gosling, and consisted of Messrs. E. Bevin, W. Palser, G. Shaw, J. Street, R. M. Bryan and F. J. Maynard (representing Mr. Robert Williams).

Mr. Ernest Bevin put the case of the Federation in a speech from which the following extracts are made:-

THE NEED FOR INQUIRY

Those who have desired to see an improvement in the Canal system have always pointed out its necessity first of all from the point of view of the social conditions of the people. I think it is the most medieval industry that is left in this country at the moment. I think that will be generally agreed, both from the point of view of the conditions of the Canals and more particularly from the mode of life that the people have to live.

I would like to explain that our view is that the subject should be separated into two parts. We think that there ought be a real inquiry, in the light of what has been done in the realms of education for the children of the country, and what is being done by the Ministry of Health, or proposed to be done, from the point of view of the living-conditions of the other people in the country. In other words, there should be a very distinctive inquiry into the whole position from the social point of view, regardless, so far as that inquiry is concerned, of whether or not it is economically sound. We feel that the human conditions ought to be inquired into, as has been done in the case of sweated trades, unhealthy trades, and all other trades, regardless of what the condition of the industry might be from an economic point of view.

EDUCATION OF THE CHILDREN

The Canals come, to a very large extent, under the Canal Boats Acts of 1877 and 1884. There is on each boat a registered certificate stating how many are allowed to reside aboard the boat, and a regulation under the Elementary Education Acts, also a subjoined article of the Order of the Local Government Board dated 20th March, 1878. We regard these things having been of great value in their day, but, like every other reform, we recognise as a Union that we are opposed to the conservatism of our own people; that possibly neither the men nor the women want the women removed from the boats. But we have to look at it from the point of view of development, and not in accordance with the prejudices of the people we want to help; so. In spite of opposition within our own Union, and the fact that we know and are conscious that our own people do not help your Inspectors at the moment, we think that this is largely due to the very bad economic wage conditions associated with the Canals. I think you will agree, as an educationalist … you cannot educate a child that is being moved about from one part of the country to another, with the very child-like idea that he is to go to school wherever the boat may find itself. That is impossible. We know the children do not attend school regularly; we know that the people, as a whole, on the Canals are the most illiterate people that we have in our Union; they are very backward, and we say, in the interest of the coming generation, that ought not to be tolerated.

DROWNING OF CHILDREN

Then again, there have been a good many cases of drowning children, and I am told by my local officials that it is always looked upon as a matter of course. Nobody worries very much about them, any more than a horse falling in the Canal. There is not that shock to the social conscience when a child is drowned in the Canal as there is when a child is run over in the street, or something similar happens, and this indicates a very bad social condition from the public point of view.

UNHEALTHY CABINS

Then the size of the cabins in which they have to sleep is a condition that I think you will agree ought not to be tolerated, and I certainly think the Ministry of Health ought to step in immediately. The living space in the cabin is very limited. The average size of the interior of a cabin is approximately 8 feet long, 5 feet high, and 6 feet wide in the widest part; the cabin runs narrower to either end. Well, now, where you have a family aboard, they have to pack in just like sardines to sleep; under those conditions everyone must agree it does not produce very good citizens, and it does not lay the foundation for any, or great, development. On the one side there is the necessary store cupboard, etc., which takes up about one-third of the space; on the other side, running the full length of the cabin, is a locker 2 feet wide and 1 ½ feet high. This serves as a seat during the day, and is used for sleeping accommodation at night. The floor space remaining is only about 2 feet wide and runs the full length of the cabin. To an ordinary outsider, it is a mystery how it is possible for a family, say, of six or seven people to sleep with any comfort at all in these cabins. How they manage to pack them in is rather a mystery.

The bed is opened out across the top end of the cabin, covering a goodly portion of the locker; as many children as possible crowd on with man and wife; the remaining children, if any, sit or lie huddled up on the remaining portion of the lockers or on the floor. The whole point is that the accommodation is bad from every aspect.

I think I have said enough from that point of view to indicate that the family living aboard a boat must be living in very unhealthy surroundings. I consider, as a general principle, it is wrong to have the women and children aboard the boat at all, especially in a country like this, where the size of the country does not warrant it; I mean they are not the great distances away from home or where homes could be built to accommodate these people.

POOR FOOD AND CLOTHING.

Then there is a very great difficulty from the point of view of food. Again I want to call the attention of the Ministry of Health to this. It must be realised, with the very limited accommodation, that the facilities they have for cooking are so limited, and the continual moving, having regard to the fact that you have to carry a family with you on board, limits them practically to the following foods. They have boiled beef, cheese, bread and margarine. This is practically their menu day to day, except, of course, I suppose they get some vegetables at times. The facilities for clothing, and all the rest of it, are of such a character that we think it merits an inquiry, for which we are prepared to ask you. We think it is of sufficient public interest for a Committee of the House of Commons. Probably, in view of its great public importance and the Departments represented, it would be wise to inquire into the whole problem publicly.

NO WAGES FOR WIFE AND CHILDREN'S WORK.

Then, of course, as I indicated, this has arisen largely from an economic point of view. The boat owner only employs a man, and he does not pay a good wage for that. These are the lowest paid people on our Federation, and the longest worked, but then he gets the services of the family and the wife for nothing. The result is that if the wife is hurt, she is not under the Workmen's Compensation Act. There is no liability for her. If a child gets drowned there is no liability, and the only liability is limited to the person employees – that is, the man. That is one of the reasons, I say, why there ought to be a very thorough inquiry by men conversant with the Canals from the social point of view, just as you have your health conditions in the schools, and your departmental representatives, I think the whole question, from the social point of view, and the coming generation, and so on, ought to be inquired into.

DOES IT PAY ?

It may be argues, and it possibly will, that if you alter these conditions the Canals would not pay. I have never yet met the industry that does, and certainly have never yet met the industry that can stand any social change. They have always argued that way.

I want to turn now to the Ministry of Transport. My view is this, Sir, that if the Committee I have referred to reports that changes in the living-conditions are essential from the citizen point of view, then it remains the business of the Ministry of Transport to use their brains to organise the Canals to give economic effect to it.

But I think it is wrong in principle to perpetuate the old system if it is producing bad citizenship. Just as sweating is wrong, and under the Trades Boards it has been directed by Parliament to say you must get rid of sweating, you must give decent living-conditions, because it is in the interests of the nation you must, whether an industry can afford it or not (and primarily I am here to urge that the social conditions of the boatmen and the children should be inquired into). I think it becomes the business of those responsible for the organisation of the industry to see that the thing can be organised, and I believe it can.

I am quite certain that if the Treasury will regard Canals as an investment instead of an expenditure, and bring them up to date, introduce modern appliances – while I am on the economic point of view I want to say this, that the recent Railway Strike demonstrates this- they will find that the Canals are capable of doing ten times the amount of traffic, or fifty times the amount of traffic, they are doing at present, with comparatively little expenditure to bring them up to date. These figures are in the Department. You have this extraordinary feature, that in those ten days, with all the thousands and thousands of tons that were carried in that emergency, in spite of that experience the Ministry of Transport will not profit by it; they simply let it go right back to the old conditions. I say our experience during the War, what has happened during the War on the Canals, what has happened during the Railway Strike, has proved that, without a very great expenditure comparatively, men can be employed instead of women. Women ought to be in the home, as every industrial worker's wife ought to be and is. That ideas is growing amongst all our workpeople, that the wife ought to be at home doing her home duties, instead of working in industry.

That is what we want, Sir, but it cannot be done, I know, at a deputation of this character. What I have in my mind is this – it is not for me to tell you who ought to be on Committees, of course, but what I have in mind is this – I think if I place my cards on the table it may help.

LEGGING.

Nobody has provided power to take the boats through the tunnels. The result is the men – and the women, too, in many cases- still "leg". Our friend is shaking his head, but I am told it still remains-men and the women lie on their backs on the top of the cargo, and with their feet push the boat through the tunnel: what we called legging the boat through. That, of course, is antiquated and out of date, and ought to be entirely wiped out. In some places little motor-boats have been put on, but when the boats have been put on, instead of supplying the power, as you would expect in any other industry, because of facilitating dispatch, and so saving charges, they want to take the cost of the tug out of the man's tonnage, out of his wages, to make him pay for it to take his cargo through. I mean it is all wrong, and therefore a man like Mr. J. Wignall, J.P., who knows all these conditions; a man like Neville Chamberlain, who, I suppose, knows Canals from end to end in the country; and public men of that type, together with your Departmental representatives, could go into the whole question, first from the social point of view, and them, I think, if they could report, as I believe they will report, that it is in the interest of the nation that these women and children should be taken off boats, that the Ministry of Health should provide housing accommodations on positions of the Canal which are the most suitable from the point of view of the halting places of the boats – I mean the terminals, the most suitable places for the people to live, having regard for the traffic; then I think the Ministry of Transport ought not to admit, as apparently everybody has admitted up till now rather, their incompetence to organise the Canals, but give effect to the social recommendations. We are quite prepared to say to the Ministry of Transport, whatever experience we have, whatever organising ability we have, we are ready to place at your disposal to assist you to develop the Canals and make them a profitable concern, provided you first admit that they must be run under humane conditions; that the women and children should be taken off, and that the whole business should be run as the railways and other industries are run, on purely an economic basis. That is our claim.

THE PRESIDENT'S REPLY.

THE PRESIDENT: Well, you have made a comprehensive, lucid statement, and a very interesting one, too. Of course I have been sensible of many of the evils to which you have drawn our attention here this morning, and I can assure you that the Government will take the matter into consideration.

As you know, a new Ministry of Transport has been established, and I will undertake to take the matter up with the Minister of Transport and see what steps can be taken to investigate the circumstances of the industry.

The Board of Education has long been sensible of the extreme difficulty, in fact the impossibility, of giving the children of the men who work on the Canals anything like an adequate education; There is a great proportion of illiterates among them. That is a great evil. How far it can be conquered, or what are the best practical steps to take, I am, of course, not in a position to say; but I think it is a matter for careful exploration, and I am much indebted to you gentlemen for having put the case before me this morning. Thank you.

The deputation then withdrew.

Committee on Living-In on Canal Boats Questionnaire 1920

Appendix A. Suggested Heads of Evidence sent to most of the witnesses

1   Can you serve the committee with the following statistics in regard to the canal boats which traverse your district:-

a)   The total number of different boats actually in use as dwellings;

b)   The number of families on these boats who have no other home;

c)   The population on these boats, divided as follows;-

Sex and age	Having no home except the boat	Having a home on shore	Total
Male Age 0-4 Age 5-14 Age 18 and upwards			
Female Age 0-4 Age 5-14 Age 18 and upwards			
Total ...			

2   Have you any information to show how the canal population compare with town dwellers of a similar social class as regards a) Health, b) cleanliness, c) education, d) morality.

3   Have you information which would enable you to say whether the presence of women on the boats conduces to the morality of the men or the reverse?

4   Can you give the Committee any information as to the confinement of women who live-in on the boats takes place?

5   As regards the children of school age who reside permanently on the canal boats, can you tell the Committee how they get their education?

6   Have you any information showing whether the children on canal boats are more liable to accidents than children of a similar class living in towns?

7   Have you any information showing whether the population living on canal boats are better or worse fed than persons of a similar class living in towns?

8   To what extent do the women and children of school age living on canal boats furnish the necessary labour for working the boats? In other words: assuming the women and children were taken off the boats, what additional hands would be required?

9   Can you tell the Committee whether a married man who takes his wife and children on the canal boat earns more money than a single man working on a canal boat?

10   Are you able to tell the Committee whether the workers on canal boats are contented with the present system of living-in?

If they are discontented, the Committee would be glad to know what you find are the particular causes of discontent and how far you consider these are remediable.

11   Do you find that the installation of motors on canal boats has the effect of driving the women and children off the boats?

Witnesses giving evidence at the Committee on Living-In on Canal Boats 1920

Name	Description
AMOS, Mr Thomas, J.P.	Owner of shop at Stoke Bruerne frequented by canal boat people.
BAGNALL, Mr William	Canal Boatman.
CHILDS, Mr. W. G. E.	Inspector of Canal Boats, Birmingham.
CLAYTON, Mr. Forrester, J.P.	Managing Director of Thomas Clayton (Oldbury), Ltd., Canal Carriers.
COLWELL, Mr. Alfred J.	School Teacher, Gloucester.
DIX, Miss Selina, M.B.E.	Head Teacher, Wheatley Street Girls' School, Coventry.
FRASER, Mr. Donald	Clerk to Runcorn Education Sub-Committee.
GRIFFITHS, Mr. John	Manager of Executors of John Griffiths, Canal Carrier
HACKETT, Mr. W. H.	Canal Boat Officer of the National Society for the Prevention of Cruelty to Children.
HAWKINS, Mr. R. T.	President of the National Association of Superintendants of School Attendance Departments for England and Wales.
HILLS, The Rev. Leonard	Vice-President of the Incorporated Seamen and Boatmen's Friend Society.
JONES, Mr. C. F.	Manager and Director of Fellows, Morton and Clayton, Ltd.
JONES, Nurse Clara.	Certified Nurse and Midwife, Brentford.
KNIGHT, Mr. R. A.	London City Missionary, working at Brentford and Paddington Basin.
LELLIOTT, Mr. E. J.	Visiting Missionary in connection with the Incorporated Seamen and Boatmen's Friend Society.
LEWIS, Mr. E. Manning	General Manager and Secretary of the Sharpness New Docks and Gloucester and Birmingham Navigation Company.
PHILLIPS, Mr. C. J.	Representing the Board of Education.
SHAW, Mr. J. T.	Inspector of Canal Boats, Runcorn.
WARD, The Rev. W	General Recording Secretary of the Incorporated Seamen and Boatmen's Friend Society.
WATTS, Mr. John I.	Director of Brunner, Mond and Company, and Honorary Secretary of the Northwich and Mid-Cheshire Branch of the National Society for the Prevention of Cruelty to Children.
*WHITTAM, Mr. W.	General Manager of the Shropshire Union Railway and Canal Company.

(*This witness was unable to appear personally before the Committee, and was therefore not examined orally).

Appendix 8

Patients problems / conditions when presenting to Nurse Ward

(Earls Barton Surgery Dressing Book)

Anatomical Site	Specific Position	Classification of presenting Problem
Upper Limb	Finger(s)	Septic +++
		Lacerations due to accident ++
		Crushed +++
		Severed End ++
		Burns
	Thumb	Wound
		Crushed ++
		Septic
		Strain
		Dislocated ++
		Rheumatic
	Hand	Accident +++
		Septic +++
		Splinter
		Dislocated ++
		Laceration
	Arm	Wound
		Wrist strain
		Colles fracture
		Carbuncle +++
		Forearm strain
		Accident
		Sting
		Scald
		Radius fracture ++
	Elbow	Injury

Head and Neck	Neck	Cyst
		Enlarged glands ++++
		Abscess ++
		Carbuncle +++
		Burn
		TB Abscess
	Scalp	Cyst
		Eczema
		Ulcer
		Injury
	Ear	Syringing +++
		Mid ear abscess ++
	Face	Cyst
		Wound / accident
		Tumour
	Chin / Jaw	Wound
		Abscess
		Dental extraction x1
	Other	Cyst of nose
		Accident forehead
Lower Limb		Leg Ulcer(s) +/- Septic
		Foot strain / sprain
		Wounds due to accident
		• Chronic
		• Acute / emergency
		Fluid on knee
		Bullous legs
		Septic toes
		Phlebitis
		Infected chilblains
		Fracture Tibia and Fibula
Skin		Eczema
		Purulent blisters
		Carbuncles
		Dermatitis
		Abscess
		Burns / scalds
Eyes		Conjunctivitis
		Foreign bodies
		Tar
		Cyst
		Injury

Others	Pregnancy related	Breast Abscess ++
		Engorged breasts
		Complex pre-natal condition
	Bee stings	+++
	Goitre	x2
	Rupture	x1
	Bites	Cat
		Dog

Committee on Canal Boat Regulations: Memorandum August 1935

TITLE: Canal Boats[515]

The Ministry have had occasion recently to review the operation of the Canal Boats Regulations of 1878 in the light of modern developments and conditions, particularly so far as they relate to the structure, equipment and arrangement of boats. The expansion of motor driven traffic has given this subject a special urgency the Ministry are aware that many new motor boats have within the last few months been built and ordered, of a new design in several respects. It therefore appears to be opportune to bring to general notice certain observations and suggestions. In so doing the Department wish to make it clear that they recognise the peculiar traditions and characteristics of the canal boat community; in fact the main features recommended below are already embodied in the design of the new boats referred to above.

These observations relate particularly to motor boats and butty-boats. A matter of the greatest concern is the risk of carbon-monoxide poisoning from the engine fumes. This risk cannot be overlooked (even from heavy oil engines) in the engine room itself, and in the cabin if there is any possibility of gas escape from the engine room, the exhaust pipes, or through the aperture between the engine room and cabin. It must be emphasised that it is a responsibility upon owners to see that adequate means are taken for disposing of exhaust gases and engine fumes, whatever is done in the way of ventilation and the provision of gastight partitions. Ventilation is another feature that calls for considerable improvement, particularly in the engine room, in view of the risk mentioned. The suggestions made for improving ventilation have the important advantage of improving natural lighting. The department have also considered the question of air space. They have come to the conclusion that the fore cabin has disadvantages as a sleeping cabin and that it would be an advantage to increase the air space in the main cabin.

The recommendations made below relate also to other features, protection against fire, latrine accommodation, increased water supply, oil wastes and bilge water. The importance of latrine accommodation arises from the less frequent stopping of the motor driven boats.

The following recommendations are made with a view to their adoption in the construction of new boats. They are grouped to correspond with the different parts of the boat:-

1) Main Cabin.

    a. Efficient gastight bulkhead (without any communicating door or opening) to be provided between the engine room and the cabin. Where controls from the engine room are taken through the bulkhead special attention to be given to rendering the sapertures gastight.

    b. For ventilation and lighting, the sides of the cabin super-structure to be provided with opening ports and the roof of it with a skylight, mushroom or other form of ventilator. Where possible, skylights to be made of steel framing with protected glass lights and to be made to open and close easily. Where a mushroom form of ventilator is installed it should be combined with some form of louvred opening at a lower level.

    c.   The cabin to be extended to a minimum length of 9 feet; this extra space to be secured at the expense of the forecabin and not of the hold. As regards design and arrangement of the cabin equipment consideration is invited to the planning of the interior of a motor trailer caravan. It is recognised, however, that the present design of cabin interior is popular with the occupants.

    d.   Provision to be made for electric generating plant and lighting equipment, driven by the main engine. This should add little to the prime cost. Where the main cabin accommodation is on the butty-boat, towed by a motor boat, provision to be made for electric lighting on the butty-boat, even when the engine of the towing boat is not running.

    e.   Where a cabin is in front of the engine room conveniently placed hand-holds to be provided for access, particularly on narrow boats.

2)   <u>The engine room.</u>

    a.   Efficient arrangements to be made for leading away the exhaust from the engine room.

    b.   Ventilation and lighting by opening ports, together with a skylight or mushroom ventilator with louvres to be provided, as for the cabin (see 1(b)).

    c.   Artificial lighting to be provided as for cabins (see 1(d)).

    d.   The engine room to accommodate a chemical closet and the moving parts of the engine to be protected.

3)   <u>Fore cabin</u> to be replaced by a compartment for stores.

4)   <u>The hold</u> to be moved a few inches forward to give room for a longer cabin.

5)   <u>Miscellaneous.</u>

    a.   The quantity of fresh water carried to be increased from 3 to 6 gallons and contained in two separate receptacles to facilitate handling.

    b.   Adequate arrangements to be made to exclude oil wastes and bilge water from the space under the cabin floor.

Ministry of Health,
Whitehall, S.W.1.
August, 1935.

Appendix 10

CONSTITUTION: Revision of Boatmen's wage rates agreement and working rules

Grand Union Canal Carrying Company and TGWU 1937[516]

CONSTITUTION

REVISION OF BOATMEN'S

WAGE RATES AGREEMENT

AND

WORKING RULES

Issued by the

Grand Union Canal Carrying

Company Conciliation Board

(Representing the Grand Union Canal Carrying Co. Ltd,
and the Transport and General Workers' Union)

HANDBOOK FOR BOATMEN

In the employ of

THE GRAND UNION CANAL
CARRYING CO. LTD.

This handbook is issued by the Grand Union Canal Carrying Company Conciliation Board (representing the Grand Union Canal Carrying Company Ltd, and the Transport and General Workers' Union) for the use and information of the boatmen and crews in the employ of the Company. They are requested to read it carefully as it is intended for their personal benefit, as well as the efficient working of their craft.

Boatmen are requested to realise that they are responsible for the safe navigation and for the upkeep and condition of their craft.

WHAT TO DO ON ARRIVAL AT BULL'S BRIDGE DEPOT.

Tie up at the berth to which you are directed and at no other place.

Have your equipment checked and report any engine defect or other complaint to the Examiner.

If you have been issued with separation cloths to carry bulk grain, return these to store and obtain a receipt.

Report to the office for settlement.

No settlement will be made unless you present a slip from the Examiner stating that your equipment is in order, and a receipt for the separation cloths.

Obtain any stores you require and sufficient oil to take you to London Docks and back to the Depot.

The Depot premises must only be entered on business; your family and mates should not enter the enclosure. The Depot staff, whilst only too willing to give you advice and assistance, must not be constantly interrupted.

When you receive orders, get to the Loading Point without delay and load strictly in turn without argument.

WHAT TO DO BEFORE LEAVING BULL'S BRIDGE DEPOT.

See that your craft are fitted with proper Fenders. Motor boats should have fenders fore and aft, and all boats and barges a fender on the fore end.

See that each boat or barge is fitted with Check Straps for both uphill and downhill working.

See that your craft have proper Head Lights.

See that you have on board a means of giving warning of approach such as a hooter, horn, or other mechanical fitting.

See that you have on board sufficient Windlasses for working the locks.

WHAT TO DO WHEN WORKING YOUR CRAFT.

Boatmen must understand that it is impossible for a motor boat and butty to be properly navigated on the Canal with less than Three Persons, that is, a Captain and Two Mates. Two handed boats must give way to properly manned crafts.

Boatmen must at all times keep to the right of the Waterway; also in tunnels. Horse drawn craft are, however, given the towpath side when meeting motor boats, to avoid the fouling of lines.

Remember when approaching a bridge, bend, or where the view is obstructed, to slow down and give warning of approach; failure to do this may cause a collision.

In the event of a *collision of any nature*, however slight and wheher or cnot damage is occasioned to craft or property, the Captain concerned must, on the specially prepared form, *notify Bull's Bridge Depot in writing within forty-eight hours.*

In the event of injury slight or serious, to any person, whether an employee of the Company or not, the Captain concerned must, on the specially prepared form, *notify Bull's Bridge Depot in writing within forty-eight hours.*

In all cases where an accident occurs, the Captain shall endeavour to obtain an independent witness as to the cause.

Failure to comply with these regulations will render the Captain concerned liable to disciplinary action.

Remember to slow down when passing other Craft or Boats Moored at wharves or other places along the Canal. Also where any canal works are in progress, particularly in Tunnels.

Boatmen must pay attention to any Special Notices which the canal company may put up, such as Working Side Ponds, Works in Progress, or Danger Notices. These are always erected for good reason and in the interests of Boatmen.

Remember that Lock-keepers are employed by the Canal Company to see that craft work through the locks properly and with the least possible delay, and boatmen must at all times obey their instructions.

Lock-keepers have instructions to call attention to any improper working, or damage done to locks, and are required to report any such occurrence to the Canal Company. Boatmen should in their own interests also report any such occurrence to the District Overseer of the Canal Company.

Boatmen unfamiliar with the working of any particular flight of Locks can always obtain any information from the Lock-keeper on duty.

Craft approaching a lock, but only when within lock distance, which is clearly indicated, should have a Lock Filler ahead to see that the lock is ready to enter. If the lock has to be filled or emptied, as the case may be, it should be done as follows:-

To fill the Lock close the lower gates, lower the bottom paddles, work the side ponds (if any) to the fullest extent before drawing upper gate paddles, which will complete the filling of the lock so that the gates can be opened to allow craft to enter lock. The same operation reversed is necessary when Emptying the Lock.

Boats overtaken by other craft outside the specified lock distance, or in a long level, must give way in all cases, allowing the overtaking craft to proceed without delay or obstruction. This rule also applies to craft navigating stern first.

Check Straps on both motor and butty boats should be ready to hand and used – do not rely entirely on th engine which may fail at the critical moment.

See that your craft are securely moored at night, and, if possible, at suitable tying up places.

ENGINES, ETC.

The attention of Captains is specifically directed to the printed card "Instructions to Captains" which must be strictly observed.

INSTRUCTIONS FOR RIVER WORKING.

Collect all river gear from Regents Dock before entering river.

Do not lay at lock gates at Regnets Dock till ordered to do so.

When on river, instructions of waterman who is responsible for craft while in his charge are to be carried out.

On arrival at respective Dock, in the absence of superintendent, Captain to report immediately at ship to ship's clerk for instructions as to time of placing boats alongside for loading.

When loaded in absence of superintendent, Captain to sign at ship's clerk's office, to take pass to Customs for Clearnace, and in event of other than P.L.A. Stevedores working ship to secure endorsement from nearest office of P.L.A. When passes are complete, Captain to proceed to lock when superintendent will arrange for waterman to take on to river for return to regent's Dock.

In the event of cargo not being stowed into boats in a proper manner, Captain should stop loading and liodge complaint with shipworker. If no satisfaction is received, take boats from ship's side and await return of superintendent.

Captain must on no account enter locks when loaded without the necessary pass signed by Customs, etc.

Do not tow under any circumstances; especially sailormen.

In the event of any bumping or accidents by any river craft, note must be tasken of name of craft, owners, time, date and position, and, if possible, lighterman's name. Any damage, however slight, to be reported at once to superintendent or office.

Captains must refrain from picking up jetsam. This is a punishable affence in the dock.

Working in harmony with stevedores and ship-workers wuill ensure good, proper and quick loading.

REFUSAL TO ACCEPT ORDERS FOR RIVER

In the event of a boatman refusing orders for the river, such boatmen shall be relegated to the end of the turn, and the orders for the river shall be given to the boatman in charge of a boat of suitable type, next in order of rotation.

WHAT NOT TO DO

Don't tamper with electrical equipment and machinery, such as Atomisers, Fuel Pumps and Govenors. These need expert attention.

Don't strap to lock gates, paddle posts, or other fittings – they are not intended for such use, and proper strapping stumps are provided at every lock.

Don't use your motor boat to force the upper gates open before the lock is full, as these are intended to be opened by hand. This practice causes serious damage to both boats and lock gates.

Don't attempt to close the lock gates by the flush of th paddles as these could be closed by hand; nor flush craft out of a lock with paddles or valves.

Don't waste water – use it carefully. A shortage, especially in short pounds, makes navigation more difficult, reduces the rate of progress and the earning power of the boatmen.

Don't try to get a pair of boats into a lock full of ice. It is much quicker to clear the ice out first. Ice hooks are provided for this purpose and must be left at the lock where found, as the boatmen following will be glad of them.

Don't throw old boat lines, snubbers or other rubbish into the waterways, as your propeller may be fouled next journey.

Don't moor craft under or close to a bridge, lock entrance, or in short pounds, and always leave the fairway clear for other craft, as they may require to work when your boats are tied up.

Don't leave your craft in a lock or in such a way to interfere with other craft using the locks on the canal.

Don't moor your craft at private wharves unless you are loading or unloading there.

Don't forget to shug swing bridges across Canal after passing through.

Don't push your craft out of dock entrances or from wharves so as to hold up other craft navigating the waterways.

Don't work loaded boats two abreast.

Failure to comply with any of the foregoing rules will rended a Captain liable to disciplinary action.

ADVANCES

Captains must present their advanced cards at the issuing office when advances are required. Unless this is done no payment can be made. With regard to "fly" working all captains on being instructed to work "fly" must obtain a written note from the person giving the instructions and no payment will be made at Bull's Bridge unless this is produced.

ISSUING OF OIL AND STORES

Captains must present their supplies cards at all issuing Depots when requiring oil or stores. Unless this is done no issue canbe made.

Captains, except when on special runs and who then fuel at Depots specially appointed, must obtain oil and stores at Bull's Bridge.

OIL AND STOCK CARDS

Captains must complete Oil and Stock Cards on the last day of each month and forward them to arrive at Bull's Bridge within forty-eight hours.

Failure to do this will render a Captain liable to Disciplinary action.

RECEIPTS

Captains must not give clean receipts unless they are certain the full quantity shown on the receipt has been loaded. If in doubt, sign for "a quantity said too be …"

After discharge at destination, Captains must obtain a receipt from consignees. This receipt must be handed in at Bull's Bridge Depot as early as possible. Unless consignees sign one copy of the consignment note, which serves as a receipt, but where Captains have not been given consignment note, they must ask for a receipt. No settlement will be made unless consignment or receipt notes properly signed and completed are handed in.

TRIP RECORD CARDS

These must be handed in for time checking at the various points mentioned, and, upon completion of the trip, returned to Bull's Bridge Depot.

PROCEDURE IN CASE OF BREAKDOWN

The following is the procedure to be adopted in the case of breakdown of craft on the sections mentioned:-

The Captain concerned will telephone, or otherwise communicate by the quickest means possible, to the Grand Union Canal Company's Depot, on the section in which a breakdown occurs, giving particulars as to the situation of craft, etc. details of Sections are as follows:-

SECTION 1

North of Lock 78, Cassio Bridge, Watford to Fenny, Lock 22 (including Aylesbury Arm).

Depot ….. Bulbourne Works, Tring. *Telephone:* Tring 261

Places on Section where repairs may be carried out:-

   Cassio Bridge Wharf

   Hunton Bridge Wharf

   Boxmoor (Fosters)

   Ravens Lane, Berkhampstead

   Cowroast

   *Bulbourne Works

   Marsworth Yard

   Cooks Wharf

   Slapton, Lock 30

   Grove Yard

   *Leighton Buzzard (L.B.Faulkner)

   Soulbury Locks

   Water Eaton Wharf

   *Fenny

SECTION II

Fenny to Braunston Turn (Including Northampton Arm)

Depot ….. Gayton Yard, Blisworth *Telephone:* Blisworth 33

Places on Section where repairs may be carried out:-

   Linford Wharf

   Cosgrove Wharf

   Stoke Bruerne (Top and Bottom)

   *Gayton Yard

   Bugbrooke

   Hayford

   Stowe Hill

   Buckby (Top and Bottom)

   *Braunston

SECTION III

Braunston Turn to Sampson Road, Birmingham, including Oxford and Coventry Canals.

Depot ……. Hatton Shops, Near Warwick. *Telephone:* Haseley Knob 46

*Places marked thus are suitable for carrying out major repairs.

Places on Section where repairs may be carried out:-

Birdingbury Wharf
*Stockton Shops
Cuttle Bridge
Welsh Road
Fosse Road
Radford (Bottom)
Leamington Basin
Cliffe Wharf
Cape (Top)
*Hatton Shops
Turners Green
Black Boy
Knowle (Top)
Barston Lane
*Sampson Road

SECTION IV

North of Sampson Road, Birmingham, and points on the Birmingham Canal Navigation.

All communications regarding breakdowns on this section to be made to Fazeley Street, Birmingham, Telephone: Birmingham Midland 5964, where the necessary arrangements will be made.

SECTION V

Leicester Section (Norton Junction to Langley Mill).

DEPOT ... Kilby Bridge, Wigston, Near Leicester. *Telephone:* Leicester 22819.

Places on Section where repairs may be carried out:-

Watford
*Crick
Yelvertoft
*Kilworth
Foxton
Kibworth Road, Lock No. 20
*Kilby Bridge
Blaby
Leicester – Public Wharf
"Hope and Anchor"

*Loughborough
Kegworth
*Trent
Sandiacre
Stanton

Broken down craft to be taken North or South in direction of travel.

SOUTH OF CASSIO BRIDGE

In cases of breakdown South of Cassio Bridge, the Captain concerned must get in touch with Bull's Bridge Depot (*Telephone*: Hayes 1178) who will make the necessary arrangements.

Break downs in Regent's Canal Dock shall be immediately reported to the Commercial Road Dock Office.

DELAYS DUE TO CAUSES OTHER THAN ENGINE TROUBLE

The captain concerned will get in touch with the local canal overseer or foreman of the district in which the trouble occurs, who will assist in making any necessary arrangements to haul the craft to some suitable tying up place.

RECREATION ROOM

A recreation room and provision store will shortly be opened at Bull's Bridge Depot. It is hoped that all Captains will make full use of the facilities provided. Any suggestions put forward will be welcomes and fully considered.

The canal runs between our two churches in the Parish, from two ...about 150 boats each way - every week.

I have been invited here to speak to you on canals. I have no claim to be an expert on subject, nor any technical qualification. I ask you please regard my remarks in a conversational manner and if any point arouses interest I hope you will frequently stop me and ask one; just to keep it conversational. By this means I may be able to tell you what you want to know which will be better than my saying a lot, of little interest to you; the whole subject to me is just a matter of daily routine. I have been employed on Canals in various capacities for 24 years which has given me knowledge of the Commercial side as well as an intimate view of the Canal Boatmen & family. I take it the latter or human side is the one to which you would prefer to listen or discuss and that you will be interested in the social life of this rather remote fraternity. This remoteness, if it is the correct word to describe them, is largely a matter of their own choice and largely due to the isolation in their manner of living. I claim to have been initiated by them or accepted by them – and approved., I hope and I see much of the internal family affairs. They like to confide their joys and sorrows and are grateful for advice or assistance. Internally they a friendly class and good neighbours – generous beyond reason, especially to help in bereavement. Their exclusiveness is partly maintained, in my opinion from the considerable intermarriages. They rarely marry ourtside the fraternity and every family seem to be some degree of cousin, or nearer, to the next one. The topical subject of conversation is Boating. Boats on passage make for convenient "tying-up places" after the day's journey and such places are general assembly points – invariably in vicinity of canal-side public houses and canal-side general shops, both of which ater especially for the canal folk. In former days-and not far back-these public houses provided stabling and fodder for boat horses.

One of these main assembly points is Hawkesbury Junc. (see map) and practically every boat, sooner of later, passes. When empty after discharge of cargo they call at my office for fresh orders and we have them again on their return from the collieries or quarries after loading. Here we have a typical boatmen's public house complete with grocery shop. Here they can be supplied with every want except meat (and that is obtainable at Longford where the local butcher will honour their Traveleers' ration cards with understanding for their special choice – somewhat different from the usual family taste). At Hawkesbury they receive their "settlement" for previous work – and perhaps some "starting money" – a canal cusatom equivalenmet to the "sub" claimed by workers in other lines. This money is usually an open cheque which is accepted and cashed at the Grocers after endorsement with a X, witnessed by the proprietor of shop. They take in perhaps a week's food or more and when it is for a large family of half a dozen children – and bread is bought by the dozen large loaves it is a sight to see them going off with bags full and all the children carrying something to the boats. Although some cannot write their signature to endorse the cheque there is no possibility of their being unfairly dealth with, they have a good knowledge of costs and calculation of money.

In the past 24 years I have seen the transition from horse-drawn to motor boats – also the radio introduced. Almost every boat carries a battery set. I think it probable that the radio and films have been greatest factor in bringing the boatmen into line with the ordinary citizen.

EDUCATION OF CHILDREN. We regard this as the worst problem of canal life. The younger married generation of canal folk are also showing some thought to the matter, but the older ones do not appear concerned. The children are healthy and happy in their freedom. It has been stated that canal boats make use of child labour – but I do not agree. All children like to be useful and help their parents in shore life as well as boats. It is better to keep them employed on the long journeys throughout the day. Children of locally employed boatmen of course attend school – and I hear they are well up to standard in intelligence and well able to hold their own in all respects.

The difficulty is with the children of long-distance canal boatmen; they stay at any given place being not more than 2/3 days. They are entitled to present themselves at any primary school near the boats if detained a day or so – provided they can produce a school-attendace book and many of them carry these books, if little use is made of them. Attendance books are issued by the Local Authority which holds the Registration of the boats on which they happen to reside at the time of application. Outr local Coventry Canal Boat Inspector – an official from the Chief Sanitary office is very co-operative and always gives immediate help with the children if a case is brought to his attention. This week he obtained books for a family of four from Daventry. Very few boats are Registered under the Coventry Authority. Some years ago we had a case of a boat boy kicked by horse resulting in blindness. His case was treated by Specialists and there came some hope of a partial restoration of sight but it was recommended that he should be treated as a blind person for educational purposes. It happened that he lived on a Coventry Registered boat. We followed up and received sympathetic consideration. He was placed in Harborne Royal Institute and today he is competent at brush and basket making, and with several musical instruments, including piano. He is living on boats during Easter vacation.

We another child at a school in Kent, an orthopaedic case.

When children attend school they cannot receive special tuition due to large size of present classes – and they are apparently just places with children of like age, so cannot understand what the lesson is about. One small boy said he had been given a penci % paper and told to draw a canal boat while the others went on with their lesson. We know a numbert of cases where children have been left with local boatmen relatives to enable them to attend school. Children are also taught by their parents where the parents have knowledge. We sometimes get a child in the office and write their names in script or capitals and give them a pencil & paper to copy it until they come back – even to be able to sign their name is an asset.

The following rather strange fact should be mentioned which is that illiterate boatmen have the ability to reckon their wages. I produce here a specimen wages sheet showing 47t.1c. @ 2/6 plus 17 ½ bonus with other credit items and deduction of insurance, etc which we have to calculate, but the boatmen would immediately detect any error in amount due. Their tonnages are usually within 2 or 4 tons difference and they memorize from former payments with allowances for the odd cwts. My company (before Nationalization) the Grand Union., have a school at Hayes, Middlesex. The class there was shewn in session in the film "Painted Boat". It is in the care of a Trained Certificated Woman Teacher from the Middlesex Education Authority. At the Depot all boats calling for refitting, refuelling, fresh orders, etc and sometimes are detained for days – durin which time children compulsorily attend school. A scheme was formulated to builkd hostels at our Depot where boatwomen could live with their children while the husband and older members of family went away on loaded trips – the scheme was principally to give children benefit of education. Whether the scheme will be furthered under Nationalization is not known at present.

Marriages. Last Saturday at Camp Hill Church, B'ham a real boatman's wedding. Neither man or woman had ever lived off boats. Vicar helpful and gave a rehearsal previous day. Guests comprised party of 50 – all boatmen & families. Reception on boat at Grand Union wharf. A long erection the whole length of boat served as table for wedding feast in the open air. They had tarpaulins or boats' top-cloths in readiness if wet. Honeymoon was a trip to H'bury to load coal for London. They duly reported to me for orders and carried straight on with work

Have personally attended many weddings and assisted to run them according to accepted procedure with a due regard to their own customs.

At a Longford Church wedding the bridggroom was unable to produce the required amount to pay fee, although he had just previously paid £5. For flowers. With some exceptions, they do not lay up for themselves treasure on Earth but live up to their earnings. Money is something to spend. Many of the weddings are financed on money advanced by the Canal Carriers for the occasion, which they afterwards work-off by stoppages. The Church wedding with it's marriage service and ceremony is strongly favoured by the majority and when we have been consulted in their plans – which has been frequent – it has been recommended and assistance given in arrangements. Mt assistant, Miss Edwards, who takes a great personal interest in their lives receives the confidences of the women. We came to conclusion that the wedding addresses to boaters was something beyond their grasp and the fact was tactfully mentioned to the Vicar – he agreed – and omitted from that time.

A number of marriages take part at the Registrars' offices and on one occasion I took two brothers and two sisters to Nuneaton Registrar for a double wedding.

One marriage incident occurred at Cov: Reg: Off: when Enoch Wenlock married Lucretia Lane. He was repeating his declaration after the Registrar and said "I Enoch Wenlock, take thee Lucretia Lane to be my (l) awful wedded wife". The Registrar without any change of expression or tone of voice said "We will gove over that again". He recorded this case within his memoirs later.

This couple, with their daughter Sarah Ann, appeared with some goof parts in the film "Painted Boat".

Immediately after all weddings they report for orders and move off to load boats – no idea of holiday or honeymoon.

Reference foregoing remarks of the care-free idea where money is concerned there are a few thrifty members. These have ambition to purchase a canal-side cottage and finish up with a job as length-man on canal. Canals employ maintenance labourers as length-men or lock-keepers at points where the mis-use of locks would have serious consequences in waste of water and these posts are mainly occupied by ex-boatmen. Another job favoured by them is that of rural district council labourers or roadmen – but the cottage they take must be near the canal. In these cases it is very probable it is the first time in their lives they have lived off the water.

I was once invited to take tea at such a cottage in Cheshire and I think to-night's circumstances permit a tale out of school to describe the experience – The walls of room were completely obscured with framed pictures and I listened to a description of every one. The largest was a photo enlargement of one of the family who had been drowned – description of this one very vivid. At tea a large centre dish on table had at least two large tins of salmon emptied thereon and I was told to cut myself some "pieces" (bread) and help myself to salmon. The tea-pot was huge and tea strong. The milk was a tin of condensed sweetened which was [assed round with a spoon in it and we all dipped & stirred and passed it on. It was an enjoyable experience and entered into in the spirit in which it was given.

MATERNITY CASES. Boatwomen invariably prefer that the event shall take place in their boat. Some of you may have heard a broadcast feature called "Midland Journey" in which a boatwoman was asked how they managed in in maternity cases and she replied "We take the boats to back of Veater's shed" her description of my office. This stretch of water is popula for the occasion. Here they have telephone facilities for midwife and midwife can also communicate with Dr if required. The midwife understands boatwomen and threatens them with hospital if consitions in boats are not up to standard required. The spot is also very convenient to the local grocer (mentioned elsewhere) and their friends and relatives on passing boats are available with assistance or care of children in fact, they feel at home there.

The impending event is always announced to us by the husband who says:- "I don't want an order as I've got to tie up". We require a certificate from midwife who frequently says they are safe for further trips and we then arrange for short jobs according to case. Boats then remain until Midwife gives a clearance and meantime we give the boatmen suitable work where he can return at night. Following her confinement, we recently asked a boatwoman into the office for some telephoniong on her behalf but she declined, saying I mustn't go in anywhere because I have not yet been churched – I am not able to say if this is peculiar to the canals. The new-borns are all christened before the boats move off again.

Here I will mention that the offices of the Church are utilised with churching, christening, marriage & funerals – but I have not heard of a case of confirmation.

CUBIC ACCOMMODATION

BOAT CONSTRUCTION. CABIN in which many are born, live all their lives, are standard in fittings in all narrow boats (except Joeys used only on local work and not for sleeping). Dimensions of ordinary butty 8'9" long by 7' wide with height of 6 ' flooring to roof. Cabin of motor being a few inches shorter, it I planned on the experience of ages of use as a bedroom, kitchen, dining room, bathroom etc. etc. Here is a cabin plan which shows the bedding cupboard wherein is contained usually a full sized mattress or bed with blankets & pillows etc. complete. The door is let down to sit on nest of drawers and forms a bed the whole width of boat – during daytime when bed nbot in use the door lifts back to the cupboard and bed cannot be seen. There is space for a single bed on the side lockers the top of which forms a bunk – generally used for children.

Crockery and eating utensils are contained in another cupboard the door of which, when let down, forms the table.

Food is kept in a ventilated lazaret cupboard at rear of steering cockpit.

A 24" cooking stove, coal fed, placed immediately below the cabin entry provides meals, warmth, etc. Decorations often show a large proportion of brass work kept well polished, crochet work and bright ribbons and frequently one or more framed mourning can … A pair of curtains usually hang to shut off the bed for use if it is required in daytime, illness, etc. They do not regard this limited space as cramping – I saw a family at Sowe Common who had been moved into a Council House, who made the living room into a typical boat's cabin with everything in one room; and made the bed up at night on the table. This was an extreme case and a visit with the local San: official and some joint advice soon obtained a great improvement.

The total length of a narrow boat is 71'6" with a beam of 7' and a depth of 4'. This is the maximum size of boat which can operate on all navigable canals due to limitation of size of locks.

The carrying capacity with dead-weight cargoes of a butty boat is up to 30 tons, usually about 28 tons. Wiuthg the motor boat cargo space is somewhat less due to length of engine room and 26 tons is a good average – but for general purposes the two nboats usually pick up 50 toms of coal or stone.

The compulsory equipment includes a 3 gall (drinking & cooking) water can replenished from water taps provided at many points. It is of a covered in pattern and always highly decorated with roses, always carried on top of cabin.

There is also a "hand bowl" - a tin bowl with long handle - easy for baling water from canal for cleaning. They cannot afford time ^ labour to carry tap water to & fro.

CANAL BOAT INSPECTOR is an appointement under the Chief Sanitary Inspector. It is not a whole time job but combined with other duties as a Sanitary Official. As mentioned under my note under Education out local officer very keen to assist. He makes surprise visits to all boats and inspects them, mainly as to state of repair and condition of paintwork, etc. He looks for overcrowding in relation to cubic space of cabins – segregation of sexes of children reaching adolescence – cleanliness. Each boat carries a copy of its Registration Certificate which must be produced to him. It shows the number of persons authorised to live in boat. Any complaint is officially passed to the boat owners and must be remedied within the specified time allowed, under threat of prosecution. He is always well received by the boatmen who understand he is there watching on their behalf. You will appreciate that this welfare service is a fine safeguard.

-   *Show Certificate of Registration*   -

MEDICAL CARE. Boatmen are not included on Doctor's panels but carry a Travelling Medical Cad which gives them benefit of National Health Insurance from any Doctor in vicinity of boat when th need occurs. Boatmen also pay voluntarily a Hospital Subscription through thei employers of about 3d p.w. which is passed on by Employers to Hospital Savings Association. In Coventry district the boatmen prefer a local Doctor who in turn appears to regard himself as the Boatmen's Doctor – a happy situation for the boatmen who receive proper treatment. This Doctor makes use of my office as a means of contact and we are thus able to arrange movement of boats to suit Doctor & Patient.

Generally speaking the boating families are a healthy community.

Sister Mary Ward, appointed by Coy to give free advice & treatment. Ward Sister Northampton Hospital, has made a speciality of canal boating families.

INCIDENTAL NOTES

Hobbies, Sport, Recreation. & C.

Have not yet heard of a boatman going to football matches, horse racing etc. A Fair is a great attraction: and they used to arrange if possible to have their boats sent to Banbury or Oxford to attend. I think the "show-booat" sort of music and the lighter coloured painting of booths appeals. They are never more proud than when their boats comes off dockl after refit, with fresh bright colours of roses, diamonds and castles. We have not been able to trace the origins of these designs.

Some of the boatmen make a hobby of painting their boats' cabin doors, following the usual designs of castles – they also paint the stereotype roses around water-cans and handbowls. We have also seen some good specimens of model canal boats.

The boatwomen take great pride in their cabin decoration and cleaning. The coaming around cockpit and stern deck are scrubbed without ceasing. Boots are wiped with the wet mop before stepping inboard.

We know a case where the boatman is not allowed to sit in cabin for meals until a newspaper has been spread for him to sit on – he has a wife and 2 daughters.

POLITICS does not interest them. Nor the 5-day week. Very few of their names appear on any register of voters. They are not rate-payers. We once found that names of 3 or 4 boatwomen had been included in register for Sutton Stop. They were schooled in voting procedure and told where we would put our cross, but they could please themselves – and then taken to polling station – all's fair in politics !!!

FAMILY AFFAIRS. Great caution necessary not to express opinion when hearing of family dissension.

NEWS is telegraphed from boat to boat when passing and travels the length of canal very quickly.

A kind of jungle telegraph

Film "Painted Boats". When showing at "Empire" Coventry we had a number of the boatmen who appeared in the picture, arrive in district for loading. I telephoned the Manager of "Empire" – result was his invitation for them to go along and some of them after being given tea went on stage – including the Wenlocks – and Enoch played his accordion – same tune as he played in the Public

House depicted in the picture.

"Painted Boats" reaction of boatmen was annoyance. They disliked the theme – their own moral standard is strict.. The women objected to the pillows shewn with the bare tick, no pillow cases. The boatmen criticised the coal-lade boat north-bound towards the collieries. The tunnel legging scene – a relic of the dark ages – was performed by a boatman who was taking over a motor-boat *(Clash of periods)*

Dress of women – The older women wore a sun bonnet of thick material, with shoulder protection, The bonnet had thick rolls running across. Have not seen this pattern worn locally in past few years but formally it was common. The women usually wear a wide leather belt to carry the windlass (used to wind up paddles at locks). I was driving through Middlewich, Cheshire, a good centre for boatmen, and saw a woman wearing the type of bonnet described – I pulled up and asked her if she knew where Tommy Kaye lived (the boatman I was seeking) but did not mention the word 'boatman' and she replied "who told you I was a boatwoman?", but she was pleased to help me.

The boatmen at the time often wore a celluloid collar with red and black vertical stripes. These also are still seen in Cheshire district.

The word "Bargees" much resented – they are canal btmn. And never refer to "Water Gypsies".

Funerals – Boatmen always expect me to view the corpse. They invariably have "death" cards with most inappropriate verse and weeping angels.

Coffin carried under top planks, claim to passage thrd locks if closed (p.12)

Boatmen telling of death of Sammy Saxon and looking at my grey or white hair – remarked "The best always go first". (back of p.11)

A matter of great convenience to the boatmen is that the local authorities recognise my signature on their required certificates as to the application being genuine. This applies to the forms for obtaining extra clothing coupons, medical travelling cards, emergency food cards in some cases of loss or absence from the London district – the "home" food office for Grand Union boatmen being Isleworth & Heston.

We mainly deal with Bedworth, Nuneaton & Atherstone Food Offices where they have a good understanding of Boatmen's problems. Bedworth in particular being most helpful. On the other hand if Bedworth requires information of any sort regarding boats & crews, they refer to my office. Police and Labour Exchange also avail themselves frequently for any contacts.

I have said my piece on behalf of boatmen in Police Court at Coventry, Nuneaton, Atherstone, Hinckley, Brentford. We have also had some interesting cases at Bedworth Labour Exchange, where Mr Maurice, the Manager, has a fine tactful manner with men. It was necessary during the war years on one or two occasions when control of labour was enforced to have to "run-in" men who refused to accept directions or orders. In these cases we did not once have to proceed to drastic measures. It can now be revealed that we always had a private discussion beforehand and a plan which always succeeded even in most obstinate cases. After I had laid the official charge – with regrets and an explanation that we had no option, Mr M. outlined the penalties which could follow and then invited me to speak on the good points of the person involved – this dual job of prosecuting & defending never failed after the summing up by the Manager.

Hawkesbury Junction practically unknown to cov people but important to the canal world & well known to canal users.

BOAT CONTROL

Before the war all boats working on canals were owned by Canal Carrying Companies or in afew cases by individuals and worked independently – free land Carrying was competitive between these Companies and my job was Midland District representative for the largest of these Companies. I was working for a keen, hard-headed Chief with a marvellous business brain, ruthless in business competition or with staff who failed to make the grade but he would employ no cheap labour. Our Coy: under his Chairmanship quickly absorbed all the best of the work on the canal; and the most efficient of the boatmen. I was sent to Cheshire, Lancashire, Nottingham, Leicester, Gloucester, etc wherever there were canals to induce or entice or collect suitable boatmen. This was a great experience which gave me a wonderful view of canals in operation. The same Chief had a revers side of great charm socially and an approach to him of a hard case received always unbounded human sympathy. One could go out in his servie with the utmost confidence knowing his support was there. Under his direction the Grand Union constructed warehouses and contracts with shipping coys: while the canals were steadily improved in all respects; including the pay and conditions for boatmen – in fact the standard of wages paid generally became based on GU rates. The came the war and his organisation was ready and in being. The Ministry of War Transport took over. One of the first acts was to institute a Boat Control for Warwickshire. All traders owning Canal Boats were directed to Pool them under the Control. Since my office was geographically –see map- obviously the best marshalling point the Control was located there. So once again the GU organization was utilized. It fell to me to be appointed as Boat Control Officer as a temporary Civil Servant of some lesser degree. Under the scheme all Traders gave me splendid co-operation and I found that the collieries immediately gave me the impression that it suited them better to deal with one office for their consignments by water than with a number of boat owners. I think it was a happy mutual agreement; and I shall always be grateful for the kindly help from every colliery. The collieries also sometime had some urgent orders to discharge which was immediately met with the man for the particular loading and destination.

First came the education of the boatmen, hitherto free, to be schooled to comply with 'directions' and it was necessary to insist with firmness, but the few difficult members soon came to heel (there were the one or two cases I mentioned as brought to notice of Labour Manager).

The system or scheme of Boat Control was to bring into use every possible boat to relieve the railways – at that time extremely short of goods wagons (large numbers of which had been sent to the Continent?) The Ministry of Fuel & Power shared out the available coal from the collieries to essential industries, particularly those on war production and where these allocations could be delivered by canal we saw to the collection. According to the canal to be traversed, quantity to be delivered, physical work involved in disposal of cargo at destination – we selected suitable boats and crews. Some boatmen have a good knowledge of one district only. Others were mananed by weaker crews. Some boat crews consisted of lady trainees and it was necessary to discriminate in giving loading orders. The control carried on through the was until the control position by Government was eased; when it officially ended. However the Canal Traders mutually and voluntarily (with the blessing of the Ministry of Transport) decided that the system was better than reverting to the old-time independence of action; so the scheme continues. The Traders pool their boats and submit them to our manipulation on their behalf.

During the war when every stranger was suspect, we taught boatmen they must report anything which might be regarded with suspicion. They were not to talk about their trips, where loaded, cargo, or destination. It must be remembered that many of their cargos were food-stuffs for dispersal throughout the buffer depots, was material from the Midland factories to the docks, etc. etc. but it was all carefully clothed up – under laced tarpaulins; and not visible to lookers-on. Our Chairman of Directors was one day at Rickmansworth and seeing a pair of his boats passing through the lock, approached the boatman and casually asked him what he was carrying – the boatman did not know the gentleman – but he retorted "Toffee apples to you, you old "so & so""

The Chairman well appreciated the reply, told him who he was, and gave him 10/- for a drink.

Bye laws ... to ... Captains of the time, one penalty for malicious damage of waterways was transportation.

Clay puddle banks are being replaced with concrete curbs, wash of motor boats a.... verhe, canal erosion – we have the tow paths – not m... for their original job –and badly maintained.

TRAFFIC.

A specimen tonnage sheet (produce) for one month carried by the Grand Union Canal Carrying Co shows that the commodities included:-

Coal, Stone, Cement, Concrete, Foodstuff, Metals, Lime-Juice, Sand, Slag, Steel, Timber, Woodpulp, Beer, totalling 18,197. Tons.

The usual run of boats is that they load one of the cargos shewn above, in the London district, for delivery in Midlands, mainly Birmingham, where the Company warehouse or distribute it. Boats then come light (empty) to the Coalfields where they come under our orders for loading (mainly) Coal to London district. These we call the long-distance boats.

Locally we employ a number of 'open' or 'joey' boats, delivering from the Collieries to Coventry factories, Power Station, Rugby, etc.

These we call the short-distance boats and they are manned by boatmen living on shore, generally.

PAYMENT is on results. Fixed rates governed by distance carried for long-distance work. Payments vary considerably in amounts, some men with a pair of boats running "fly" which means practically non-stop from London to B'ham with special cargos, which they can do in under 60 hours, have been earning £20.p.w. On the other hand slow workers with a pair of boats probably average down to £6.

P.w. If work is not available for some reason beyond the boatman's control a minimum wage is paid for a 2-boat man of £5.10. p.w. and £3. For a single-boat worker.

LADY TRAINEES.

During the War a Women's Training Scheme for work on Inland Waterway's was introduced by the Ministry of War Transport. The first two entrants were trained by a Boatman and his wife and proved successful. These two ladies then became Instructresses and took over crews of lady volunteers, making several round trips through the Grand Union system, London to Birmingham, to Coalfields and back to London. The Chief Instructress, Miss Gayford, was very keen on the work and remained at the job throughout, being the last to return to her private occupation. She was in her boats in London when they were struck by 'flying bomb' and received injuries, but kept to the work. She was awarded decoration of M.B.E.

The ladies were a mixture of efficiency & otherwise and a number gave the work only a short trial.

The present Duchess of Grafton, (then Mrs Curry, widow of a Naval Commander) was one of the Traineed.

These ladies were mainly of the University Student Class.

They all took copious notes apparently with the notion of getting their experiences into print. We heard that when Mrs Wolfitt (wife of Donald Wolfitt, Shakespearian Actor) managed to get her book published "Idle Women" she queered the pitch publications by others, since the subject matter would have been much repetition. The ladies included members from Australia, New Zealand and Ireland.

One remains. She married a boatman. This unusual match has survived over two years and is going very well.

The ladies outvied the boatmen in their "show-boat" colours; brasses, etc. and complied with all the customs.

The WORK of a normal trip.

A round trip on which a boatman is paid, according to the weight and commodity carried. Specimen rates London to Birmingham:-

Iron & Steel	3/- per ton	plus 50%
General Cargo	3/5	
Spelter	3/4	
Strawboards	3/8	
Copper lead Alum:	3/6	

Light money B'ham to Coalfields 12/6

Coal to London District   2/6 or 2/9 London East

Boats load in London – and usually deliver in B'ham on 5th day. Then after discharge follow track shown on map to Hawkesbury. Receive orders for coal loading at one of the Collieries and return to London.

50 tons Northbound at ¾ obtains credit of	£12.10.0
Light money to coalfields	12/6
50 tons coal to London	9.7.6
	£22.10.0

Including loading time London, Discharge at B'ham. Loading time at Collieries and discharge of coal in London, the time occupied in approximately 20 days; many are much faster and earn the same money in a shorter time.

The work involved in such a round trip is a distance of

Brentford to B'ham	135 miles	with	150 locks
B'ham/Coalfields	62		52
Coalfd / London BB	109		92
	306		294

Foregoing is based on good travelling conditions – but there are times of drought in dry seasons when conservation of water may require boats to be delayed while water is made up in higher reaches and use of locks is under strict supervision. In winter we contend with ice. Ice breakers keep traffic moving – sometimes in convoy as long as possible., but in Feb:47 all movement stopped for 6 weeks. Special arrangements then made for maintenance of crews, outside work

Old men in union - rate as union rate. First T&GW Union conciliation board Ernie Bevan & 4 others. "Gave me something to go back to men with" (back of p.18)

LOCKS.

Different from road and rail where gradients can be used, the canal must travel on the horizontal. Where a change of level becomes necessary the ascent or descent from a level stretch must be made abruptly by some device for lifting or lowering.

The lock is not a modern invention – there are indications they were used in the 15th century in Italy, Holland & Germany. The earliest record of a lock in England is one on the Exeter canal, made to retain tidal waters at low tide, was constructed in 1539. This lock has been kept in use since those days.

In principle, a lock is a chamber, enclosed by gates at each end, constructed at a point separating two reaches at different levels. Conduits or sluices are provided to pass the water from the upper reach into the chamber or lock, and again for the water inside to pass out of the lower reach until level with that reach is obtained. So that any boat floating in the water can be raised or lowered from one level to the others as required. The gates are water-tight etc. etc.

Locks on Grand Union, London/Birmingham main line have been reconstructed by being doubled in width. They take a pair of boats together – being 83 feet long and 15 ft wide with a depth over sill of 6 feet. The intention when made was to enable 14 ft beam barges to travel direct from London to Birmingham. The locks on Coventry & Oxford Canals average 72 feet long by 7 ft beam with a draught of 3'6". This is the minimum size to accommodate a narrow boat and is as economical as possible in use of water. The locks in London district are capable of taking 100 ton barges. The same simple system is in use with the enormous locks of 600 x 80 feet of Manchester Ship Canal, but the largest locks ever constructed are in Panama Canal 1000 x 110 feet.

For canal locks the normal rise at one lift varies from 4 to 10 feet. At Hatton the 21 locks lifts boats 146 feet over a total distance of 2 miles.

Where the amount of traffic does not warrant the construction of duplicate locks which would take part of the water used, instead of the loss of the complete lock of ater with each boat – a dummy lock is often constructed – called a side pond lock. Before the opening of the sluice for emptying or lowering level of lock, the water is run off into the side pond until a mean level is obtained. This water is saved until lock is again used for lifting a boat. When the bottom gate is closed this amount of water can be run in and a corresponding lesser amount from the top is thus required to bring boat to top level. Theoretically this should save one third of a lock at each operation.

Other systems of raising boats to higher levels of water have been in operation but with the exception of the Anderton lift on the River Weaver in Cheshire, lifting boats into the Trent & Mersey Canal, they have now been discarded for the simple lock system. This is a lift of over 50 feet. Boat floats into a wrought-iron tank which is raised by wire ropes passed over pulleys with compensating iron counter-weights. Formerly hydraulic but now worked electrically.

Variations in levels of canals – a few specimens

Bentford ....   30 ft above sea level

Bletchley   235

Braunston   358

Leamington   176

Birmingham   379

Tring   395

The water supply is maintained by use of reservoirs andnatural feeders (brooks and rivers).

Where water from reservoirs cannot reach the higher levels, water is pumped. One pump at Braunston lifts 200.000 gallons per hour.

Use of a double lock on Grand Union drops 56,000 gallons to a lower level

Map – show reservoir – Weston Turville in Wendover. Reservoir 368 & 30th ... water lifted to canal summit 393, 15, 25

The canals were originally constructed where engineers could of choice cut into level land, or through cuttings on a rise of land. This was an easier method than crossing valleys with the need for an artificial embankment, which would be a costly business. Fior this reason it can be seen that many canals winf through the country, instead of the direct line.

At Wolverton the canal crosses the Ouse Valley over an aqueduct which was constructed in 1802/7

Bridgewater canal from Manchester to Worsley collieries boats actually loaded in tunnels at coal face 1760.

A normal trip to South ½ .

"Go as we please – no one behind with a whip"

Boat loads at Baddersley Colliery with coal for Nestles Food Products, Hayes Mddx. During loading Steerer's wife will have completed her shopping at Atherstone. *Monday 2.30* Boats are clothed-up (tarpaulins spread) up 5 locks to Hartshill through Nuneaton, near Bedworth and arrive Hawkesbury, 6-0 p.m. Here boats are gauged – the canal system of ascertaining weight carried. Method – dry inches – water to gunwale. These dips are taken at 4 given marks on boat. Figures obtained applied to chart or boat table (previous the boat has had weights placed and readings taken) Boats are "permitted" with a Permit form showing that tolls have been calculated and charged. *6-0.a.m. Tuesdy.* Boats are now on Oxford canal and secure for night Boats leave Hawkesbury proceeding via Ansty 7-15 Brinklow 8-30. Newbold tunnel 9-30. Rugby 10-0. Hillmorton ascend 3 locks, top 11-30 – dinner while boats carry on. Braunston 2)o. leving Ox Canal and joining G.U.Canal. Passing Nurser's Dock (where Painted Boat was prepared). Up 6 locks and enter braunston Tunnel 2042 yds – 25 minutes of darkness – emerged at back of Daventry. Passed Norton Junction where boats are check-gauged for official recording of passing on Grand Union. Through Buckby Whf, down 7 locks into the 14 mile pound through to Stoke Bruerne. At 7.30 tied uop for night at Heyford. The day's work being 13 ½ hours and worked through 34 miles with 16 lks. *Wednesday.* Off at 6.30 a.m. through Gayton Junc with Northmp Arm 7.30 and then approached Blisworth Tunnel 3056 yards. With 45 minutes of darkness. Boats under electric head lights which reveal the slimy wet brickwork. There are ventilating shafts at intervals but protective clothing required as rain water or springs drop a cascade down these shafts. Boatwomen steering put up umbrellas. We emerge at Stoke Bruerne and descend 7 locks. Where Painted Boat was filmed. *Sister Ward.* We pass Wolverton 2.0 p.m. and arrive Fenny Stratford, Soulbury and then Leighton Buzzard 7-o p.m. We end the day at Marsworth 9.30. The days work was 43 miles with 20 locks in 16 hours.

Thursday. At 5.30. a.m. we begin to mount with 7 adjoining locks reaching the Tring Sunnit, the highest level on trip 393 feet a.s.l. On the summit we passed through a chalk sided cutting about 3 miles in length and about 30 to 40 feet deep. All canal water at this level is pumped from Wendover Reservoir (368 feet). Now being over the Chilterns the locks are down-hill to the Thames. The days work took us through Berkhampstead, Boxmoor, Kgs Langley, Watford to Uxbridge and on toi Hayes. Arriving 9.30 p.m. and alongside the Cocoa Factory. Days work, 33 miles with 54 locks. The journey has taken us 3 days from Hawkesbury.

Extract from John Thorpe (2002) Sister Mary's property

The front door opened directly onto a squarish room with a broken-tiled floor. A somewhat rusty range stood on the left and facing us were two doors with latcheswhich gave access to the stairs and a kitchen area so small that only one person at a time could fit into it. The whole cottage smelt musty and rather damp and a sadly forlorn air of abandonment hung about it .... It had stood empty for lack of tenant or purchaser. Unhelpfully the cottage had a closing order on it; essentially this measnt that certain work had to be carried out before the local council would pass it as being fit for human habitation …

Lifting the latch on the door at the back of the room we found ourselves climbing up a curving wooden spiral staircase to the first floor. Here a thin wooden partition divided the available space giving about two-thirds of the floor area to a front bedroom facing out onto the canal and the remaining third to a bathroom which was in reality, empty except for a pedestal sink. The bathroom project had clearly got no further than the arrival of the sink as neither water nor drainage was yet laid on to this floor. A back window gave a view over a neglected looking yard with rusting tin-roofed open-fronted barn opposite providing parking space for a couple of cars. Immediately below the cottages was a small block of brick-bui9lt toilet cubilcles, one for each cottage, in which resided the Elsan bucket. Mains sewerage had not reached the village at that time, the buckets being emptied on a weekly basis by the council's sanitation truck.

To the left a weedy and nettle-strewn area about ten yards wide led from yard between stone walls right through to Chapel Lane, about seventy-five to eighty yards away. … the ropewalk, where many years before … Mr Amos, had manufactured lines of various length … the ropewalk had fallen into utter disrepair …

Beside the ropewalk a blue gate gave entry to a large and very neglected orchard which also backed onto Chapel Lane. All of this yard, together with the orchard and ropewalk, still belonged to Sister Mary and the little access lane, running along from the bridge and passing behind her house and garden, was legally a shared access for her and the residents of the four cottages. It also afforded access onto land behind the empty Mill … owned by British Waterway's … the ground floor for storage of stop-planks and other material … The whole area behind the cottages was in a very sorry state of benign neglect, exuding an air of melancholy charm as it slumbered in the sunshine.

An identical latched door gave on to a further spiral staircase which led up to a large top-floor bedroom whose low sash window offered a superb view of the canal. A weatcher here could see right across the bridge to the second lock and the curve of the waterway beyond

The room was the largest of all occupying the full length and width of the house, damp stains marked the old fashioned wallpaper on the outside wall and the ceiling bowed ominously … … back down the wooden stairs … emerged into the sunshine before turning down the narrow cobbled path between Sister Mary's house and the cottage.

This was known as the *jetway*, so named because of the propensity of water to rush down it from the towpath under conditions of heavy rain, The jetway admitted us to the rear of the cottage and toi the dilapidated yard … The canal was embanked as it approached the top-lock and this had allowed a fourth room to be included in the form of a cellar, accessible only from below.. Originally this had served as the wash-house and a broken rusting washtub, heated by an adjacent coal-fire, stood forlornly in one corner covered in layers of dust and festooned with spiders webs … The cellar had a very dusty earth floor with black cobwebs draped along thye walls and ceiling and looked as if it hadn't been swept out for a century. Two of the cottages only were favoured with a railed-off flight of steps giving additional entry from the front, an odd arrangement …

End Notes

1   Rolt. L. T. C. (1950) *The Inland Waterways of England* . London. George Allen and Unwin Ltd. (p.191).

2   **Evidence Based Family History:** The family historian using this approach doesn't add claims unless they have the evidence to support the claim. Evidence coming from CREDIBLE SOURCES which are built up over time, leading the historian to a system of cross-referncing of materials / claims, always working with an open approach to new evidence which cumulatively adds to the richness of the (never) final account (Lorna York).

3   **Triple Nurse:** A term used in relation to *Rural Nurses* who c1940's–70's were qualified as a Registered Nurse, Registered Midwife and Registered Health Visitor, who in the course of their day to day work performed all three roles. My aunt, Nurse Elsie May Moore was a Triple Nurse as well as a Queen's District Nurse, in the Worcestershire village of Pershore. Aunty Elsie / Nurse Moore lived in a County House with an attached Surgery where she treated patients, ran baby clinics, provided ante and post-natal care. At the bottom of Aunty Elsie's garden ran the River Severn, which as a child I recall it often overflowing (Della Sadler-Moore).

4   **Willis, P. and Trondman, M, (2000) Manifesto for ethnography.** *Ethnography.* **1(1), pp. 5-16.**

The first sixty years.

5   Pratt, E. A. (1906) *British Canals: Is their resuscitation practicable ?.* London. John Murray.

6   With the caveat the existing Oxford Canal Company agreeing Grand Junction Canal traffic could use its' upper part of their line from Braunston to Napton, subject to tolls (Christopher M Jones).

7   NRO: G3954/1. His Grace the Duke of Grafton to the Grand Junction Canal Company Conveyance of Land: Blisworth, Stoke, Ashton for railway, canal, tunnel, road, wharfs, lock houses (1794).

8   Ibid: 20th May 1794 £600. 25th September 1798 £643 13s. 13th October 1807 £1,479 5s 7d.

9   Plot numbers correspond with map shown in Figure 6.

10   At Stoke Bruerne there was a Water Mill / Wind Mill. The Water Mill was still in use when the Grand Junction Canal was promoted in the early 1790's, it was powered by the stream (NRO: Canal Deposit Plan number 7). The Water Mill was abandoned shortly after the canal arrived and disappeared by 1820's. The Wind Mill (NRO: G.2525) appeared on the plan for the Grand Junction Canal. Francis Wood bought the Wind Mill in 1862 at a cost of £80, but later sold it to the Grafton Estate, who put it back in order. By the 1880's it had been demolished (NRO: G.3893 ff 220-9).

11   NRO: RoP. 690. Hatley. V. A. (1966) *Northamptonshire's First Railway: The Blisworth Hill Railway 1800-1805.* Northampton Historical Series. No2.

12   Faulkner, A. H. (1972) *The Grand Junction Canal.* David and Charles. Newton Abbott.

13   The original paintings by Brian Collings are on permanent display in The Canal Museum, Stoke Bruerne.

14   *Morning Post.* Grand Junction Canal. June 18th 1801.

15   Blagrove, D. (2005) *Two Centuries of Service. The story of the canal at Stoke Bruerne and Blisworth.* Wharfside Publications. Northants. Chapter 3: Blisworth and Stoke Bruerne must have taken on the appearance of small ports.

16   *The London Gazette.* Melancholy Accident. 22nd October 1803.

17   Blagrove, D. (2005) *Two Centuries of Service. The story of the canal at Stoke Bruerne and Blisworth.* Wharfside Publications. Northants.

18   *Northampton Mercury.* The Grand Junction Canal. March 30th 1805.

19   NRO: Kelly's Trade Directory (1854) Northamptonshire's two divisions: Northern and Southern, divided into 20 hundreds and a number of parishes. Stoke Bruerne being in Towcester, in the Southern Division.

20   NRO: Stoke Bruerne Parish Register. Volume 11. 1776-1813 (microfiche). Copy of both deaths available in Sherwood K B (1979) *Stoke Bruerne: A documentary account of the impact of the canal on a village community.* Using the Environment. No 4: Northamptonshire Waterway's. Stoke Bruerne. Nene College Northamptonshire. Document 10. (Lorna York Collection also available Northampton Central Library).

21   Ibid

22   NRO: Saint Mary the Blessed Virgin. Stoke Bruerne. Transcripts 1813-1920.

23   Hassell J (1819) *A tour of the Grand Junction Canal in 1819*. Cranfield and Bonfiel Books. London. Chapter 4: Stoke Bruerne to Braunston. p.47.

24   This 1819 colour view by Hassell of the Grand Junction at Stoke Bruerne shows the original flight of locks from Stoke Bruerne bridge. Although some aspects of the view have been altered, presumably to make a more picturesque composition, the basic layout of the canal is still as it is today even though the locks were duplicated after this image was drawn. The artist is positioned in the lock-keepers garden looking south-east towards Grafton Regis, and the bridge is now double-arched with the bed of the canal beneath the arch shown now filled in. The present day lock 14 is out of the picture to the extreme left. An early map of 1794 indicates a short basin just the other side of the road although not as large as the one shown. Next to the cottage on the right is lock 15, then beyond the double bend should be lock 16 next to the lock-keepers cottage in the middle distance, followed by four more locks either side of the Northampton to Stoney Stratford turnpike road bridge, non of which is shown (Christopher M Jones). *For a further interpretation of the picture see Blagrove. D, (1990) Waterway's of Northamptonshire. Northamptonshire Libraries and Information Services. Northamptonshire. pp 92-93.*

25   Hassell's 1819 view from the Northampton to Stoney Stratford turnpike road bridge of lock 18, 17 and 16, the latter with its adjacent lock house clearly shown in the middle distance. The towpath runs either side of the locks with the path nearest the viewpoint being the former course of the Blisworth Hill tramway. On the left are common fields upon which a man is creating stooks of wheat. Beyond that in the distance is Stoke church. The boat appears to be a wide-beam craft with features akin to Thames western barges, a once common but now extinct type of vessel which often had a canvas shelter at the stern for her crew (Christopher M Jones). *For a further interpretation of the picture see Blagrove. D, (1990) Waterway's of Northamptonshire. Northamptonshire Libraries and Information Services. Northamptonshire. pp 92-93.*

26   *Northampton Mercury.* Casual Leggers. 31st July 1819.

27   NRO: 3954/3: Duke of Grafton conveyancing of land for the construction of duplicate locks and additional canal related structures. 28th November 1837.

28   Account by Christopher M Jones.

29   Evidence used in this drawing is from written descriptions such as in John Hollingshead's account in 'On the Canal' in *Household Words.* 1858. Also from a view of a cabin interior shown on the cover of *The Graphic.* March 20th, 1875 (Christopher M. Jones).

30   Ale houses sprang up along the towing path, and due to the problem of clean water, drinking ale or 'small beer' as an alternative to water, was a reflection of the land based labouring population of the time, by the 1840's clergymen were remarking on the 'generality of drunkenness' within the boatmen, who drowned too often due to drunkenness (tremendous benders) with canal staff (Christopher M. Jones).

31   NRO: 303p/67.

32   The *Child's* family history (Lorna York).

33   1841 Census. Stoke Bruerne: George Smith age 46, William Gardner age 35, George Dimpsey age 20, William Frost age 62, Walter Childs age 30, James Webb age 40, Thomas Dempsey age 50, Thomas Gostick, age 50, Joseph Dyke age 20, John Carter age 35, John Childs age 36.

34   Jenkins, E. (1999) *Victorian Northamptonshire Vol.2 Scandals and Surprises of 1840-41.* W. D. Wharton, Wellingborough, Northants. At the time the major landowner was the Duke of Grafton, with three other landowners in Stoke Bruerne; The Sheppard family (100 acres), the Church (69 acres) and the GJCC (20 acres), the Duke commenced the process with his agent John Gardner.

35   *Northampton Mercury.* The verdict on the young man … Accidental Death. 14th October. 1843.

36   Joseph Ebbern b.1810 in Sowe, Warwickshire, one of nine children born to Thomas (Canal Boatman) and Sarah Ebbern (Family History. Lorna York).

37   The Last Will and Testament of Thomas Ebbern 27th December 1842 (Lorna York Collection). The Will of Thomas Ebbern as proved in the Prerogative Court of Canterbury 1842 (interpretation of Thomas Ebbern's will by David Blagrove). On the death of Thomas Ebbern his son Joseph Ebbern was released from the money owed to his father and received monies during probate.

38   *Northampton Mercury.* Ebbern's Wharf. Stoke Bruerne. October 12th 1844.

39   NRO: V2796. Duke of Grafton Inclosure Map (1844).

40   Marriage Certificate: Joseph Ebbern and Caroline Bailey 8th December 1846. All Saint's Church. Northampton.

41   **George Savage**. Baptised on 7th November 1813 at Whittlebury, the son of William and Ann Savage, his father being a butcher in Whittlebury. On June 19th 1835 George Savage married Elizabeth Brice by special license at St Matthews, Bethnal Green, Elizabeth's father being a surveyor. On the 1841 Census George and Elizabeth Savage are living at the Toll House on the A5, George in the occupation of Butcher / Shopkeeper and Toll Collector. They have three children; George age 5, Elizabeth Caroline age 3 (at her grandparents on the census return) and Sarah Ann age 4 months. On the birth of George Savage junior his fathers occupation when baptised is given as *Huckster*. No specific date is available when the Savage family arrived in Stoke Bruerne, although their fourth child William Thomas was born in 1844 and baptised at Pattishall, his fathers occupation given as Butcher living in Heathencote. Three children were born to George and Elizabeth in Stoke Bruerne Georgina in 1847, father's occupation given as publican, Henry Alfred in 1848, fathers occupation publican and farmer and Caroline Isabella in March 1850 fathers occupation the same as in 1841 (Family History Lorna York).

42   NRO: G 4081/8.

43   NRO: Saint Mary the Blessed Virgin. Stoke Bruerne. Transcripts 1813-1920. Georgina Jane Savage baptised 2nd July 1846. Alfred Henry Savage baptised 17th July 1848.

44   **Edwin Chadwick.** b.1832. Served on a royal commission investigating the effectiveness of the Poor Laws which led to the 1834 Poor Law Amendment Act. Whilst investigating the living conditions of the poor, Chadwick became interested in the sanitation and as a believer in miasma theories he was convinced active measures such as cleaning, drainage and ventilation would lead people to be healthier and less dependent on welfare. Epidemics of cholera, influenza and typhoid prompted government to ask Chadwick to carry out an enquiry into sanitation. In *The Sanitary Conditions of the Labouring Population* (1842), Chadwick demonstrated the direct link between poor living conditions, disease and life expectancy using quantitative methods. These findings stimulated government to introduce the 1848 Public Health Act, with a general Board of Health of which Chadwick was appointed director.

45   At Parliamentary level investigation into *Sunday Trading* had up to this point comprised the Lords Day Bill and Amendment Bills debated in the Lord's between 1837-1838. No resolution was achieved during the debates so a Select Committee was convened. *The sessional papers of the House of Lords presented by Royal Command in the session 4 & 5 Victoriae (20th January – 22nd June) 5 Victoriae (19th August – 7th October) 1841 – Vol xxi.* Reports from the Select Committee and Evidence *Sunday Trading on Canals appointed to inquire into the expediency of 'Restraining the Practice of Carrying Goods and Merchandise on Canals, Navigable Rivers and railways on Sundays' and to report to the house evidence and index laid before your lordship.

46   *House of Lords Hansard.* Lords Sitting of Friday April 23rd 1841. Victoria year 4 1017-1022. Third Series, Volume 57. Canal Traffic on Sunday's.

47   *London Morning Post.* Sunday Trafficking on Canals. 27th April 1841.

48   Rev. Davies was not the only witness who gave evidence to the Select Committee to condem the working conditions of the boatmen and it's effects on their character and wellbeing (Della Sadler-Moore).

49   **Divine Service:** In this context Bouverie was referring to a specific time when the church held it's Sunday Evening service. His suggestion being not to stop traffic on the canal all day on a Sunday, but only between certain hours, so boater's could attend a church service.

50   *London Standard.* Boatmen's Pastoral Instruction Society. Report of the General Committee. 9th September 1841.

51   The 1848 act was the first time the term *Public Health* appeared. For an account of the effects of the Public Health Act 1848 see Sram I and Ashton J (1998) Millenium report to Sir Edwin Chadwick. *British Medical Journal.* 29th August. pp.592-596 and Calman K (1998) The 1848 Public Health Act and its relevance to improving public health in England now. *British Medical Journal.* 29th August. pp.596-598.

52   The main purpose of which was the building of Sanitary Systems, in particular water supplies and sewage management systems.

53   *Northampton Mercury.* A Boat Society. Long-Buckby. 22nd February. 1840.

54   *London Gazette.* Ebbern William and Joseph general canal carriers, Stoke upon Trent and South (Sic) Bruerne. Debts

by William Ebbern. June 4th. 1847

55 Family History Lorna York

56 NRO: Saint Mary the Blessed Virgin. Stoke Bruerne. Transcripts 1813-1920.

57 *Northampton Mercury.* Accidental Death. 1st August 1835.

58 *Northampton Mercury.* Drowned Stoke Bruerne. 13th May 1843.

59 *Northampton Mercury.* Stoke Bruerne,- Another Man drowned. 12th January 1850.

60 1841 Census: Wharf Locks, Long Buckby. Thomas Amos - occupation Lock Keeper.

61 Marriage Certificate: John Amos and Elizabeth Ireson November 5th 1849. Naseby Parish Church.

The Amos family arrive in Stoke Bruerne.

62 1851 Census: Stoke Bruerne. John Amos, occupation Rope Maker.

63 Hemp being considered the best rope-making material, used extensively by the navy and fishing industry, whilst cotton was considered to handle better than hemp although not as strong or water-resistant (Christopher M. Jones).

64 Account of rope and it's use in farming and boating (Christopher M Jones)

65 Three original account books of Blacksmith John Pettifer (In the private ownership of Brian Collings).

66 NRO: *Kelly's Trade Directory* (1854) sheds light on the hustle and bustle of the village.

67 1851 Census: Stoke Bruerne.

68 *Northampton Mercury.* Stoke Bruerne and Blisworth Brick Yards. 2nd December 1854.

69 NRO: CAM 796 a and b, CAM 798, CAM 799, CAM 800 a and b, CAM 801, CAM 802. The Personal and family papers of Major Christopher A Markham. FSA of Northampton.

70 *Northampton Mercury.* Roger Fellows V. Joseph Ebbern. May 21st 1853. Between November 1850 and December 1851, for which the plaintiff Mr Roger Fellows, Draper, had only received £9 by instalments over the said period.

71 *Northampton Mercury.* Joseph Ebbern Auction of Property, Stoke Bruerne. 25th February 1854.

72 **Joseph Ebbern.** Following his leaving Stoke Bruerne Joseph married 60 year old Jane Charlesworth in 1858 licensee of The Tyndall Arms, King Edward Road, Birmingham, after the marriage the license was transferred to Jospeh. In 1868 Joseph Ebbern's adopted son Peter Tite was a 21 year old boatman, who appeared in court for stealing a horse from his father (the prosecutor) which he sold for £7 10s in Wolverhampton. The prisoner was discharged because the ownership of the horse could not be proven by the prosecutor. On the 1871 census Joseph Ebbern was a lodger in Leighton Buzzard, his occupation given as boatman. He died in 1874 age 64 (Family History Lorna York).

73 In urban communities high death rates continued in relation to the labouring population. The 1854 outbreak of Cholera around London's Broad Street was investigated by John Snow which enabled him to expand his theory on the communication of Cholera. Tthe Crimean War (1853-1856) resulted in thousands of lives lost (1,933 killed in action, 2,312 died from wounds, 15,398 deaths from disease). The Thames continued to receive raw sewage, and London experiencing *The Great Stink*, which continued into 1858 at which point it caused the Houses of Parliament to close its windows. A new Public Health Act was issued in 1858 followed by amendments to the Local Government Act in 1861. This resulted in a requirement for Local Authorities to purify sewage before discharging it into natural waterways. The Sanitary Act of 1864 required Local Authorities to make and enforce regulations. These legislative developments marked the beginning of *Sanitary Reform*, although sanitation was not the only ill to affect the population at this time as Tuberculosis (TB) continued to be associated with high deaths rates. It was suggested TB was a communicable disease, but this suggestion was received with *disbelief and derision*.

74 *Northampton Mercury.* Inquest Stoke Bruerne. 28th October 1854.

75 Conversion of warehouse to Steam Mill by George Savage. Date indicated in George Pettifer Blacksmith Records (Brian Collings Private Collection).

76 Hollingshead J (1854) *A narrative of a voyage from London to Birmingham in 1858.* Published by The Waterway's Museum. Stoke Bruerne, 1973.

77 NRO: V665. Courteenhall Grammar School Attendance Record Book.

78   1861 Census: Stoke Bruerne.

79   *Northampton Mercury.* Frightful Accident in a tunnel on the Grand Junction Canal. Two men killed and three men injured. September 14th 1861. *Northampton Herald.* Two men suffocated in the Blisworth Tunnel Accident. 14th September 1861. For a more technical account of the incident see: Blagrove, D. (2005) *Two Centuries of Service. The story of the canal at Stoke Bruerne and Blisworth.* Wharfside Publications. Northants. pp.59-63. For a transcript of the Northampton Herald article see www.steamerhistorical.co.uk/steamers_accidentreport01.htm

80   O'Rourke R (1970) Some Northamptonshire Brickworks. *Bulletin of Industrial Archaeology in CBA Group 9.* Number 13. pp. 8-27.

81   *Northampton Mercury.* Stoke Bruerne Floral Fete and Harvest Festival. 19th September 1863.

82   *Northampton Mercury.* Fatal Accident Stoke Bruerne Mill. 30th July 1864.

83   *Northamptonshire Mercury.* The Bankruptcy Act, 1861. 27th November 1869.

84   *Northampton Mercury.* A boy drowned in the canal at Stoke Bruerne. 23rd December 1865.

85   1871 Census: Stoke Bruerne.

86   These were often from carriers issuing loading or delivery orders to their men. The clerks would also write letters for boaters if they were not able to do it themselves, and as the boaters knew these clerks over a long period of time they were trusted and would understand their illiteracy. Colliery offices also dealt with letters between boaters and carriers as the colliery agents acting for the colliery or a coal factor, often organised the loading of boats through these offices. Carriers would also send postal orders for tolls or starting money as well to be handed over only after boats were loaded and ready to leave. Post offices near the canal were also used to cash postal orders or to receive and post mail, probably more so if the post master was well known to the boaters (Christopher M Jones).

87   A member of one of the authors boating family (Della Sadler-Moore).

88   Family History Lorna York.

89   Family History Lorna York.

90   The 1870's saw an influenza pandemic and widespread outbreaks of Smallpox, which led to tens of thousands of dead across England. Government responded by creating the Local Government Board (LGB), which took over from Urban Poor law Board's, but had extended responsibilities for local sanitation. In rural areas health administration was devolved to Rural Sanitary Authorities, under the aegis of the Poor Law Board of Guardians (Della Sadler-Moore).

91   George Smith F.S.A (December 1875) *Our Canal Population: The sad conditions of the women and children,-with remedy. An appeal to my fellow country men and women.* London: Haughton and Co., (Accessed From The British Library Document Supply. 9th April 2014. Ref. 331.7656 N500). Transcript of Smith's letter October 1873: *Boatmen and Their Children._ An Appeal.* pp 15-16.

92   For a detailed account of George Smith's life see Bristow A (1999) *George Smith. The Children's Friend.* Chester. Imogen.

93   Ibid. Transcript of article: Life on the Canals. *The Potteries Examiner.* 1st November 1873. pp 18-20.

94   Ibid. pp 20-25.

95   Ibid. pp.87-88.

96   *Northampton Mercury.* The Regent's park Explosion. 19th October 1874.

97   George Smith F.S.A (December 1875) *Our Canal Population: The sad conditions of the women and children,-with remedy. An appeal to my fellow country men and women.* London: Haughton and Co., Accessed from The British Library Document Supply. 9th April 2014. Ref. 331.7656 N500. pp 93-110.

98   Sherwood K B (1979) *Stoke Bruerne: A documentary account of the impact of the canal on a village community.* Using the Environment. No 4: Northamptonshire Waterway's. Stoke Bruerne. Nene College Northamptonshire. Document 20 Log Book. Stoke Bruerne Primary School. (Lorna York Collection also available from Northampton Central Library, History Centre).

99   NRO: ZA 6834. Malin E M (1953) Roade Village Scrapbook. Compiled by a committee drawn from the Women's Institute and Parish Council.

100   Payne E A (1938) *Roade Baptist Church 1688-1938. The story of a Northamptonshire Church during two and a half centuries.* Wyman and Sons. Ltd., London.

101 *Northampton Mercury.* Baptist Bazaar at Roade. 29th July 1871.

102 Women's Institute and Parish Council (1953) *Roade village scrapbook.* Roade History Society.

103 NRO: 1879 *Register of Voters. Southern Division of The County of Northamptonshire. Towcester Polling District N0.VII.* At a time when the 1867 Representation of the People Act was passed (although still a time when suffrage was restricted), the 1868-69 Towcester District poll books reveals six men eligible to vote in Stoke Bruerne plus three under the Peoples Act 1867, it is not until 1870 John Amos first appears as eligible to vote, besides his entry it states *house and garden as occupier, near the canal.*

104 *Death Certificate:* William Ireson Amos, age 22 years. 20th June 1873. Cause of Death: Rheumatic Fever, Pericarditis.

Thomas Amos … following in fathers' footsteps

105 *Northampton Mercury.* Band of Hope Concert – Corn Exchange. 19th February 1877.

106 *Marriage certificate:* Thomas Amos and Sarah Ellen Hollowell. 23rd April 1878. Wellingborough Road Chapel.

107 *Northampton Mercury.* Mrs T Amos. Member of Noted Templar Family Dead. The Good Samaritan. 27th July 1928.

108 Marriage Records: Mary Ann Amos married William Wilson Mitchell. Saint Mary the Blessed Virgin. Stoke Bruerne. 29th September 1879 (Lorna York).

109 Marriage Records: Elizabeth Amos married George Chalmers b. Forfar, Scotland. Roade Baptist Church (Lorna York).

110 *President.* Fleet Number 195, built at Saltley Dock and launched June 1909. Steamer Registered at Birmingham on 23rd June 1909 to Captain James Woodfield (see Richard Thomas web site www.steamershistorical.co.uk Family History Lorna York).

111 *Northampton Mercury.* Towcester. July 3rd 1875

112 1881 Census: Stoke Bruerne.

113 John Henry Amos b.1856 (Thomas Amos's brother / Sister Mary's Uncle) in 1871 was a rope-maker in Stoke Bruerne. John Henry married Georgina Ellen Platt on June 13th 1891 in West Gorton, Manchester, they moved to Bolton and had five children. On the 1901 census John is a tea salesman in Eccles, on the 1911 census John is a smallwares dealer in Bolton. John died in 1926 age 70 (Family History. Lorna York).

114 *Northampton Mercury.* Stoke Bruerne. Pride of the Valley Lodge. 23rd February 1889. Quote: … *a fruit banquet was provided, the table being tastefully set out by Sisters Amos and Wilkins. After the good things were disposed of addresses were given by Brothers Gardiner, Abbott and Amos. A good number were present, and a most enjoyable evening spent.*

115 *Northampton Mercury.* Stoke Bruerne.- Church of England Temperance Society. 7th April 1883.

116 *Northampton Mercury.* Good Templary. 8th August 1885.

117 *Northampton Mercury.* Northamptonshire Temperance and Band of Hope Union. 24th October 1885.

118 Birth Certificate. Ellen Hollowell Amos. b. 4th April 1885. Stoke Bruerne.

119 George Smith F.S.A (December 1875) *Our Canal Population: The sud conditions of the women and children,-with remedy. An appeal to my fellow country men and women.* London: Haughton and Co., (Accessed from The British Library Document Supply. 9th April 2014. Ref. 331.7656 N500).

120 PRO: MH 25/27. Local Government Board miscellaneous correspondence and papers 1876.

121 Bristow A (1999) *George Smith. The Children's Friend.* Chester. Imogen.

122 **Canal Association.** For an account of the association see Cleasby P (2012) The Canal Association 1855-1947. A brief survey. *Journal of the Railway and Canal Historical Society.* Number 213 (March), pp.8-14.

123 *Hertfordshire Record Office:* Roy Fidoe collection. Circular letter from the LGB prescribing the initial list of boat registration authorities and layout and design of the various forms for the implementation and administration of the Canal Boats Act 1877, together with rules and regulations as created by the LGB. 17th May 1878.

124 Cubic Air Space in relation to the Canal Boat Act 1877 (Christopher M Jones).

125 George Smith of Coalville (1881) *Canal Adventures by Moonlight.* London: Hodder and Stoughton. (Accessed from The British Library Document Supply. 7th May 2014. Ref. W19-1513). pp 44-45.

126 NRO: LG 33/1. Towcester Sanitary Committee Meeting Minutes. 13th November 1879.

127 *Northampton Mercury.* Canal Boat Inspection. 6th December 1879.

128 George Smith of Coalville (1881) *Canal Adventures by Moonlight.* London: Hodder and Stoughton. (Accessed From The British Library Document Supply. 7th May 2014. Ref. W19-1513). pp 90-92.

129 Ibid: pp.97-98.

130 Ibid: p.160.

131 Report from the Select Committee. The Canal Boats Act (1887) Amendment Bill; together with the proceedings of the committee, Minutes of Evidence, and Appendix. July 1884 (263). Henry Hansard and Son, London.

132 At the session it became obvious the 1877 Act had resulted in difficulties with enforcement because *registration authorities were not bound to do so, and the LGB had no powers to force them to do so* (Della Sadler-Moore)

133 Account of narrow boat *back cabin changes* after the Canal Boat Amendment Act (Christopher M Jones).

134 NRO: LG 33/1. Towcester Rural Sanitary Authority Minute Book. 9th December 1884

135 William Woodward was a publican at the Boat Inn, he also operated as a canal carrier hauling mainly coal, building stone, clay, sand, lime, bricks, timber and slag, the latter coming from Northampton. He may have sold horse feed to the boaters as well. The first recorded evidence of his boat ownership comes from the Towcester Canal Boat Register started under Canal Boats Acts of 1877 and 1884, in which his first boat was entered as entry number one in February 1885. This was a second hand craft named *Indian Chief*, said to have been bought from a man named Kilminster. Two other craft followed, the first was named *Frank* in January 1887, most likely bought from boat builder William Nurser at Braunston Wharf. The second was named *Ada* bought in May 1890. William died in the summer of 1891 aged 45, his widow Annie took over both as landlord and the canal carrying business. Apart from inheriting the three existing craft, Annie also started buying other boats to increase the size of her small fleet or to replace older craft (Christopher M Jones).

136 NRO: LG 33/1. Towcester Rural Sanitary Authority Minute Book. 3rd February 1885

137 Ibid.

138 C.4515 Fourteenth Annual Report of the Local Government Board 1884-85 (1885)

139 C.4844. Fifteenth Annual Report of the Local Government Board 1885-86 (1886)

140 C.5131. Sixteenth Annual Report of the Local Government Board 1886-87 (1887)

141 NRO: LG 33/2. Towcester Rural Sanitary Authority Minute Book. 12th October 1886

142 NRO: LG 33/2. Towcester Rural Sanitary Authority Minute Book. 18th January 1887

143 NRO: LG 33/2. Towcester Rural Sanitary Authority Minute Book. 1st March 1887

144 NRO: N 17b. Diagram of the Sanitary Districts in Northamptonshire also showing Civil Parishes 1888

145 C.6141. Nineteenth Annual Report of the Local Government Board 1889-90 (1890)

146 C.6745. Twenty First Annual Report of the Local Government Board 1891-92 (1892)

147 *Northampton Mercury.* Sad death of a boatman. 14th March 1885

148 Ibid: A verdict in accordance with the medical evidence was returned

149 *Northampton Mercury.* Attempted Triple Murder and Suicide at Stoke Bruerne. 7th March 1885.

150 *Northampton Mercury.* The Stoke Bruerne Tragedy. 2nd May 1885.

151 *Northampton Mercury.* Summer Assizes. 4th July 1885.

152 *Northampton Mercury.* Stoke Bruerne. Liberalism. May 2nd 1885. *Northampton Mercury.* Stoke Bruerne. Liberal Meeting. 27th February 1886

153 *Northampton Mercury.* Selection of Liberal Candidate for South Northamptonshire. Enthusiasm and Unanimity. 21st April 1888.

154 *Northampton Mercury.* Bi-centenary of Roade Baptist Chapel. 29th September 1888.

155 NRO: B/RoBC/10 to 1938. Roade Baptist Church. 8th January 1890.

156 NRO: ML 2471. Roade School Board Manager Minute Book. 7th May 1895.

157 NRO: ZB 701/2. Temperance and Band of Hope Union Speakers Plan January-June 1890. Thomas Amos speaker number 112.

158 Family History (Lorna York).

159 NRO: B/RoBC/10 to 1938. Roade Baptist Church meeting minutes. 7th November 1892.

160 NRO: LG 33/2. Towcester Union Sanitary Authority Meeting Minute book. 23rd January 1894.

161 *Northampton Mercury.* Mrs T Amos. Member of Noted Templar Family Dead. The Good Samaritan. 27th July 1928.

162 *Northampton Mercury.* Board of Guardians Meeting, Towcester Rural Sanitary Authority meeting. 19th October 1894.

163 C.7867. Twenty Fourth Annual Report of the Local Government Board 1894-95 (1895)

164 NRO: Towcester Rural District Council Sanitary Officers Letter Book 1894 to 1898: Letter from Wm. Whitton to T. Amos, Stoke Bruerne. 17.10.1894 p.75.

165 *Northampton Mercury.* Towcester Board of Guardians Meeting, followed by Rural Sanitary Authority meeting of the committee. 19th October 1894.

166 NRO: Towcester Rural Sanitary Authority / Rural District Council Minute Book 1894 to 1898 - 13.11.1894. p.23:

167 NRO: Towcester Rural Sanitary Authority / Rural District Council Minute Book 1894 to 1898 - 27.11.1894. p.24:

168 NRO: Towcester Rural District Council Sanitary Officers Letter Book 1894 to 1898 - 27.11.1894. p.88:

169 NRO: Towcester Rural District Council Sanitary Officers Letter Book 1894 to 1898: Letter from Wm. Whitton to Fellows, Morton & Co., Lower Fazeley St., Birmingham. Re: Small-Pox case at Stoke Bruerne. 29.11.1894. p.89. *'I will bring your letter under the notice of the Guardians at their next meeting. I suppose you understand that the Guardians have nearly £30 to pay over and above the amount mentioned in my letter to you for compensation to Mr. Amos for things destroyed'.* 11.12.1894 p.28: '*The clerk produced a letter from Messrs. Fellows, Morton & Co. re - the Small Pox case at Stoke Bruerne stating the amount the man Humphreys was asked to pay was more than they were led to believe would be demanded and they did not think it likely that the man could pay it out of his earnings'.*

170 *Northampton Mercury.* The Good Samaritan. 27th July 1928.

171 *The Bristol Mercury.* Great Battle of the Bargees: By an eye-witness. 12th September 1896.

172 NRO: George Freestone Collection (Uncatalogued).

173 Ibid: 1st September 1896

174 Ibid: 11th September 1896

175 Ibid: 2nd November 1896

176 *Northampton Mercury.* Towcester Divisional Petty Sessions. 7th May 1897.

177 *Northampton Mercury.* Towcester Divisional Petty Sessions. The Theft of Postal Orders. 21st May 1897, p.3

178 *Northampton Mercury.* A Bad Indictment. 2nd July 1897.

179 *Northampton Mercury.* Jubilee at Stoke Bruerne Park. June 24th 1897.

180 *This is Your Life.* c.c. Telerecording No. 35/T/4676. Sunday, 7th September 1958. Television Theatre. Sister Mary Ward. Stoke Bruerne. Running order script (David Blagrove collection).

181 Ibid.

182 *Northampton Mercury.* Found Drowned at Stoke Bruerne. 4th November 1882.

183 *Northampton Mercury.* Drowned at Stoke Bruerne. 26th August 1892.

184 *Northampton Mercury.* Boatman Found Drowned at Stoke Bruerne. 27th October 1899.

185 NRO: B/RoBC/10 to 1938. Roade Baptist Church meeting minutes.

186 Family History Lorna York

187 MacLeod R M (Dec 1966) Social Policy and the Floating Population. The Administration of the Canal Boats Acts 1877-1899. *Past and Present.* 35. pp.101-132. This in-depth paper documents Brydone's work as the first Chief Inspector of Canal Boats, in which is a damning account of the way Mr Brydone was treated by the Ministry of Health.

188 C.8978. Twenty Seventh Annual Report of the Local Government Board 1897-98 (1898)

189 NRO: LG 33/4. Towcester Rural District Council meeting minutes 28th March 1899. Letter from Mr Amos was read tending his resignation of the Office of Canal Boats Inspector. Mr Young gave notice that at the next meeting he would propose Mr Geo Ed Phipps be appointed Canal Boats Inspector at a Salary of £10 per annum.

190 NRO: LG 33/4. Towcester Rural District Council meeting minutes 11th April 1899. Mr Phipps appointed.

191 *The (Northampton) Herald.* Death of Mr George Savage of Stoke Bruerne. 16th September 1899

192 Warwick County Record Office: No. 10183 Grand Junction Canal Company Boat Gauging Table. 3rd July 1872

193 Published books by Rev Hirst Hollowell: *National Elementary Education* (1888) and *Education and Popular Control* (1898).

194 Ireton K (1899) *Ritualism Abandoned or A Priest Redeemed.* London, James Clarke and Co. British Library Holdings: BV 181.H6. Chapter xi: Sorrow at the Manse, Chapter xii: Severely Boycotted, Chapter xiii: Cheque Enclosed, Chapter xvi: A Coffin Refused, Chapter xv: I've come to stay, Chapter xvi: The Undertaker Undertaken. pp.68-104.

195 Ibid. p.88.

196 **Owen John Llewellyn.** b.1870. Son of Evan Henry Llewellyn, MP. Educated at Lancing College and Radley, awarded a BA from Trinity College Cambridge in 1891. Inspector at the Board of Agriculture 1895-1899 (Venn J ed 1951 Alumni Cantabrigienses. Cambridge University Press. New York).

197 Sherwood K B (1986) The canal boatmen's strike of 1923. *Journal of Transport History.* 3rd Ser. 7 (1986/7) pp.61-79.

198 Cd.292: Twenty-ninth report of the Local Government Board 1899-1900 (1900)

199 *Northampton Mercury.* Two Barges Sunk. 29th December 1899.

The Watershed continues for the Amos family

200 *Northampton Mercury.* Good Tempars' Grand Lodge. Friday 20th April 1900. The conference resolutions related to the *Sale of Drink to Children Bill,* a demand for *entire Sunday Closing without compensation* and, in view of the approaching general election the Good Templars reaffirmed their determination to only give electoral support to candidates … *willing to entrust the people with the power to prevent the issue of licenses in localities and not to support anyone directly engaged in the manufacture or sale of intoxicants.*

201 1901 Census: Stoke Bruerne

202 NRO: B/RoBC/5 17-19. Roade Board School. School attendance book.

203 NRO: B/RoBC/10 to 1838. Roade Baptist Church Meeting Minutes. Notes from meeting Monday November 18th 1901.

204 Charles being the only other member of the second generation Amos children to stay in Northamptonshire. Brother John Henry Amos moved to Bolton, and sister Elizabeth Mitchell moved to London, until her death at 47 in 1906 (Family History Lorna York).

205 …there never was a time when there was more need than there was at the present time for every man who called himself a Liberal to stand by the Liberal cause. [I am] very glad to see that Liberalism had a good deal of life in it at Blisworth … [I only] wished that the Liberalism of the Liberal leaders in the Houses of Parliament was as healthy. [I] wished the leaders felt as united as the Liberals were in the constituencies. If only the Liberals in the constituencies remained united, [I] did not think that the day would be far distant when a transformation would occur and the country would see back in power those men whom Liberals believed to be the most capable men to govern the British Empire. *Northampton Mercury.* Liberal Meeting at Blisworth. 28th February. 1902.

206 *Northampton Mercury.* Liberal Meeting at Blisworth. 28th February 1902.

207 *Northampton Mercury.* South Northamptonshire Liberals. 5th August 1904.

208 Death Certificate: Mary Hollowell Amos. Registered 10th April 1902. Age 17. Father present at the death.

209 NRO: B/RoBC/10 to 1838. Roade Baptist Church Meeting Minutes. Accepted as a member of Roade Baptist Church 10th July 1904. Sisters baptised 7th August 1904.

210 *Northampton Mercury.* Stoke Bruerne Parish Meeting. 11th March 1904.

211   NRO: George Freestone Collection (Uncatalogued) Letter from T W Milner . 23rd March 1905.

212   *Northampton Mercury.* Stoke Bruerne. A dangerous spot. Concert. 15th April 1904.

213   Ibid.

214   *Northampton Mercury.* Singular Fatality at Stoke Bruerne. 6th May 1904.

215   *Northampton Mercury.* Stoke Bruerne. Fatal Injuries. 13th May 1904.

216   NRO: LG 33/5. Towcester Rural Sanitary Committee Minute Book. April 1903-January 1905.

217   Birth Certificate: Charles William Shepherd Perry. Bath, Somerset. 5th January 1869.

218   In 1881 Charles aged 12 was living with his family in St Giles artillery barracks in Colchester, his step father a serving soldier, by the age of 21 he was unmarried, and a Clothiers Packer living with his family in Leeds (Family History Lorna York).

219   *Northampton Mercury.* Oldest Soldier in the British Army. 1st December 1944.

220   Marriage Certificate. Charles William Ward and Emma Parkinson. September 3rd 1898.

221   *Northampton Mercury.* Stoke Bruerne Parish Meeting. 11th March 1904. At the meeting the following were elected Parish Concillors: Mr Thomas Herbert Savage, Mr John Abbott, Mr John Charles Tew, Mr John Valentine, Mr Bertie Wentworth Vernon, Mr Thomas Young, anf Mr Joseph Woodward.

222   *Northampton Mercury.* Daventry: Divisional Petty Sessions. 15th January 1904.

223   Death Certificate. Emma Ward. 2nd February 1906. Death due exhaustion following labour and operation.

224   *Northampton Mercury* Death of Mrs C. Ward 9th February 1906.

225   *Northampton Mercury:* Ward-Amos. 28th November 1906.

226   Marriage Certificate. Charles William Ward and Ellen Hollowell Amos. 28th November 1906. The Baptist Chapel, Hardingstone.

227   NRO: B/RoBC/10 to 1838. Roade Baptist Church Meeting Minutes. In 1906 Roade Baptist Church sent a letter of introduction for Mrs Ward (nee Nellie Amos) to Herne Bay Baptist Church. No records survive for Herne Bay Baptist Church (email correspondence with Church Secretary 2014).

228   Sherwood K B (1986) The canal boatmen's strike of 1923. *Journal of Transport History.* 3rd Sep. 7 (1986/7).

229   1011 Census. Ernest and Rosie with their 2 year old son Thomas Arthur Amos were visitors residing at the home of Mr Gordon Gray (manager of picture hall) in Durham. Their occupations given as variety artists, also residing in the household were the Bailey Family, father, mother and daughter also recorded as variety artists (Family History Lorna York).

230   *Northampton Mercury.* IOGT. 8th January 2009.

231   Birth Certificate. Olive Mary Winifred Ward. b. 22nd April 1909. Moreton Pinkney.

232   *Northampton Mercury.* Liberal Meeting Stoke Bruerne. 31st December 1909.

233   *Northampton Mercury.* The Radical Workers. Friday 7th January 1910. p.5.

234   Marriage Certificate. Ethel Margaret Amos to Francis Cecil Grant. 23rd December 1909. New Cross Road Wesleyan Methodist Chapel. Lewisham.

235   Sutton, C W. Durthoys. Rev. M C (2004) *Hollowell, James Hirst (1851-1901).* Oxford Dictionary of National Biography, Oxford University Press.

236   Hirst Hollowell, J,. Rev,. (1901) *What Nonconformists Stand For.* London. Arthur H. Stockwell.

237   *Northampton Mercury.* Mr. Hollowell's Funeral. 31st December 1909.

238   Hunt. C., (1911) James Hirst Hollowell. *The United Methodist.* April 27th. p.361.

239   1911 Census: Stoke Bruerne.

240   Family History Lorna York.

241   *Northampton Mercury.* In the Market. 19th May 1911.

242   *Northampton Mercury.* Roade. 23rd February 1912.

243   Payne E A (1938) *Roade Baptist Church 1688-1938.* Wymand & Sons Ltd. London.

244 Ibid. 30th January 1912.

245 NRO: LG 33/7. Towcester Sanitary Minute Book. 24th March 1912. p.285.

246 NRO: LG 33/7. Towcester Sanitary Minute Book . 28th January, 19th May 19th 1913.

247 The reasons why were not given but she might have had losses due to that constant bain of coal boating, delays loading at the collieries. It isn't clear what happened to all of Annie Woodward's boats. One ended up sunk in the arm at the bottom of Stoke locks and the GJC had to chain it up so as not to cause a hazard to navigation. She was asked to remove it. This was most likely *Indian Chief*. *Providence* was sold to owner boatman John Woodward of Gloucester in April 1913 and renamed *You Never Know* and *Charybdis* was sold to another owner boatman John Grantham of Banbury at the same time. Their boatmen moved on to other employers. Thomas Woodward appears to have gone to work for the GJC, but was discharged from his employment as a boatman due to drunkeness and being absent from work during a stoppage. George Callow went to work for Thomas Clayton (Oldbury) Limited steering their boat *Cromford* (Christopher M Jones).

248 *Northampton Mercury*. Temperance Worker's Death. The late Mr. Richard hollowell, Northampton. 6th March 1914.

249 PRO: ED 11/40. The Sixth Annual Report of the Canal Boatmen's Mission and Day School, 7, Brentford End.

250 Ibid.

251 Cd.746: Thirtieth report of the Local Government Board 1900-1901 (1901)

252 Ibid.

253 Cd.1231. Thirty-first report of the Local Government Board 1901-1902 (1902)

254 Ibid

255 Cd.2214. Thirty-third report of the Local Government Board 1903-1904 (1904)

256 Cd.3105. Thirty-fifth report of the Local Government Board 1905-1906 (1906)

257 Cd.3665. Thirty-sixth report of the Local Government Board 1906-1907 (1907)

258 Sherwood K B (1986) The canal boatmen's strike of 1923. *Journal of Transport History*. 3rd Ser. 7 (1986/7) pp.61-79.

259 *Northampton Mercury*. State Insurance for 15,000,000 workers. A gigantic scheme. May 12th 1911.

260 For a resume of the scheme see *Northampton Mercury*. State Insurance for 15,000,000 workers. A gigantic scheme. May 1911.

261 Majority of the following section from 'Boating Through World War One' by Christopher M. Jones in NB Summer 2014.

262 1911 Census: Stoke Bruerne: Post-Mistress Mrs Anne Mary Cakebread

263 As the Shropshire Union Railway and Canal Company (SUR&CC) had 17 horses in the stables with no boaters to use them, and Fellows, Morton and Clayton Limited (FMC) had similar complaints (Christopher M Jones).

264 NRO: B/RoBC/18. Roade Baptist Sunday School. 1909 attendance records.

265 NRO: George Freestone Collection (Uncatalogued)

266 *This is Your Life*. c.c. Telerecording No. 35/T/4676. Sunday, 7th September 1958. Television Theatre. Sister Mary Ward. Stoke Bruerne. Running order script. Section 27-29. p.8 (David Blagrove collection).

267 Account by Christopher M Jones.

268 For an account of boaters in World War I see Appendix 4 (Christopher M Jones).

269 *Birmingham Daily Post*. Need for Boys' labour on canals. The Board of Education's opposition. 10th May 1916.

270 Ibid.

271 *Northampton Mercury*. N.C.O.'s and Men. Killed. 1st December 1916.

272 *Northampton Mercury*. Private W. G. Batchelor. 10th November 1916.

273 *Northampton Mercury*. Wounded at Stoke Bruerne. 13th August 1915. *Northampton Mercury*. Stoke Bruerne. Entertaining the wounded. 13th July 1917.

274 *Northampton Mercury*. Blisworth By-Election. 24th October 1919.

275 Waterway's Archive: Grand Junction Canal Company, World War 1 (1914-18) Roll of Honour. Contains the names

of all those in the employ of the Company who joined His Majesty's Forces during the Great War. Eighty six men are named alphabetically, including The Rt Hon Visc G C V O Churchill, Director of the Company. The name of those men who gave their life for their country are marked with a *. Fifteen men did not return. The Roll of Honour is on permanent display at the Canal Museum. Stoke Bruerne.

276   Jones C. M. (2014) Boating in World War II. *Narrowboat.* Summer. pp.22-29.

277   Sherwood K B (1986) The canal boatmen's strike of 1923. *Journal of Transport History.* 3rd Ser. 7 (1986/7) pp.61-79.

278   PRO: ED 11/89. Waterway's Archive: Dock, Wharf, Riverside and General Workers' Union of Great Britain. Canal Workers. Report of Deputation. Extracts from the speech made by Ernest Bevan to the President of the Board of Education, who was accompanied by a representative of the Ministry of Transport and the Ministry of Health, on Wednesday, November 12th.

The inter-war years ... father calls

279   NRO. G3988. Sale of The Wakefield Estate, short summary of lots. Tuesday October 14th 1919. Brochure.

280   The Laurels being a property to let in Stoke Bruerne by Miss Wrighton. *Northampton Mercury.* To Let. 20th June 1913.

281   *Northampton Mercury.* Freehold Brickyard for Sale. 30th April 1920.

282   Regarding Figure 70. The account included about the picture is taken from an article by Blagrove D (2014) Picturing the past. Stoke Bruerne. *NarrowBoat.* Autumn. pp.24-26.

283   Stewart. S,. (1993) *Ramlin Rose: The Boatwoman's Story.* Oxford University Press. Oxford. p.128.

284   *Northampton Mercury.* A Popular Service in Northampton Picture Palace. January 9th 1920.

285   NRO: B/RoBC/10 to 1838. Roade Baptist Church Meeting Minutes. February 1921.

286   Ibid. February 1922.

287   *Northampton Mercury.* Stoke Bruerne Fire. 4th February 1921.

288   NRO: George Freestone Collection (uncatalogued). Letter to W. Yates Esq from T.W. Milner, July 2nd 1923.

289   *Northampton Mercury.* Lock-keeper's death. Fell from the gates at Stoke Bruerne. 12th September 1924.

290   No reports had been issued since 1913.

291   Cmd.923. First annual report of the Ministry of Health 1919-1920 (1920)

292   During the war government control of canals [and railways] bought unions closer together. In June 1920 the NTWF voted in favour of an amalgamation of transport unions, following the balloting of individual members eleven unions met in May 1921 and decided to merge into the National Union of Transport and General Workers (Sherwood 1979).

293   Cmd.1446. Second annual report of the Ministry of Health 1920-1921 (1921)

294   Waterway's Archive. Weaver Navigation. *Committee on Living-In on canal boats. Minutes of evidence taken before the Departmental Committee appointed to Inquire into the practice of living-in on canal boats in England and Wales, and to report whether any alteration in the practice is desirable* (1921). London. HMSO. Mr. Thomas Amos, J.P., of Stoke Bruerne, paragraphs 1080-1142

295   Ibid. Nurse Clara Jones, paragraphs 1934-1983.

296   Ibid. Minutes of evidence. pp.63-64.

297   Ibid. Evidence index. pp. 90-100.

298   Waterway's Archive. Weaver Navigation. *Committee on Living-in on Canal Boats. Ministry of Health. Report of the Departmental Committee Appointed to Inquire into the practice of living-in on canal boats in England and Wales, and to report whether any alteration in the practice is desirable* (1921). London. HMSO.

299   Ibid. p.2. It is interesting to note the report included an indication of the costs incurred in conducting the enquiry. The sstimated grpdd cpost of the preparation of the appended Report (including the expenses of the Departmental Committee) is £179 5s 2d of which £7 15s 0d represents the gross cost of the pinting and publishing of this Report. Signed. Christopher Addison, Minister of Health. 11th August, 1920.

300   The **schooling of boat children** was a recurring issue throughout commercial carrying, this subject area has been researched extensively by other authors. *It has not been the intention in this research project to separate families into their constituent parts ie. Boatwomen, Boat children or Captains / Boatmen.* For additional material see the following published

material. Freer W (1995) *Women and Children of the cut.* Railway and Canal Historical Society. Mold, Clwyd.

301 Cmd.1713. Third annual report of the Ministry of Health 1921-1922 (1922)

302 Sherwood K B (1986) The canal boatmen's strike of 1923. *Journal of Transport History.* 3rd. Ser. 7 (1986/7) pp. 61-79.

303 Ibid.

304 *Northampton Mercury.* Barge Boy's funeral. Impressive scenes at Braunston. 31st August 1923.

305 Family History Lorna York.

306 *Northampton Mercury.* Barge Boy's funeral. Impressive scenes at Braunston. 31st August 1923.

307 Family History Lorna York.

308 *Northampton Mercury.* Boatmen's Concert. 2nd November 1923.

309 Account of Boatman's strike (Christopher M Jones June 2015).

310 Samuel Barlow (Tamworth) Ltd. Minutes of Directors meeting. 24th September 1920 (Chris R Jones).

311 Samuel Barlow (Tamworth) Ltd. Minutes of Directors meeting. 23rd July 1923 (Chris R Jones).

312 Samuel Barlow (Tamworth) Ltd. Minutes of Directors meeting. 27th September 1923 (Chris R Jones).

313 Samuel Barlow (Tamworth) Ltd. Minutes of Directors meeting. May – June 1924 (Chris R Jones).

314 PRO: HLG 52/139. MoH Canal Boats Amendment Regulation. 30th September 1925.

315 PRO: HLG 52/139. Statutory Rules and Orders, 1925, No.843.

316 Cmd.2724. Seventh annual report of the Ministry of Health 1925-1926 (1926)

317 Cmd.3185. Ninth annual report of the Ministry of Health 1927-1928 (1928)

318 Dr Baird admitted to Edinburgh Obstetrical Society in 1906.

319 Marriage Certificate. William Joseph Baird and Mary Palmer. 23rd September 1905. St Barnabus Church. London.

320 *The London Gazette.* 22nd June 1915. p.6017

321 *Northampton Mercury.* Home Nursing. March 1st 1918.

322 NRO: Register of Electors 1918. Polling District of Earls Barton.Numbers 997 and 998.

323 NRO: Earls Barton electoral register 1925.

324 The employment of a Nurse in a General Practice in the 1920's is an illusive topic in the nursing literature see Royal College of General Practitioners (1968) *Reports from General Practice. No 10, The Practice Nurse.* London.

325 Earls Barton (EB) *Surgery Dressing Book.* An overview of the content of the book is given in Appendix 1.

326 Ibid.

327 Plucknett F (1922) *Introduction to the Theory and Practice of Boot and Show Manufacture.* Longmans, Green and Co. London. In the index to this textbook just looking at the entries for the letter 'A' reveals a range of products used in the manufacture of Boots and Shoes: Abrasives. Acetic Acid. Acid Bath. Adhesives. Alumina, sulphate of. Amazeen. Amber varnish. Ammonia. Ammonium ferric sulphate. Aniline dyes. Asbestos. Astragalum. pp.315-322.

328 Earls Barton (EB): *Surgery Dressing Book* . p. 88. Female total 54 times legs dressed.

329 Midwifery care was highly regulated via legislative mechanisms. The Midwife's role being to care for women during their pregnancy, confinement and for the ten day's following birth.

330 Earls Barton (EB) *Surgery Dressing Book.* pp. 11 & 18.

331 *Northampton Mercury.* Earls Barton. An interesting lecture. 21st September 1928.

332 *Northampton Mercury.* Earls Barton. 20th March 1931.

333 *Northampton Mercury.* Earls Barton. Club meeting. 7th February 1930.

334 *Northampton Mercury.* Earls Barton. 20th April 1934.

335 *Northampton Mercury.* Womens Institute. 18th February 1927.

336 *Northampton Mercury.* Earls Barton. 17th January 1930.

337 *Rushden Echo.* Spiritualist Rally at Rushden. 20th May 1927. www.rushdenheritage.co.uk/churches/spiritualistMoorRd.html

338 *Northampton Mercury*. Liberal Meeting. 4th July 1930.

339 *Northampton Mercury*. Earls Barton. 17th October 1930.

340 *Northampton Mercury*. Motor cycle death of John Palmer Baird age 15. 6th April 1928.

341 *Northampton Mercury*. Earls Barton Hospital Fete. 12th February 1932. *Note Miss Olive Ward with Miss Eva Essom and Mr Eric Drage tastefully decorated the hall. p.6.*

342 *Northampton Mercury*. Country dancing by old folk. Happy evenin g at Earls Barton. Prizes in guessing competition. 27th January 1933. p.14.

343 *Northampton Mercury*. Fancy dress dance. Earls Barton help the heroes. 29th November 1929.

344 *Marriage Certificate*: Eric Arthur Drage and Olive Mary Winifred Ward July 1st 1933.

345 *Mercury and Herald*. Miss M.P. Baird. Married. Daughter of Earls Barton Doctor. Four attendants. July 1934 … *The maiden's wore blush pink georgette dresses were trimmed with silver at the waist, the skirts and short sleeves being frilled. They wore pink mittens and silver shoes, and wide jewelled bracelets, the gifts of the bridegroom. Pink roses formed their bouquets.*

346 Earls Barton (EB): *Surgery Dressing Book*. Last entry by Nurse Ward.

347 *Northampton Mercury*. A loss to Blisworth. Death and funeral of Mrs. C. Amos. 11th may 1928.

348 *Northampton Mercury*. Mrs T Amos member of noted Templar family dead. The Good Samaritan. 27th July 1928.

349 *Northampton Mercury*. Mrs Amos. Funeral at Roade on Saturday. A large congregation. August 3rd 1928. (Front page).

350 *Northampton Mercury*. Former County Councillor. Death of Mr T Amos. 1st July 1938.

351 Cmd.3362. Tenth annual report of the Ministry of Health 1928-1929 (1929)

352 Cmd.3937. Twelfth annual report of the Ministry of Health 1930-1931 (1931)

353 PRO: Ministry of Health Circular 1211. Canal Boats Act, 1884. 4th August 1931.

354 NRO: 303p/510. Parish Council meeting book Stoke Bruerne. United Parish Councils Meeting Stoke Bruerne and Shutlanger. 14th January 1930.

355 NRO: Roade Baptist Church meeting minutes. February 21st 1934.

356 *This is Your Life*. c.c. Telerecording No. 35/T/4676. Sunday, 7th September 1958. Television Theatre. Sister Mary Ward. Stoke Bruerne. Running order script. Section (David Blagrove collection).

357 Stewart. S,. (1993) *Ramlin Rose: The Boatwoman's Story*. Oxford University Press. Oxford. p.154.

358 Sherwood K B (1979) *Stoke Bruerne: A documentary account of the impact of the canal on a village community*. Using the Environment. No 4: Northamptonshire Waterway's. Stoke Bruerne. Nene College Northamptonshire. p.68. (Lorna York Collection also available from Northampton Central Library, History Centre).

359 Ibid. p.69.

360 PRO: HLG 52/1636. Committee on canal boat regulations minutes of meetings 1934-1941.

361 Ibid. Report of the committee on canal boat regulations. 21st June 1935. Appendix A Old Type Horse Drawn Narrow Barge, Appendix B New Type Mechanically Propelled Narrow Barge (MoH June 1935).

362 Account by Christopher M Jones.

363 PRO: HLG 52/1636. Memorandum 'Canal Boats': Ministry of Health. August 1935.

364 **Industrial Nursing.** It was not until October 1932 the Royal College of Nursing (RCN) became interested in 'tuked away' industrial nurses, they formed a committee 'to consider the position of nurses in industry'. Industrial nurses at the time were emerging from their seclusion, many 'tucked away' for years in a surgery, perhaps only tolerated because the factories act required a responsible person trained in first aid to be available for accidents. The RCN performed a survey, the findings indicated an assorted number of grades, not all registered / trained. Although they also found some amusing discoveries during the survey … for example a humble boilerman was charging 2d for a dry dressing and 6d for a hot fermentation. The first course of training commenced in 1934 with the The Times publishing an article Nurse's working on their own (1936). With the introduction of the Factoruies Bill 1937 scope was given to the developing role of the industrial nurse, Industrial Nursing was a sub-committee of the Public Health section memorandum to the Royal Commission on Workmens Compensation which recommended employment

of Nurses in factory First Aid Departments etc be more widely extended under statutory orders. World War II then effected the availability of Nurses … courses were shortened, eventually becoming a correspondence course during the war. The transference of the Factory Department of the Home Office was transferred to the Ministry of Labour and National Service in 1940 (Ernest Bevan). For a more detailed account see Charley I H (1954) *The Birth of Industrial Nursing*. London. Bailliere Tindall.

365   NRO: 303p/501. Stoke Bruerne Parish Council Meeting Book. 28th April 1936.

366   Earls Barton / Stoke Bruerne case book (SDB) 1936 entries pp.156-183 (See appendix 1).

367   Ernest James Veater was originally employed as the Chief Toll Clerk of the Oxford Canal Company at Hawkesbury Junction from 26th January 1924. His appointment was not without controversy as he was new to canals; it was normal for someone to have a good deal of experience, usually as a toll clerk for some years, before reaching such a senior position. In this case the Chief Toll Clerk did not just collect tolls, but assisted the Oxford canal's own traffic agent organise the finding of coal cargoes from the Warwickshire and Leicestershire collieries, and cargoes of roadstone from quarries in the Hartshill district for boatmen contractors and some carriers. This also included assisting to organise loading of their boats as he was in daily telephone contact with many of these firms. After the formation of the GUCCC in 1934 they started to use the office of Chief Toll Clerk to assist their boatmen, which put such a strain on the Oxford company that in 1935 they gave permission for the GUCCC to set up their own boat control office at Hawkesbury Junction (Christopher M Jones).

368   Public Health Act, 1936. [26 GEO. 5. & 1 Edw. 8. Ch. 49.]

369   NRO: 303p/501. Stoke Bruerne Parish Council Meeting Book 15th March, 5th May, 27th October 1937:

370   NRO: B/RoBC/21. Subscription and attendance sessions 1935-1936. C W Ward.

371   ie 2 cylinder engine, electric lights, larger cabin, fleet increased from 14 to 100 pairs eventually totalling 180 pairs, although only 100 were in service at any time, 'Sculptor' being an example of the 1st tranche, 'star class' boat (Christopher M Jones).

372   Waterway's Archive: CONSTITUTION Revision of Boatmen's wage rates agreement and working rules. GUCCCo Conciliation Board Issued by the Grand Union Canal Carrying Company Concilliation Board (Representing the Grand Union Canal Carrying Company Ltd and the Transport and General Workers' Union): 1937.

373   *Mercury and Herald.* High Above Villages and Churches! A trip on the Grand Union Canal. Stoke Bruerne's Seven Locks. August 20th 1937.

374   *Northampton Mercury.* Canal Boatpeople wed. Honeymoon on floating home. Four bridesmaids. 31st December 1937.

375   *Northampton Mercury and Herald.* Former County Councillor. Death of Mr T Amos. 1st July 1938.

376   *Northampton Mercury.* Funeral of Mr T. Amos. Son-in-law officiates at Roade. 8th July 1938 p.3.

377   Rolt L T C (1944) *Narrow Boat.* Eyre and Spottiswoode. London. pp.66-67.

378   Stewart. S,. (1993) *Ramlin Rose: The Boatwoman's Story.* Oxford University Press. Oxford. p.154.

379   Ibid. p.153.

Sister Mary, World War II and boating on the Grand Union Canal

380   NRO: Kelly's Trade Directory Northamptonshire. 1940.

381   NRO: 303p/501. Stoke Bruerne Parish Council meeting minutes … 22nd May 1941.

382   Blagrove, D. (2005) *Two centuries of service. The story of the canal at Stoke Bruerne and Blisworth.* Wharfside Publications. p.94

383   Eric Smith became foreman bricklayer for British Waterway's recounted his childhood memories of Sister Mary's fire watch brigade during the *This is Your Life* broadcast (David Blagrove collection).

384   RX indexed WW II Ledger. Inventories (David Blagrove collection).

385   *Northampton Mercury.* Good Blackout. 27th October 1939.

386   Sherwood K B (1979) *Stoke Bruerne: A documentary account of the impact of the canal on a village community.* Using the Environment. No 4: Northamptonshire Waterway's. Stoke Bruerne. Nene College Northamptonshire. Document

20 Log Book. Stoke Bruerne Primary School. (Lorna York Collection also available from Northampton Central Library, History Centre).

387 *Northampton Mercury.* Oldest Soldier in the British Army. 1ˢᵗ December 1944.

388 Hadfield C (1950) *British Canals an illustrated history.* David and Charles. Newton Abbot.

389 In May 1940 Frank Pick produced a major report on inland waterways and their contribution to the war effort, including in-depth studies of several canals and navigations.

390 Brigadier Sir Henry Osborne-Manse (1875-1966) see St Anthony's College Oxford biography https://www.sant.ox.ac.uk/mec/MEChandlists/GB165-0200-Mance-Collection.pdf

391 Stewart. S,. (1993) *Ramlin Rose: The Boatwoman's Story.* Oxford University Press. Oxford. p.152.

392 Ibid.

393 PRO: HLG 52/1636. Canal Boat Regulations. Letter from Mr Legge to Colonel Clayton. 8ᵗʰ June 1941.

394 Ibid. Note from Forrester Clayton to Mr Legge. 9ᵗʰ June 1941.

395 Ibid. Letter from Mr Legge to Colonel Clayton. 11ᵗʰ June 1941.

396 A boat owned by her brother Christopher March, built by Frank Nurser (Braunston) as a pleasure boat before the war.

397 Gayford E (1973) *The Amateur Boatwomen. Canal Boating 1941-1945.* David and Charles. Newton Abbot. p.47.

398 Ibid. p.47.

399 Ibid. p.47.

400 PRO: HLC 52/1094: Central Canal Control Committee Minutes. Friday 12ᵗʰ September 1941.

401 PRO: MT 52/102. Letter to Miss March signed Sgt S W Nelson. 20ᵗʰ October 1941.

402 Ibid. Letter from Daphne March to Sgt Nelson … *I have told Mrs Traill of this project and she is much interested; but she has accepted this hospital job and feels she cannot back out of it now. She said however that if anything definite was arranged she would consider coming back if the hospital would let her.* October 21ˢᵗ 1941.

403 Ibid. Typed note dated October 31ˢᵗ 1941 re Mrs Traill's visit.

404 Ibid. Letter from Sgt Nelson to J Miller. 6ᵗʰ November 1941.

405 Gayford E (1973) The Amateur Boatwomen. Canal Boating 1941-1945. David and Charles. Newton Abbot. p. 53.

406 Ibid. p.78.

407 Boatwomen's Training Scheme documents can be seen at http://www.unionhistory.info/workerswar/narrativedisplay.php?irn=59

408 *Northampton Mercury.* Children's First Aid. 12ᵗʰ September 1941.

409 In what has been described as one of the most important class based analyses of society, Marjery SpringRice conducted the largest survey in regard to the health and conditions of working-class wives (publishing the product of her labour in 1939). Without going into too much detail, the essence of the study was a survey to a large number of working-class, working women, the findings identified SEVEN ailments of greatest significance affecting the working women: *Anaemia, *Headaches, * Constipation (with or without haemorrhoids), * Rheumatism, * Gynaecological trouble, *Carious teeth and toothache, *Leg problems; varicose veins, ulcerated legs, white legs, phlebitis. Reviewing Sister Mary's case books all these ailments were common amongst the boatwomen. See. SpringRice M (1939) Working-Class Wives. Their Health and Conditions. Penguin Books Limited. Harmondsworth, Middlesex.

410 Hanson, H. (1978) *Canal People.* David and Charles. Newton Abbot. Quoting from Manchester Guardian 28ᵗʰ January 1925.

411 It was reported by the BDA there were 12,000 dentists in the UK and many still unqualified. The Beveridge report included a recommendation that as part of free health care this should include dental care, with one caveat *to ensure careful use, it is reasonable that part of the cost of renewal of dentures be borne by the person using them.* In 1944 the Inter-departmental committee on dentistry (cmd 6565) issued an interim report drawing attention to the poor dental conditions of the population (Della Sadler-Moore).

412   Woolfit S (1947) *Idle Women.* M & M Baldwin. London. pp.69-71.

413   *Northampton Mercury.* Northants Friend of Sir A. Conal Doyle Dies. Mrs W J Baird's interest in psychic research. Foresaw R101 Disaster. 30th June 1939. NB: Marjorie Baird taught in concentration camps for Boer prisoners during the South African War, and was also a close friend of the late Sir Arthur Conan Doyle, whose interest in psychic research she shared. Following an accident in the village about six months ago, when she fell fro a bus and broke her leg she had constantly failing health. She died suddenly at Eastcote where she was staying with her daughter.

414   *Waterway's Archive:* BW 201. Letter from Sister Mary Ward to Mr and Mrs Merchant. June 10th 1944.

415   Lacken G (1945) *The Story of Penicillin.* Pilot Press Ltd. London. (Della Sadler-Moore collection). Although Penicillin had been discovered in 1928, it was not until World War II in the North African battlefields it was tested on wounded soldiers.

416   Starns, P. (2000) *Nurses at War. Women on the front-line 1939-45.* Sutton Publishing. Somerset.

417   Lacken G (1945) *The Story of Penicillin.* Pilot Press Ltd. London. (Della Sadler-Moore collection). In previous battles thousands of soldiers died from gas-gangrene and other bacterial infections.

418   Waddy F F (1974) *A History of Northampton Hospital 1743-1948.* The Guildhall Press (Northampton) Limited. Northampton. pp.129-130

419   Red and Blue (RB) Case Book: Entry 11th September 1943 (David Blagrove collection)

420   Waterway's Archive. BW 953/96 H.R. Dunkley Collection. E. J. Veater Lecture Notes 1948.

421   PRO: MT 52/102. Letter from Hugh Beaver to Sir Osborne Mance. 2nd Novemebr 1942.

422   PRO: MT 52/102. Letter to Sir Osborne Mance from Mrs H Butson. 6th November 1942.

423   Ibid

424   PRO: MT 52/102: Letter Sir Osborne Mance: Women's Training School for Boat Crews. 26th January 1943.

425   Ibid. Typed document. 24th March 1943.

426   PRO: MT 52/134 Types notes from a meeting with Mrs Traill at The Ministry of War Transport. 11th May 1943.

427   Ibid.

428   PRO: MT 52/134: Typed notes from Mrs Traill's meeting with the Parliamentary Secretary and Sir Osborne Mance on 10th June, typed notes dated 11th June 1943.

429   PRO: MT 52/134. Handwritten letter from Mollie Traill to Sir Osborne Mance. June 21st 1943.

430   Family History Lorna York .

431   PRO: MT 52/134. Typed notes of meeting between Mollie Traill and Sir Osborne Mance. 6th July 1943.

432   Gayford E (1973) The Amateur Boatwomen. Canal Boating 1941-1945. David and Charles. Newton Abbot. p.122.

433   Mollie's Grand-son writing TUC web site http://www.unionhistory.info/workerswar/narrativedisplay.php?irn=59

434   Philip Noel-Baker Parliamentary Secretary at the Ministry of War Transport from February 1942. Received the Nobel Prize for Peace in 1959.

435   Mollies grand-son has Mollie's scrapbook of her time on the canal http://www.unionhistory.info/workerswar/narrativedisplay.php?irn=59

436   PRO: HLC 52/1094 and MT 52/134: Letter from Ministry of War Transport to Ministry of Health. 23rd August 1943.

437   PRO: HLC 52/1094: Ministry of Health handwritten notes 26th August – 10th September 1943.

438   PRO: MT 52/134. Minutes of the meeting held at the Ministry of War Transport with representatives from the Ministry of Health. 14th September 1943.

439   PRO: HLC 52/1094. Typed notes made by the Ministry of Health regarding the meeting with Sir Osborne Mance. 21st September 1943.

440   PRO: MT 52/134. Letter from Sir Osborne Manse to Ministry of Health. 21st September 1943.

441   PRO: HLC 52/1094: Typed and handwrittem memos. 10th November 1943

442   Ibid. In addition, the Ministry of Health compiled a short bibliography to inform Sir Osborne of the way the Ministry and Local Government Boards had discharged their function in relation to canal boats and how they had *kept themselves*

informed on this issue. The internal investigation was underway when a Miss Puxley reported *it is for us to satisfy ourselves all not well before taking any active steps.*

443 PRO. HLC 52/1094. Ten page Ministry of Health report. 31ˢᵗ January 1944.

444 Fellows Morton and Clayton had been approached by the Ministry to see if they had a similar scheme, but Directors informed them of the complexities of identifying quantities of packages and locations for distribution, whereas the GUCCCo had overcome these issues by managing distribution and quantity of packages using a large map in their office and moving a flag representing a boat each day to show the movement of the vessels (Della Sadler-Moore).

445 PRO: HLC 52/1094: Letter from Ministry of Health to Joint Secretary Regional Joint Councils. November 1944.

446 PRO: MT 52/134. Undated report of informal meeting. Loopholes in Acts of Parliament in regard to transport workers.

447 PRO: MT 52/134. Formal noted from meeting 23ʳᵈ June 1944.

448 PRO. HLC 52/1094. Ten page Ministry of Health report. 31ˢᵗ January 1944.

449 This picture was taken by Thomas Monnington who after a successful career as an artist joined the Ministry of Defense's Camouflage team in 1939. Thomas was chiefly responsible for designing camouflage for aircraft production fields, from 1943 he flew as an official war artist. During his work at the camouflage department he took a series of photographs along the Grand Junction Canal, one of which is Figure 101 showing Evelyn Hunt with Sister Mary. Monningtons wife died on February 7ᵗʰ 1947, and on December 6ᵗʰ 1947 he married the daughter of a mining engineer and silver prospector, Evelyn Jane Hunt. Walter Thomas Monnington was Knighted in 1967. Source. Egerton J (2015) Monnington, Sir (Walter) Thomas. Oxford Dictionary of National Biography. http://www.oxfordddnb.com/printable/31455 *Evelyn Hunt was one of the recruits to the all women boat crews on the Grand Union Canal during World War II. Possibly Sister Mary, seen in the picture with Evelyn knew love was in the air on the day Thomas took the picture (Della Sadler-Moore).*

450 PRO: HLC 52/1094. Letter to Mr Batterbury. 18ᵗʰ February 1944.

451 *Northampton Mercury.* Northants Attracts Film Producers. 9ᵗʰ June 1944.

452 Waterway's Archive. BW 953/96. H.R. Dunkley Collection. E. J. Veater Lecture Notes 1948.

Sister Mary post-war …

453 For a recent academic interpretation of the employment of the all women boat crews during World War II see Hately-Brown B and Moore B (2014) Chapter 12. *IDLE Women: Challenging gender stereotypes on Britain's Inland Waterways during the second World War* in Andrews M and Lomas J eds. *The Home Front in Britain.* Palgrave Macmillan. Hampshire.

454 NRO: SC 308. *Auction Catalogue. Stoke Bruerne Park and Associated Properties.* 1947. On the sale of Stoke Park two Lots were sold in Stoke Bruerne.

455 *Northampton Mercury.* Water, Water Everywhere. But not a tap to turn. Friday 17ᵗʰ May 1946.

456 Death Certificate: Charles William Shepherd Perry Ward. 28ᵗʰ September 1946.

457 *Northampton Mercury.* Oldest Soldier in the British Army. 1ˢᵗ December 1944.

458 *The Daily Mirror.* The Lady of the lamp – 1946 style. November 8ᵗʰ 1946.

459 *Ibid*

460 *Nursing Mirror.* Canal Nurse. 3ʳᵈ May 1947.

461 Also, the National Insurance Act (c67) established the Welfare State with compulsory contributions to cover unemployment (except for the self-employed), sickness, maternity, funeral grants and finally widows and old-age benefits. The same year The National Insurance (Industrial Injuries) Act c62 brought into being benefits for those who sustained injuries at work and for industrial disease *and during absences from work due these causes at rates higher than benefits payable for absence due other illness.*

462 After the start of World War Two costs and wages started to rise for all canal carriers, but tight Government control prevented them increasing their rates to prevent losses. The Government paid a subsidy from June 1940 on 50% of the tolls to relieve pressure on businesses, but Fellows, Morton and Clayton (FMC) was such an important carrier the Government took control of it in July 1942, and not only paid its carrying losses but also guaranteeing income to the point that FMC could still pay a dividend to its shareholders. This continued after the war until the end of 1947 with the canals being nationalised, but once released from this safety net FMC had to pay its own way (Christopher M.

Jones: Source: A. H. Faulkner 2010 *FMC.* Belmont . pp. 99 -102).

463   Waterways Archive. *Lock & Quay.* Lock and Quay Encounters. No. 1 Sister Mary. October 1949.

464   Waterways Archive. *Lock & Quay.* Best kept lock competition. November 1949.

465   *Northampton Mercury.* Prize presented. 28th October 1949.

466   *Lock and Quay.* Letters page. March 1950.

467   British Pathe. Bargee Doctor. Available at <u>http://www.britishpathe.com/video/stills/bargees-doctor</u>

468   Sherwood K B (1979) *Stoke Bruerne: A documentary account of the impact of the canal on a village community.* Using the Environment. No 4: Northamptonshire Waterway's. Stoke Bruerne. Nene College Northamptonshire. Document 20 Log Book. Stoke Bruerne Primary School. (Lorna York Collection also available from Northampton Central Library, History Centre).

469   Waterway's Archive. *Lock & Quay.* Family spirit at Bulls Bridge. February 1950.

470   From 1924 Mr Veater who had a naval background worked as Chief Toll Clerk for the Oxford Canal Company when in 1936 he was poached by the GUCCCo to be Midland Representative at Sutton Stop boat control office, where he stayed throughout the war years (Christopher M. Jones).

471   Waterway's Archive. *Lock & Quay.* Mr Veater retirement. June 1950.

472   Waterway's Archive. BW 953/96. H.R. Dunkley Collection. E. J. Veater Lecture Notes 1948.

473   Waterway's Archive. *Lock & Quay.* South Eastern Division. July 1950.

474   Mr Dick Dyke was born in the cottage at the bottom of Stoke flight of locks, later moving to the rented canal side cottage where he remained for over thirty years. In 1925 Dick applied for the vacancy of tunnel tug driver and was interviewed and appointed by Mr Millner, Section Engineer for the Grand Union Canal Company, he got the job and worked the tug till it was finally withdrawn in 1936 (Sherwood K 1979).

475   *Northampton Independent.* Canal Nurse's Honour. January 5th 1951.

476   *The British Journal of Nursing.* British Empire Medal. January 1951, p.3.

477   *Northampton Mercury.* Friend of Boatmen and their Families. 5th January.

478   *Nursing Times.* Family Welfare for Water Gypsies. February 17th 1951. pp. 163-166.

479   *Northampton Mercury.* Changes on the canal. 29th August 1952.

480   Watereway's Archive. *Lock & Quay.* Canal Trip for the Flood Relief Fund. April 1953.

481   *Northampton Mercury.* Grand Send Off. 27th February 1953.

482   *Northampton Mercury.* Northants man runs festival cruises. January 23rd 1953.

483   PRO: HLG 52/1412: Conditions of Sanitation and ventilation in canal boats. Letter from The Sanitary Inspectors Association to Ministry of Housing and Local Government. 20th March 1952

484   PRO: HLG 52/1412: Conditions of Sanitation and ventilation in canal boats. Letter from The Sanitary Inspectors Association to Ministry of Housing and Local Government. 12th February 1953.

485   Hauldren A. B. (1955) The Hygienic and Welfare aspects of waterways transport. *The Royal Sanitary Institute Journal.* 75(5).

486   In 1956 Sanitary Inspectors had a Change of Designation Act passed which introduced the title *Public Health Inspector* . Brimblecombe P. (2003) Historical Perspectives on Health: The emergence of the sanitary inspector in Victorian Britain. *The Journal of The Royal Society for the Promotion of Health.* 123 (2). pp.124-131.

487   Waterway's Archive. BW 201/1/3: Letter to friend May 11th 1954.

488   *Northampton Mercury.* Cover-age. 27th August 1954.

489   Names of Boats transcribed from Sister Mary's Willow Wren (WW) Case Book (David Blagrove collection)

490   Ibid. July 8th 1955.

491   Some of those in the picture were identified by boaters during the research: On the front row is *Young Carter*, on the second row with the head scarf is *Mrs Alf Best*, fourth from the right is *Lou Carter*, fourth from the left is *Diane Jackson*, third from the left *Mrs P Ward*.

492   Waterway's Archive. *Waterway's.* Staff Magazine of British Transport Waterways. Sister Mary Ward.

493 Existing Case Book: Only a small number of case books have come to light during the research, and these do not cover all the years Sister Mary was providing her canal-side surgery in Stoke Bruerne. See Appendix 1 for an overview of the years covered in the surviving case books, from which the detailed accounts in this book have been reported from (Della Sadler-Moore).

494 Letter reproduced from Hanson H (1978) *Canal People.* David and Charles. Newton Abbot. p.169.

495 Thorpe J (2002) *Windlass in my belt. A canal adolescence.* Waterway's World. Ltd. Burton-on-Trent.

496 This is Your Life. From left to right. *Lesley N. Morton* (Manager, Willow Wren Canal Carrying Co & one time Manager GUCCCo. *Jack Monk*, Captain Willow Wren. *Roy Peters. Mrs Lilian Monk* and partly concealed by *Neil Ingram* . Behind Sister Mary *Mr and Mrs Williamson.* On Sister Mary's left, daughter *Olive Drage.* Next behind her is *Eric Smith* late foreman bricklayer for BW. *Alf and Francis Best* from BW pair Sudbury and Argo. *Bill and Doris Bellingham* from BW pair Alton and Slinfold. Mrs *Anna Ingram*, mother of Neil. *Beatrice Woodward* from the Boat Inn (Adapted from Blagrove D 1990 *Waterways of Northamptonshire.* Northamptonshire Libraries and Information Services. Northampton. pp.196-197).

497 Waterway's Archive: British Waterways Progress Report 1955-1960: Welfare and Amenities. pp.36.

498 Waterway's Archive. *Waterway's.* Staff Magazine of British Transport Waterways. Stoke Bruerne wins Ritchie Rose Bowl. November 1960. 5(48). pp.8-9.

499 Waterway's Archive. *Waterway's.* Staff Magazine of British Transport Waterways. Jack does it again! Ritchie Trophy stays at Stoke Bruerne. October 1961. 6 (59) pp.10-11.

500 McKnight, H. (1984) Up the Cut with George Harris. *Narrowboat.* May. pp.36-41.

501 Waterway's Archive. *Waterway's.* Staff Magazine of British Transport Waterways. Mother Christmas at Stoke Bruerne. October 1960. 5 (47). p.4.

502 *The Times.* Sister Mary Not Deterred. January 8th 1962.

503 Birmingham Central Library Archive: MS 4000/2/85. Cry from the Cut. Production book, scripts, correspondence. Broadcast BBC home service. Tuesday 13th February 1962, 7.30-8.30 pm.

504 *Waterways World.* Letter. July 2002 p.91.

505 Della Sadler-Moore collection.

506 *Northampton Independent.* Sister Mary leaves the canal. August 1962. p.18.

507 Blue Line Canal Carriers was formed from the remaining Samuel Barlow Coal Company Limited fleet, and Willow Wren Canal Transport Services Limited from the Willow Wren Canal Carrying Company. Several other firms appeared which were basically groups of enthusiasts, but was to no avail and in 1970 long distance canal carrying on the Grand Union by professional boating families was finished (Christopher M Jones).

508 Thorpe J (2002) *Windlass in my belt. A canal adolescence.* Waterway's World. Ltd. Burton-on-Trent. p.46.

509 Probate records of Edward Thomas Gibson 1963 (Family History Lorna York).

510 Waterways Archive. *Waterway's.* Staff Magazine of British Transport Waterways. What a treasure house this Waterways Museum is! 1963.

511 Death Certificate. Mary Ellen Winifred Ward. 22nd March 1972. Colindale Hospital. Hendon. Cause of death: 1a) Congestive heart failue 1b) Ischaemic Heart Disease. Informant Timothy J Drage, Grandson.

512 *Chronicle and Echo.* Florence Nightingale of canals' dies. March 22nd 1972

513 Glynn. J,. (2014) Sister Mary Ward. *Narrow Boat.* Winter Edition. pp.12-13.

514 Stewart. S,. (1993) *Ramlin Rose: The Boatwoman's Story.* Oxford University Press. Oxford. p.154.

515 PRO: HLG 52/135. Ministry of Health Circular August 1935.

516 Waterway's Archive: GUCCCo Handbook 1937.